Nutrition and Chronic Conditions

Nutrition and Chronic Conditions

Special Issue Editor

Omorogieva Ojo

MDPI • Basel • Beijing • Wuhan • Barcelona • Belgrade

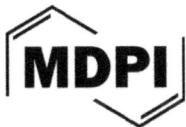

MDPI

Special Issue Editor
Omorogieva Ojo
University of Greenwich
UK

Editorial Office
MDPI
St. Alban-Anlage 66
4052 Basel, Switzerland

This is a reprint of articles from the Special Issue published online in the open access journal *Nutrients* (ISSN 2072-6643) in 2018 (available at: https://www.mdpi.com/journal/nutrients/special_issues/ nutrition_and_chronic_conditions)

For citation purposes, cite each article independently as indicated on the article page online and as indicated below:

LastName, A.A.; LastName, B.B.; LastName, C.C. Article Title. *Journal Name* **Year**, *Article Number*, Page Range.

ISBN 978-3-03897-602-8 (Pbk)
ISBN 978-3-03897-603-5 (PDF)

Contents

About the Special Issue Editor

Omorogieva Ojo has a Ph.D. in nutrition from the University of Greenwich, London, a post-graduate diploma in diabetes from the University of Surrey, Roehampton and a graduate certificate in Higher Education from the University of Greenwich. Prior to these qualifications, Dr. Ojo was awarded his BSc and MSc in animal science from the University of Ibadan, Nigeria. He is currently a Senior Lecturer in Diabetes Care and Management in the Faculty of Education and Health, the University of Greenwich and he teaches across a range of courses and programmes. He was previously a nutrition specialist at the Home Enteral Nutrition Team, Lewisham Primary Care Trust, London, a post-doctoral research fellow in the School of Science, University of Greenwich, London, and taught at the College of Agriculture, Asaba, Nigeria. He is an internationally acclaimed expert in nutrition and diabetes and these are the primary focus of his teaching and research activities, including Ph.D. supervision. Dr. Ojo has been a keynote speaker at international conferences and he is on the Editorial Board of many international journals including *Nutrients*.

Preface to "Nutrition and Chronic Conditions"

This book on Nutrition and Chronic Conditions aims to provide insight into the effect of nutrition in the development, care, and management of chronic conditions. This is in recognition of the impact that nutrition has on chronic conditions, such as diabetes, cardiovascular disease, dementia, stroke, and inflammatory bowel disease, which continues to generate interest among researchers. There is evidence that diet is a modifiable risk factor for these diseases, which manifest either as single entities or in co-morbid states in individuals and populations around the world. In particular, the prevalence of diabetes and cardiovascular disease is on the increase, especially in developed countries, but also in developing economies, partly due to lifestyle changes, including diet. For example, ischaemic heart disease is the leading cause of death globally. When combined with stroke, these conditions accounted for 15 million deaths in 2015 and are the world's greatest killers. In addition, there were an estimated 422 million adults who were living with diabetes in 2014 compared to 108 million in 1980.

These chronic conditions and their associated complications have significant implications for morbidity and mortality, and incur huge costs to the health services around the world. The composition of the diet, the proportion and types of macronutrients and micronutrients present in the diet are major contributors to these diseases. In addition, the beneficial effects of nutritional interventions have been well documented although differences remain among researchers with respect to their overall impact. The evaluation of the role of nutrition in chronic conditions draws on its effect on body weight and body composition, glycaemic and insulin excursions, vascular remodeling, and gastro-intestinal dysfunction.

Internationally acclaimed experts in the field of nutrition and chronic conditions have contributed chapters to this book that should provide the evidence base for practice and research. Therefore, this book is aimed at patients, students, and healthcare professionals, including nurses, doctors, public health practitioners, and dietitians/nutritionists. The book has sixteen chapters covering original research and reviews, which should guide healthcare professionals in their areas of practice. These include evaluations of the effects of various nutritional interventions, dietary and lifestyle modifications on cognitive decline, anthropometric parameters, metabolic syndrome, diabetes, and glycaemic control. In addition, assessment of food consumption, knowledge, attitudes, and practices related to salt, dairy intake and acne vulgaris, food perceptions, and dietary changes in chronic conditions are the key topics of interest in this book.

Omorogieva Ojo
Special Issue Editor

nutrients

MDPI

Review

The Effect of Dietary Glycaemic Index on Glycaemia in Patients with Type 2 Diabetes: A Systematic Review and Meta-Analysis of Randomized Controlled Trials

Omorogieva Ojo [1,*], Osarhumwese Osaretin Ojo [2], Fajemisin Adebowale [3] and Xiao-Hua Wang [4]

[1] Department of Adult Nursing and Paramedic Science, University of Greenwich, London SE9 2UG, UK
[2] Healthcare, Care UK, HMP Wormwood Scrubs, London W12 0AE, UK; Osarhumwese.Ojo@careuk.com
[3] Department of Animal Production and Health, Federal University of Technology, PMB, Akure 704, Ondo State, Nigeria; debofajemisin@yahoo.co.uk
[4] The School of Nursing, Soochow University, Suzhou 215006, China; wangxiaohua@suda.edu.cn
* Correspondence: o.ojo@greenwich.ac.uk; Tel.: +44-020-8331-8626; Fax: +44-020-8331-8060

Received: 31 January 2018; Accepted: 15 March 2018; Published: 19 March 2018

Abstract: Background: The increasing prevalence of diabetes in the United Kingdom and worldwide calls for new approaches to its management, and diets with low glycaemic index have been proposed as a useful means for managing glucose response. However, there are conflicting reports and differences in the results of studies in terms of their effectiveness. Furthermore, the impact of low-glycaemic index diets and their long-term use in patients with type 2 diabetes remains unclear. Objectives: The objective of this study was to conduct a systematic review and meta-analysis of the effect of low-glycaemic index diets in patients with type 2 diabetes. Methods: Search methods: Randomised controlled studies were selected from a number of databases (EBSCOHost with links to Health Research databases, PubMed, and grey literature) based on the Population, Intervention, Comparator, Outcomes and Study designs (PICOS) framework. The search terms included synonyms and Medical Subject Headings (MeSH) and involved the use of Boolean operators (AND/OR) which allowed the combination of words and search terms. Selection criteria: As per the selection criteria, the following types of articles were selected: studies on randomised controlled trials, with year of publication between 2008 and 2018, including patients with type 2 diabetes. Thus, studies involving patients with gestational and type 1 diabetes were excluded, as were observational studies. Nine articles which met the inclusion criteria were selected for the systematic review, whereas only six articles which met the criteria were included in the meta-analysis. Data collection and analysis: Studies were evaluated for quality and risk of bias. In addition, heterogeneity, meta-analysis, and sensitivity tests of the extracted data were carried out using Review Manager 5.3 (Review Manager, 2014). Results: The findings of the systematic review showed that the low-glycaemic index (low-GI) diet resulted in a significant improvement (<0.05) in glycated haemoglobin (HbA1c) in two studies: low-GI diet Δ = −0.5% (95% CI, −0.61% to −0.39%) vs. high-cereal fibre diet Δ = −0.18% (95% CI, −0.29% to −0.07%); and low-GI legume diet Δ = −0.5% (95%, −0.6% to −0.4%) vs. high-wheat fibre diet Δ = −0.3% (95% CI, −0.4 to −0.2%). There was a slight improvement in one study (low glycaemic response = 6.5% (6.3–7.1) vs. control = 6.6% (6.3–7.0) and no significant difference (p > 0.05) in four studies compared with the control diet. Four studies showed improvements in fasting blood glucose in low-GI diets compared to higher-GI diets or control: low-GI diet = 150.8 ± 8.7 vs. higher-GI diet = 157.8 ± 10.4 mg/dL, mean ± SD p = 0.43; low-GI diet = 127.7 vs. high-cereal fibre diet = 136.8 mg/dL, p = 0.02; low-GI diet = 6.5 (5.6–8.4) vs. standard diabetic diet = 6.7 (6.1–7.5) mmol/L, median and interquartile range p > 0.05; and low-GI diet = 7.3 ± 0.3 vs. conventional carbohydrate exchange diet = 7.7 ± 0.4 mmol/L, mean ± SEM (Standard Error of Mean) p < 0.05. The results of the meta-analysis and sensitivity tests demonstrated significant differences (p < 0.001 and p < 0.001, respectively) between the low-GI diet and the higher-GI diet or control diet in relation to glycated haemoglobin. Differences between the low-GI diet and higher-GI diet or control were significant ($p < 0.05$) with respect to the fasting blood glucose following meta-analysis. Conclusion: The low-GI diet is more effective in controlling glycated haemoglobin and fasting blood glucose compared with a higher-GI diet or control in patients with type 2 diabetes.

Keywords: glycaemic index; glycated haemoglobin; fasting blood glucose; type 2 diabetes; randomised controlled trials; meta-analysis; systematic review

---

1. Introduction

The increasing prevalence of diabetes and its impact on morbidity and mortality have become global problems [1,2]. About 422 million adults worldwide were reported to live with diabetes in 2016, and the global prevalence rose from 4.7% in 1980 to 8.5% in 2014 [1]. In the United Kingdom, the prevalence of type 2 diabetes more than doubled from 2.39% in the year 2000 to 5.32% in 2013 [2]. The management of type 2 diabetes and its related complications, including retinopathy, kidney dysfunction, neuropathy, and foot problems accounts for about 10% of the entire National Health Service (NHS) budget in the UK [2]. Presently, 11% of U.S. adult population has diabetes and the total estimated costs associated with the condition in 2012 were US $245 billion due to direct medical costs and reduced worker productivity [3]. Several factors, including genetic predisposition and environmental factors, have been implicated in the aetiology of diabetes [3,4]. This is particularly true in the case of type 2 diabetes, which accounts for over 90% of all forms of diabetes and where lifestyle has a profound effect on its manifestation [5]. Usually, lifestyle factors such as diet and physical activities can be modified in terms of the choices that individuals make. The composition of diet with respect to the quality of the nutrients including carbohydrates, protein, fats, minerals and vitamins is important in determining nutritive value and usefulness in human health [6].

1.1. Description of the Intervention

Foods that are composed of carbohydrates which break down quickly during the process of digestion (such as white bread) and that are rapidly absorbed into the blood stream are often termed as foods with high glycaemic index (GI) [7–9]. Foods with high GI not only rapidly increase blood glucose, but also insulin responses following the consumption of food [10]. In contrast, foods with a low glycaemic index such as legumes, lentils, and oats usually contain carbohydrates which break down slowly during digestion and are slowly assimilated [8,9]. Therefore, these foods have a slower impact on blood glucose levels and insulin response.

The GI is a measure of the percentage of the area under curve (AUC) with respect to 2-h blood glucose following the ingestion of a test diet compared with a standard diet (usually glucose or bread) [7]. It can also be viewed as a reflection of the relative rate of digestibility of the available carbohydrates of the food compared with a reference food, which is often glucose [11,12]. Differences exist in literature as to what constitutes a low-GI diet and a high-GI diet. Values such as GI ≤ 40 and GI ≤ 55 for the low-GI diet and GI ≥ 70 for the high-GI diet have been reported [7,13].

1.2. How the Intervention Might Work

The GI value of food is not based on the characteristics of the individual that consumed it, instead, it depends on the food consumed [9,14,15]. Therefore, dietary management approaches which target weight loss and improved glycaemic control (including glycated haemoglobin and fasting blood glucose) in patients with type 2 diabetes may rely on the use of diets with low glycaemic index instead of using standard low-fat diet [16]. The foods with low GI may contribute to glycaemic control compared to foods with high GI through the promotion of insulin sensitivity, reducing fluctuations in blood glucose levels and reducing daily insulin requirements [8]. While glycated haemoglobin

(HbA1C) provides a measure of the average glycaemia over the preceding 3 months, the fasting blood glucose is a measure of blood glucose level following at least 8 h of fasting, and is usually taken before breakfast [17].

1.3. Why It Is Important to Do This Review

Strategies for managing diabetes often rely on lifestyle modifications, including dietary interventions and pharmacological approaches. There is also evidence that the consumption of diets with high glycaemic index and glycaemic load over a long period of time may have implications for metabolism and health, including chronic hyperglycaemia and hyperinsulinaemia, which can lead to insulin resistance and diabetes [14]. In addition, studies involving populations in China and the USA have shown that women with a high intake of food with a high glycaemic index were more at risk of developing type 2 diabetes compared with women on diets with low glycaemic index [14,18,19]. However, there are inconsistencies and controversies with respect to the use of GI of food as a guide in the selection of foods for patients with diabetes [8,12,20–22]. Evidence from previous studies on the role of diets with low GI on health and health-related outcomes have produced mixed results [16]. While some studies have found the high-GI diet to be related to poorer short-term metabolic outcomes, greater hunger, less satiety, and greater food intake [10], the results from other studies have been different, either not finding the same association or finding an inverse relationship [12,23]. Jung and Choi [13] demonstrated the beneficial effects of low-GI diet on glucose control in relatively short-term trials in patients with type 2 diabetes, although the long-term effects of low-GI diets remain unclear. This view is further reinforced by Thomas and Elliott [8] who noted that the effects of low-GI diets in managing patients with diabetes have demonstrated mixed results, from small but clinically useful effects on the medium-term glycaemic control in diabetes, to only modest secondary benefit. The review by Thomas and Elliott [8], which was published more than 7 years ago and involved patients with type 1 and type 2 diabetes, found that there was a significant decrease in HbA1c in a low-GI diet compared with control. Some of the studies included in this review involved children, and the primary outcome measures were HbA1c and fructosamine. Another review on glycaemic index and type 2 diabetes included only observational studies [22].

However, the current systematic review is based only on randomised controlled trials and involves only adults with type 2 diabetes, and the outcomes of interest are HbA1c and fasting blood glucose. In addition, there is currently no globally agreed form of diet for managing patients with diabetes [8]. Therefore, research on how best to understand the quality and composition of carbohydrates and other nutrients in foods will be essential in developing diets that will one day be useful to patients with diabetes and acceptable to the global community.

1.4. Objectives

This is a systematic review and meta-analysis which evaluates the effect of the low-glycaemic index diet in patients with type 2 diabetes

Research question: Is a low-GI diet effective in improving glycaemia in patients with type 2 diabetes compared with a higher-GI diet?

2. Methods

2.1. Types of Studies

Only studies involving randomised controlled trials were selected for this review (Table 1).

2.2. Types of Participants

The participants in the studies selected were adult patients with type 2 diabetes (Table 2).

2.3. Types of Interventions

The effect of low-glycaemic index diet was compared with higher-glycaemic index diet or control (conventional carbohydrate exchange, high-cereal fibre diet, high-wheat fibre diet, standard diabetic diet, American diabetes association diet) in adult patients with type 2 diabetes. The higher-GI or control diets were classified as having a higher glycaemic index based on the lower GI values of the intervention diets (low-GI diet).

2.4. Types of Outcome Measures

The following were the outcome measures of interest:
Blood glucose parameters: Glycated haemoglobin (%), fasting blood glucose (mg/dL).

Search Methods for Identification of Studies

The Population, Intervention, Comparator, Outcomes and Study designs (PICOS) framework was used to identify articles in the various databases [24,25]. The search terms included synonyms and Medical Subject Headings (MeSH) and involved the use of Boolean operators (AND/OR) which allowed the combination of words and search terms (Table 1).

Table 1. Search terms and search strategy.

Patient/Population	Intervention	Comparator	Study Designs	Combining Search Terms
Patients with diabetes	Low-glycaemic index diet	Higher-glycaemic index diet or control	Randomised controlled trial	
Patients with diabetes OR type 2 diabetes OR diabetes OR diabetes complications OR diabetes mellitus, type 2 OR diabetes mellitus	Glycaemic index OR glycemic index OR glycaemic load OR glycaemic indices or glycaemic index number or glycaemic index numbers		#1 Randomised controlled trial OR controlled clinical trial OR randomized OR placebo OR drug therapy OR randomly OR trial OR groups #2 "Animals" NOT "Humans" #3 #1 NOT #2	Column 1 and Column 2 and Column 3

2.5. Electronic Searches

A number of research databases were used to search for relevant articles for this review. These included EBSCoHost research databases with links to Health Research databases which incorporate Academic Search Premier, Medline, the Psychology and Behavioural Sciences Collection, PSYCInfo, and the Cumulative Index to Nursing and Allied Health Literature (CINAHL) Plus. In addition, Pubmed was searched for useful articles (Figure 1).

2.6. Searching Other Resources

The Web of Science database which encompasses the BIOSIS citation index was searched for conference papers, and the reference list of articles were also searched.

2.7. Selection of Studies

Only primary research on randomised controlled studies carried out between 2008 and 2018 were included in this review (Table 2). This period was chosen because the search period for the previous systematic review and meta-analysis by Thomas and Elliot study [8] ended in March 2009. Earlier search conducted from 2009 to 2018 did not yield enough studies for the current review.

In addition, only studies involving adults with type 2 diabetes and the use of the dietary glycaemic index were included. Studies written in English from across the world have been included as diabetes is a worldwide problem.

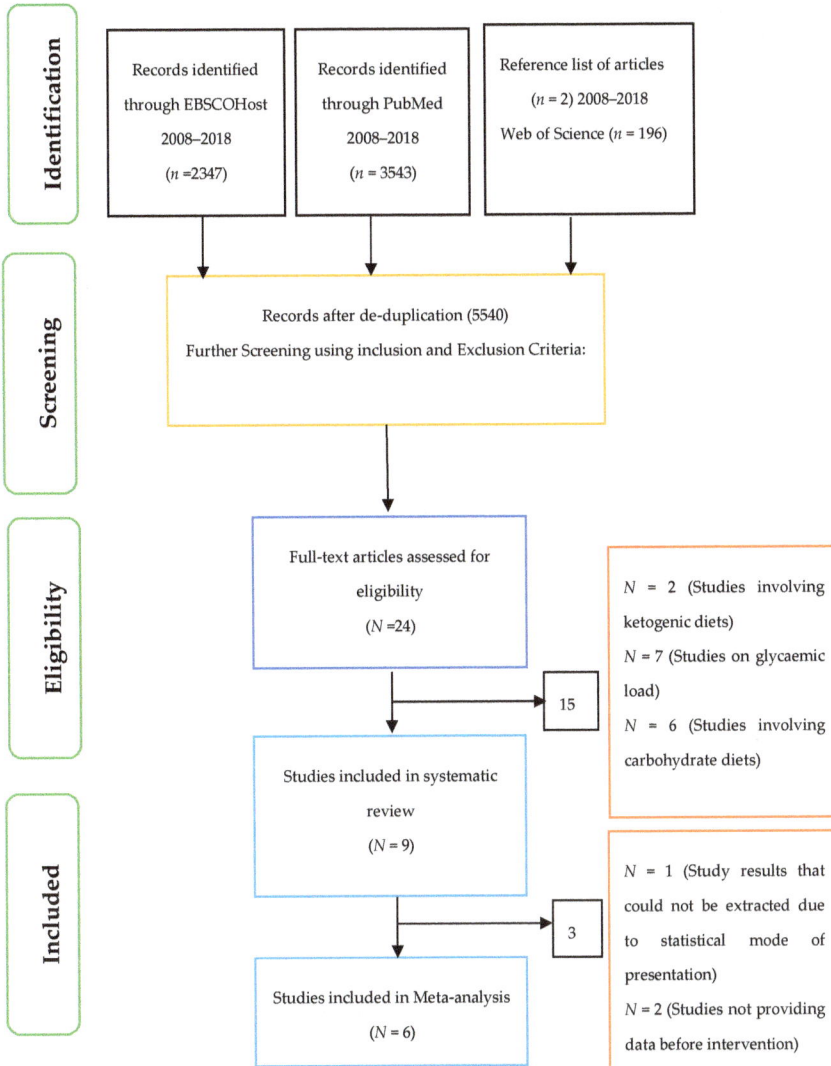

Figure 1. PRISMA flow chart showing the selection of articles.

Therefore, other studies involving patients with type 1 diabetes or gestational diabetes and animal studies were excluded from this review (Table 2). Similarly, studies involving children with diabetes or healthy adults without diabetes were also excluded. Studies which were not randomised and those involving dietary supplements have been excluded from this review.

Table 2. Criteria for considering studies for the review based on the Population, Intervention, Comparator, Outcomes and Study designs (PICOS) structure.

	Inclusion Criteria	Exclusion Criteria
Population	Adult patients ($\geq$18 years) with type 2 diabetes	Studies involving patients with type 1 diabetes or gestational diabetes and animal studies. Studies involving children with diabetes or healthy adults.
Intervention	Low-glycaemic index diet	Studies involving dietary supplements
Comparator	Higher-glycaemic index diet and/or control	Studies involving additional supplements
Outcomes	Blood glucose parameters: Glycated haemoglobin, fasting blood glucose	Qualitative outcomes
Types of study: quantitative	Randomised controlled trials	Observational studies Letters Comments Reviews

2.8. Evaluation of Quality

The quality of the peer-reviewed articles was evaluated using the checklists for quantitative studies [26] and the experience of the authors.

2.9. Data Extraction and Management

Data from the selected articles were extracted separately by all the authors based on an agreed framework and verified by all the authors following completion.

2.10. Meta-Analysis Methods

The meta-analysis of data was carried out using Review Manager (RevMan) 5.3 software [24]. Changes in means and standard deviations between the baseline values and final results for each outcome of interest in the low-GI diet and the higher-GI diet or control for the different studies were determined. In addition, the number of participants in the intervention and control groups in each study were included in a table and entered into the RevMan software for analysis. A heterogeneity test was carried out in order to evaluate the evidence of variability of the intervention effects [27]. For the heterogeneity test, a p value of 0.1 was used to determine statistical significance [27]. The heterogeneity statistic I^2 value was <50 and this indicated low heterogeneity for the studies included in both the glycated haemoglobin and fasting blood glucose analyses. Therefore, the fixed effects model was used for both the meta-analysis and the sensitivity tests.

A fail-safe number was also calculated for both outcomes of interest. A sensitivity analysis involving a repeat of the meta-analysis of studies that were definitely known to be eligible was also conducted [27]. This process involved removing some of the studies from the primary analysis in order establish that the findings from the systematic review were not dependent on unclear decisions [27]. In this case, the sensitivity tests were carried out for both glycated haemoglobin and fasting blood glucose by repeating the meta-analysis after removing the studies with the most weight in order to confirm whether the results were stable.

2.11. Assessment of Risk of Bias in Included Studies

The assessment tool used for evaluating the risk of bias was a domain-based evaluation tool [27]. The process involved the separate critical assessment of the various domains including the random sequence generation (selection bias), allocation concealment (selection bias), blinding of participants and personnel (performance bias), blinding of outcome assessment (detection bias), incomplete outcome data (attrition bias), selective reporting (reporting bias), and other bias [27]. The risk of bias was assessed by Review Manager 5.3 software [24].

3. Results

With respect to the systematic review, only nine articles [28–36] met the criteria for inclusion (Table 3). However, six of these studies [28–31,35,36] were used for the meta-analysis to test the effect of low-GI diet on glycated haemoglobin and fasting blood glucose in patients with type 2 diabetes. The others were excluded as they did not meet the criteria for meta-analysis such as reporting their results in the form of median and interquartile or not providing data before intervention.

The length of study ranged from 2 weeks to 22 months. In terms of the interventions, these involved comparing the low-GI diet with the higher-GI diet or control (conventional carbohydrate exchange, high-cereal fibre diet, high-wheat fibre diet, standard diabetic diet, American diabetes association diet) (Table 3).

In most of the studies [28,30,34–36] that reported dietary glycaemic index values, the low-GI diet had significantly ($p < 0.05$) lower values than the higher-GI diet or the control. The study by Jenkins et al. [29] also showed that the low-GI diet resulted in lower GI values than the high-cereal fibre diet, although the level of statistical difference was not stated (Table 3). However, differences in dietary GI values were not significant ($p > 0.05$) in one study [31], while data were not available in two of the studies [32,33] although the authors stated that the intervention diets involved low glycaemic index or low glycaemic response.

In studies reporting on the effect of dietary GI on the HbA1c levels, diets with low GI were shown to result in a significant improvement ($p < 0.05$) in HbA1c levels in two studies [29,30] compared with the higher-GI diet or the control. One study [33] reported slight improvement in HbA1c in the low-GI diet group compared with control, while differences between low-GI diet and higher-GI diet or control were not significantly different in four studies [31,34–36].

The effect of low-GI diets on fasting blood glucose compared to higher-GI diets or control diets was evident in seven of the studies selected [28–30,32–34,36]. While four studies [28,29,34,36] showed a greater improvement in fasting blood glucose in the low-GI diet compared with higher-GI diet, some of the differences were not statistically significant. Furthermore, there was a lower fasting blood glucose level in the higher-GI diet or control compared with low-GI diet in two studies [30,33]. The fasting blood glucose levels were not significantly different in the low-GI diet compared with control in one other study [32].

Table 3. Summary of studies included in the systematic review.

Citation	Length of Study	Study Type	Sample Size	Age (Years)	Diabetes Duration (Years)	Interventions	Glycated Haemoglobin (HbA1c) %	Blood Glucose	Dietary Glycaemic Index
Gomes et al. [28]	1 month	Parallel Design	20	# 42.4 ± 5.1	# Low-GI (Glycaemic Index) diet (4.8 ± 1.5) higher-GI diet (4.9 ± 1.6)	Low-GI diet versus higher-GI diet	No data	*# Baseline Low-GI diet = 148.9 ± 8.2 vs. higher-GI diet 147.8 ± 10.7 30 days Low-GI diet = 150.8 ± 8.7 vs. higher-GI diet = 157.8 ± 10.4 $p = 0.43$	## Baseline Low-GI diet = 63 ± 6 vs. higher-GI diet = 66 ± 4 30 days Low-GI diet = 54 ± 4 vs. higher-GI diet = 72 ± 3 $p = 0.005$
Jenkins et al. [29]	6 months	Parallel Design	210	# Low-GI diet = 60 (10) High-cereal fibre diet = 61 (9)	# Low-GI diet = 8.3 (6.5) High-cereal fibre diet = 7.2 (5.9)	Low-GI diet versus high-cereal fibre diet	Low-GI diet Δ = −0.5% (95% CI, −0.61% to −0.39%) vs. high-cereal fibre diet Δ = −0.18% (95% CI, −0.29% to −0.07%) $p < 0.001$	* (Mean) Week 0 Low-GI diet = 138.8 vs. high-cereal fibre diet = 141.2 Week 24 Low-GI diet = 127.7 vs. high-cereal fibre diet = 136.8 $p = 0.02$	### Week 0 Low-GI diet = 80.8 (79.6–82.0) vs. high-cereal fibre diet = 81.5 (80.4–82.7) Week 24 Low-GI diet = 69.6 (67.7–71.4) vs. high-cereal fibre diet = 83.5 (82.4–84.7)
Jenkins et al. [30]	3 months	Parallel Design	121	## Low-GI legume diet = 58 (1.3) High-wheat fibre diet = 61 (1.0)	## Low-GI legume diet = 9.2 (8.0) High-wheat fibre diet = 8.6 (0.8)	Low-GI legume diet vs. high-wheat fibre diet	Low GI legume diet Δ = −0.5% (95%, −0.6% to −0.4%) vs. high-wheat fibre diet Δ = −0.3% (95% CI, −0.4 to −0.2%) $p < 0.001$	#### Baseline Low-GI legume diet = 141 (135–147) (95% CI) vs. high-wheat fibre diet = 134 (127–141) (95% CI) End of study Low-GI legume diet = 132 (126–138) (95% CI) vs. high-wheat fibre diet = 127 (121–133) (95% CI) $p = 0.001$	#### Baseline Low-GI legume diet = 80 (79–82) (95% CI) vs. high-wheat fibre diet = 78 (77–80) (95% CI) End of study Low-GI legume diet = 66 (64–67) (95% CI) vs. high-wheat fibre diet = 82 (81–83) (95% CI) $p < 0.001$
Ma et al. [31]	12 months	Parallel Design	40	# 53.53 ± 8.40	# 9.32 ± 9.66	Low-GI diet vs. American Diabetes Association diet (ADA)	## Baseline Low-GI diet = 8.74 ± 0.29% vs. baseline ADA diet = 8.1 ± 0.28% 12 months Low-GI diet = 8.39 ± 0.30% vs. 12-month ADA diet = 7.67 ± 0.28% $p = 0.08$	No data	## Baseline Low-GI diet = 79.35 ± 1.36 vs. ADA diet = 82.03 ± 1.31 12 months Low-GI diet = 76.64 ± 1.46 vs. ADA diet = 80.36 ± 1.40 $p = 0.07$

Table 3. *Cont.*

Citation	Length of Study	Study Type	Sample Size	Age (Years)	Diabetes Duration (Years)	Interventions	Glycated Haemoglobin (HbA1c) %	Blood Glucose	Dietary Glycaemic Index
Gonçalves Reis and Dullius [32]	2 weeks	Cross-over study	12	# 60 ± 8	# 12 ± 7	Low-GI diet vs. higher-GI diet	No data	*# Low-GI diet first day (127 ± 30) vs. higher-GI diet (148 ± 62) (p < 0.05) By the second day FBG levels had the same average value (132 mg/dL) (p = 0.78)	No data
Stenvers et al. [33]	22 months	Cross-over study	20	# 60 ± 7	### 5 (1–9)	Low-GR (Glycaemic Response) liquid formula versus free choice (control)	### Baseline Low-GR = 6.5% (6.1–6.9) Control = 6.5% (6.2–6.9) 12 weeks Low-GR = 6.5% (6.3–7.1) Control = 6.6% (6.3–7.0)	**### Baseline Low-GR = 7.3 (6.4–8.1) Control = 6.8 (6.1–7.4) 12 weeks Low-GR = 7.2 (6.5–7.7) Control = 7.0 (6.7–7.8)	No data
Visek et al. [34]	3 months	Cross-over study	20 (12 men + 8 women)	# 62.7 ± 5.8	# 7 ± 4.1	Low-GI diet versus standard diabetic diet	### Low-GI diet = 6.63 (6.08–7.0)% Standard diabetic diet = 6.45 (6.18–6.91)% (p > 0.05)	**### Low-GI diet = 6.5 (5.6–8.4) Standard diabetic diet = 6.7 (6.1–7.5) (p > 0.05)	### Low-GI diet = 49 (48–51) Standard diabetic diet = 68 (61–72) (p < 0.01)
Wolever et al. [35]	12 months	Parallel Design	162	Low-GI diet = 60.6 ± 1.0 Higher-GI diet = 60.4 ± 1.1	No data	Low-GI diet vs. higher-GI diet	## Baseline Low-GI diet = 6.2 ± 0.8% Higher-GI diet = 6.2 ± 1% Outcomes Low-GI diet = 6.34 ± 0.05% Higher-GI diet = 6.34 ± 0.05% p > 0.05	No data	## Baseline Low-GI diet = 60.3 ± 0.4 Higher-GI diet = 61.5 ± 0.4 Study Low-GI diet = 55.1 ± 0.4 Higher-GI diet = 63.2 ± 0.4 p < 0.001
Yusof et al. [36]	12 weeks	Parallel Design	100	53.5	No data	Low-GI diet vs. conventional carbohydrate exchange (CCE)	## Baseline Low-GI diet = 7.68 ± 1.13% CCE = 7.51 ± 1.24% Week 12 Low-GI diet = 7.2 ± 0.1% CCE = 7.2 ± 0.2% p > 0.05	**## Baseline Low-GI diet = 7.33 ± 2.23 CCE = 7.01 ± 1.79 Week 12 Low-GI diet = 7.3 ± 0.3 CCE = 7.7 ± 0.4 p < 0.05	# Week 12 Low-GI diet = 57 ± 6 Week 12 CCE = 64 ± 5 p < 0.001

Abbreviations: ADA (American Diabetes Association); CCE (conventional carbohydrate exchange); FCB (fasting blood glucose); glycated haemoglobin (HbA1c); GI (glycaemic index); GR (glycaemic response); low-GR (low glycaemic response); * (change); ** (FBG, mg/dL); ** FBG (mmol/L); # (Mean ± SD); ## (mean ± SEM); ### (Median) (25th–75th percentile); #### (Mean and 95% CI, confidence interval).

3.1. Assessment of Risk of Bias in Included Studies

In terms of the selection bias (random sequence generation and allocation concealment) 100% of the studies showed low risk of bias (Figures 2 and 3). With respect to the other risks of bias (blinding, incomplete outcome data, selective reporting and other potential sources of bias), all the studies demonstrated 100% low risk of bias or unclear risk of bias (Figures 2 and 3) except for the Gomes et al. study [17] which demonstrated high risk of bias in relation to the blinding of participants and personnel.

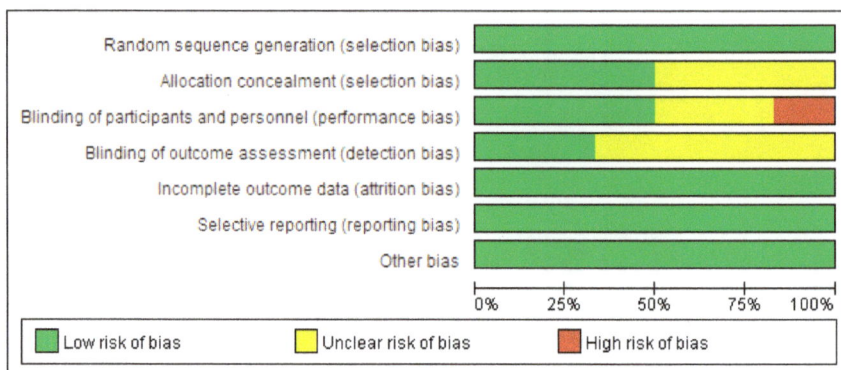

Figure 2. A risk of bias summary.

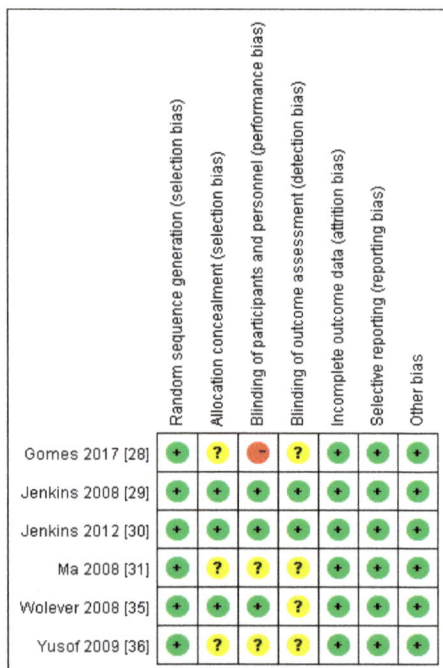

Figure 3. A risk of bias graph.

3.2. Effect of Low Glycaemic Index on Glycated Haemoglobin

The test of the overall effect of the low-GI diet compared to higher-GI diet or control on HbA1c showed that the low-GI diet was more effective both in the meta-analysis ($p < 0.001$) and in the sensitivity test ($p < 0.001$) (removing the study with the most weight) (Figure 4).

There was low heterogeneity ($p = 0.33$) in the studies used to evaluate the effect of low-GI diet on glycated haemoglobin. The I^2 test showed $I^2 = 13\%$ for meta-analysis and $I^2 = 33\%$ for the sensitivity test, again, confirming low heterogeneity of the studies included.

The result of the sensitivity test (Figure 4) showed that the effect of the low-GI diet on glycated haemoglobin was reliable. According to $N_{fs0.05} = (\sum Z/1.64)^2 - S$ (Z representing the Z value of each single study; S representing the number of all enrolled studies) to calculate the fail-safe number ($N_{fs0.05}$)[24], the $N_{fs0.05}$ was 16. That is, another 16 negative studies would be needed to reverse this result, thus indicating that the result is stable.

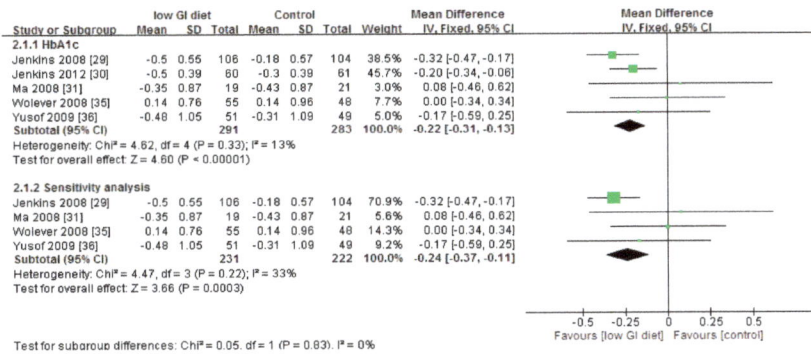

Figure 4. A forest plot showing the effect of low-GI diet on glycated haemoglobin (%).

3.3. Effect of Low Glycaemic Index on Fasting Blood Glucose

With respect to evaluating the effect of the low-GI diet on fasting blood glucose compared to the higher-GI diet or control diet, the meta-analysis favoured the low-GI diet. However, while the differences were significant in the meta-analysis ($p < 0.05$), this was not so in the sensitivity test ($p = 0.15$) (removing the study with the most weight) (Figure 5). These sensitivity results (Figure 5) indicate that the effect of the low-GI diet on fasting blood glucose was not very reliable. The fail-safe number ($N_{fs0.05}$) with respect to fasting blood glucose was 5.

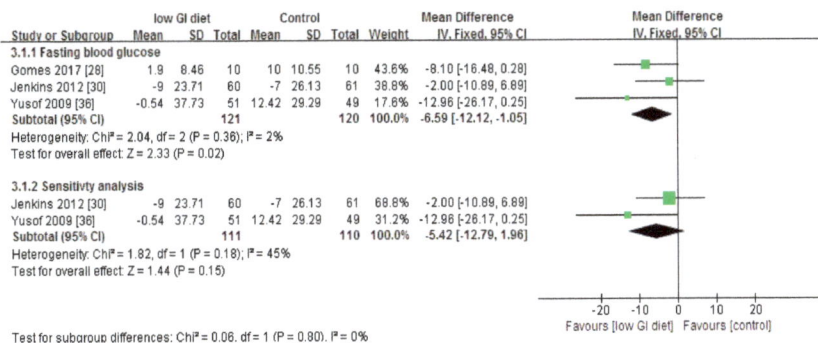

Figure 5. A forest plot showing the effect of low-GI diet on fasting blood glucose (mg/dL).

Regarding the heterogeneity test, the high p value ($p = 0.36$) and the chi-squared statistic (2.04) relative to the degree of freedom (2) would suggest that there was low heterogeneity between the studies. This was confirmed by the results of the I^2 test. The heterogeneity test for fasting blood glucose showed $I^2 = 2\%$ for meta-analysis and $I^2 = 45\%$ for the sensitivity test, indicating low heterogeneity of the studies included.

4. Discussion

Based on the findings of the systematic review, the low-GI diet resulted in greater improvement in glycated haemoglobin [29,30] and fasting blood glucose [28,29,34,36] compared to higher-GI diet or control in patients with type 2 diabetes. In the study by Yusof et al. [36], although the effect on HbA1c was not significantly different between the low-GI diet and the higher-GI diet or control, the improvement within the low-GI group was more pronounced and of clinical benefit. However, compared with the American Diabetes Association (ADA) diet, the low-GI diet achieved equivalent control of HbA1c using less medication [31] and for patients on diet alone with optimal glycaemic control, long-term HbA1c was not affected by altering the GI [35]. The findings of this systematic review confirm the results of earlier systematic review by Thomas and Elliot [8] which suggests that lowering the glycaemic index of food may improve glycated haemoglobin in patients with diabetes. However, the difference between this review and the Thomas and Elliot [8] study is with respect to the second outcome measure. While fasting glucose was the outcome of interest in this review, it was fructosamine in the review by Thomas and Elliot [8]. Regarding the risk of bias, 100% of the studies showed low risk of selection bias while all the studies demonstrated 100% low risk of bias or unclear risk of bias in relation to blinding, incomplete outcome data, selective reporting, and other potential sources of bias except for one study that showed a high risk of bias with respect to the blinding of participants and personnel.

There was no statistically significant difference between the low-GI and higher-GI diets in relation to HbA1c and fasting blood glucose in the study by Visek et al. [34]. Acute glycaemic control was variable over the 3-day period in the study by Gonçalves Reis and Dullius [32] following the adoption of low-GI diet. While the first day of the study demonstrated a significant difference in acute glycaemic control, differences were not significant on the second or third day [32]. Stenvers et al. [33] found no beneficial effect of the low-glycaemic response liquid meal with respect to fasting blood glucose. The differences observed between these studies in terms of their results may be due to the limitations of using HbA1c in identifying the daily changes in glycaemia [17]. The use of HbA1c may not detect the harmful effects of excessive postprandial hyperglycaemic excursions and the risk of hypoglycaemia [7]. According to Chiu and Taylor [7], the contribution of postprandial glucose may be up to 70% in daily hyperglycaemia, and the contribution of fasting glucose increases as glycaemic control worsens. This may explain why the association between dietary GI and HbA1c is not consistent across studies [7]. Therefore, the use of a meta-analysis of both fasting blood glucose and HbA1c levels to evaluate the effect of dietary GI in patients with diabetes is a useful strategy of eliminating the limitation of using HbA1c to assess GI exposure. Other factors to consider include the nature of the starch, particle size, pH, the amount of fibre, fat, and protein, and the cooking method and time, which may affect the GI of food and its effect on blood glucose response, and lead to differences in outcomes of studies [15]. The differences in the classification of low- and high-GI diets may also have effect on outcomes of studies [37].

The Food and Agricultural Organisation [9] has recommended the use of the glycaemic index of foods in clinical applications in patients with diabetes, and that the glycaemic index be used as a useful indicator of the impact of food on the blood glucose response. Recently, the American Diabetes Association (ADA) [38] recommended that patients with diabetes consume carbohydrates from vegetables, fruits, legumes, whole grains, and dairy products. The ADA [38] also recommended that emphasis should be placed on foods which are higher in fibre and lower in glycaemic load as opposed to other sources, especially those with added sugar. The glycaemic load is the product of the glycaemic index of food or diet and the grams of available carbohydrate in that food or diet divided by 100 [9,15]. These recommendations are in line with the findings of the current systematic review and meta-analysis, which showed that low-GI diets were more effective in controlling glycated haemoglobin than higher-GI diets. The position of the ADA [38] with respect to the mixed results of glycaemic index or glycaemic load in patients with diabetes is also true in relation to the findings of the studies included in this review. Foods with low GI have demonstrated beneficial effects on glucose control in short-term trials in patients with type 2 diabetes [13]. However, the higher intake of sucrose or fructose and the long-term use of high-GI diets can place higher metabolic demands on the body in relation to higher insulin requirements [6,39,40].

5. Strengths and Limitation of the Study

This review used a systematic approach and meta-analysis to provide contemporary evidence on the positive effects of low glycaemic index diet on fasting blood glucose and glycated haemoglobin. The limitation is in the number of studies included in the meta-analysis. In addition, most of the studies had relatively small sample sizes. The availability and inclusion of more studies would have increased its wider application.

6. Conclusions

The findings of this systematic review and meta-analysis have shown that low-GI diets are more effective in controlling HbA1c and fasting blood glucose compared with higher-GI diets or control diets in patients with type 2 diabetes. Although the outcomes of the individual studies were sometimes different with respect to the variables of interest, the results of the meta-analysis and sensitivity tests have demonstrated significant differences ($p < 0.001$ and $p < 0.001$, respectively) between low-GI diets and higher-GI diets or control diets in relation to glycated haemoglobin. In addition, differences between the low-GI diet and the higher-GI diet or control were significant ($p < 0.05$) with respect to the fasting blood glucose following meta-analysis.

7. Perspectives for Future Research

It will useful to evaluate the long-term effectiveness of low-glycaemic index diet in patients with type 2 diabetes.

Author Contributions: The concept for this article was agreed upon by O.O., O.O.O., F.A. and X.-H.W. O.O. O.O.O., F.A., and X.-H.W. participated in the searches and in extracting data from the articles reviewed. O.O. and X.-H.W. carried out the data analysis. O.O. wrote the initial draft, which was reviewed and revised by O.O., O.O.O., F.A., and X.-H.W.

Conflicts of Interest: The authors declare no conflict of interest.

References

1. Zghebi, S.S.; Steinke, D.T.; Carr, M.J.; Rutter, M.K.; Emsley, R.A.; Ashcroft, D.M. Examining trends in type 2 diabetes incidence, prevalence and mortality in the UK between 2004 and 2014. *Diabetes Obes. Metab.* **2017**, *19*, 1537–1545. [CrossRef] [PubMed]
2. Sharma, M.; Nazareth, I.; Petersen, I. Trends in incidence, prevalence and prescribing in type 2 diabetes mellitus between 2000 and 2013 in primary care: A retrospective cohort study. *BMJ Open* **2016**, *6*, e010210. [CrossRef] [PubMed]
3. Haynes-Maslow, L.; Leone, L.A. Examining the relationship between the food environment and adult diabetes prevalence by county economic and racial composition: An ecological study. *BMC Public Health* **2017**, *17*, 648. [CrossRef] [PubMed]
4. Hill, J. Management of diabetes in South Asian communities in the UK. *Prim. Health Care* **2007**, *17*, 49–55. [CrossRef]
5. National Collaborating Centre for Chronic Conditions (NCCCC). *Type 2 Diabetes: National Clinical Guideline for Management in Primary and Secondary Care (Update)*; Royal College of Physicians: London, UK, 2008.

6. Russell, W.R.; Baka, A.; Björck, I.; Delzenne, N.; Gao, D.; Griffiths, H.R.; Weickert, M.O. Impact of Diet Composition on Blood Glucose Regulation. *Crit. Rev. Food Sci. Nutr.* **2016**, *56*, 541–590. [CrossRef] [PubMed]
7. Chiu, C.; Taylor, A. Dietary hyperglycemia, glycemic index and metabolic retinal diseases. *Prog. Retin. Eye Res.* **2011**, *30*, 18–53. [CrossRef] [PubMed]
8. Thomas, D.E.; Elliott, E.J. The use of low-glycaemic index diets in diabetes control. *Br. J. Nutr.* **2010**, *104*, 797–802. [CrossRef] [PubMed]
9. Food and Agricultural Organisation (FAO). *Carbohydrates in Human Nutrition. Report of a Joint FAO/WHO Expert Consultation*; FAO (Food and Nutrition paper–66); FAO: Rome, Italy, 1998. Available online: http://www.fao.org/docrep/w8079e/w8079e00.htm (accessed on 16 January 2018).
10. Chang, K.T.; Lampe, J.W.; Schwarz, Y.; Breymeyer, K.L.; Noar, K.A.; Song, X.; Neuhouser, M.L. Low Glycemic Load Experimental Diet More Satiating Than High Glycemic Load Diet. *Nutr. Cancer* **2012**, *64*, 666–673. [CrossRef] [PubMed]
11. Mohan, V.; Anjana, R.M.; Gayathri, R.; Ramya Bai, M.; Lakshmipriya, N.; Ruchi, V.; Sudha, V. Glycemic Index of a Novel High-Fiber White Rice Variety Developed in India—A Randomized Control Trial Study. *Diabetes Technol. Ther.* **2016**, *18*, 164–170. [CrossRef] [PubMed]
12. Similä, M.E.; Valsta, L.M.; Kontto, J.P.; Albanes, D.; Virtamo, J. Low-, medium- and high-glycaemic index carbohydrates and risk of type 2 diabetes in men. *Br. J. Nutr.* **2011**, *105*, 1258–1264. [CrossRef] [PubMed]
13. Jung, C.; Choi, K.M. Impact of High-Carbohydrate Diet on Metabolic Parameters in Patients with Type 2 Diabetes. *Nutrients* **2017**, *9*. [CrossRef] [PubMed]
14. Ikpotokin, O.S.; Adeleye, O.S.; Aliu, E.D.; Osayande, A.B. Ehiabhi, S. Dietary factors in fasting blood glucose levels and weight gain in female Sprague Dawley in rats. *J. Clin. Nutr. Diet.* **2017**, *3*, 2. [CrossRef]
15. Esfahani, A.; Wong, J.W.; Mirrahimi, A.; Villa, C.R.; Kendall, C.C. The application of the glycemic index and glycemic load in weight loss: A review of the clinical evidence. *IUBMB Life* **2011**, *63*, 7–13. [CrossRef] [PubMed]
16. Fabricatore, A.N.; Ebbeling, C.B.; Wadden, T.A.; Ludwig, D.S. Continuous glucose monitoring to assess the ecologic validity of dietary glycemic index and glycemic load. *Am. J. Clin. Nutr.* **2011**, *94*, 1519–1524. [CrossRef] [PubMed]
17. Dunning, T. *Care of People with Diabetes a Manual of Nursing Practice*, 4th ed.; Wiley Blackwell: Hoboken, NJ, USA, 2014.
18. Villegas, R.; Liu, S.; Gao, Y.; Yang, G.; Li, H.; Zheng, W.; Shu, X.O. Prospective study of dietary carbohydrates, glycemic index, glycemic load, and incidence of type 2 diabetes mellitus in middle-aged Chinese women. *Arch. Intern. Med.* **2007**, *167*, 2310–2316. [CrossRef] [PubMed]
19. Krishnan, S.; Rosenberg, L.; Singer, M.; Hu, F.B.; Djoussé, L.; Cupples, L.A.; Palmer, J.R. Glycemic index, glycemic load, and cereal fiber intake and risk of type 2 diabetes in US black women. *Arch. Intern. Med.* **2007**, *167*, 2304–2309. [CrossRef] [PubMed]
20. Ludwig, D.S. The glycemic index: Physiological mechanisms relating to obesity, diabetes, and cardiovascular disease. *JAMA* **2002**, *287*, 2414–2423. [CrossRef] [PubMed]
21. Sacks, F.M.; Carey, V.J.; Anderson, C.M.; Miller, E.; Copeland, T.; Charleston, J.; Appel, L.J. Effects of high vs low glycemic index of dietary carbohydrate on cardiovascular disease risk factors and insulin sensitivity: The OmniCarb randomized clinical trial. *JAMA* **2014**, *312*, 2531–2541. [CrossRef] [PubMed]
22. Greenwood, D.C.; Threapleton, D.E.; Evans, C.L.; Cleghorn, C.L.; Nykjaer, C.; Woodhead, C.; Burley, V.J. Glycemic Index, Glycemic Load, Carbohydrates, and Type 2 Diabetes. *Diabetes Care* **2013**, *36*, 4166–4171. [CrossRef] [PubMed]
23. Fabricatore, A.N.; Wadden, T.A.; Ebbeling, C.B.; Thomas, J.G.; Stallings, V.A.; Schwartz, S.; Ludwig, D.S. Targeting dietary fat or glycemic load in the treatment of obesity and type 2 diabetes: A randomized controlled trial. *Diabetes Res. Clin. Pract.* **2011**, *92*, 37–45. [CrossRef] [PubMed]
24. The Nordic Cochrane Centre. *Review Manager (RevMan) [Computer Program]*; Version 5.3.; The Nordic Cochrane Centre, The Cochrane Collaboration: Copenhagen, Denmark, 2014.
25. Moher, D.; Liberati, A.; Tetzlaff, J.; Altman, D.G.; The PRISMA Group. Preferred Reporting Items for Systematic Reviews and Meta-Analyses: The PRISMA Statement. *Ann. Intern. Med.* **2009**, *151*, 264–269. [CrossRef] [PubMed]
26. Critical Appraisal Skills Programme (CASP). Randomised Controlled Trial Checklist. 2017. Available online: http://docs.wixstatic.com/ugd/dded87_4239299b39f647ca9961f30510f52920.pdf (accessed on 18 January 2018).

27. Higgins, J.P.T.; Green, S. *Cochrane Handbook for Systematic Reviews of Interventions*; Wiley-Blackwell: Hoboken, NJ, USA, 2009.

28. Gomes, J.G.; Fabrini, S.P.; Alfenas, R.G. Low glycemic index diet reduces body fat and attenuates inflammatory and metabolic responses in patients with type 2 diabetes. *Arch. Endocrinol. Metab.* **2017**, *61*, 137–144. [CrossRef] [PubMed]

29. Jenkins, D.A.; Kendall, C.C.; McKeown-Eyssen, G.; Josse, R.G.; Silverberg, J.; Booth, G.L.; Leiter, L.A. Effect of a low-glycemic index or a high-cereal fiber diet on type 2 diabetes: A randomized trial. *JAMA* **2008**, *300*, 2742–2753. [CrossRef] [PubMed]

30. Jenkins, D.A.; Kendall, C.C.; Augustin, L.A.; Mitchell, S.; Sahye-Pudaruth, S.; Blanco Mejia, S.; Josse, R.G. Effect of legumes as part of a low glycemic index diet on glycemic control and cardiovascular risk factors in type 2 diabetes mellitus: A randomized controlled trial. *Arch. Intern. Med.* **2012**, *172*, 1653–1660. [CrossRef] [PubMed]

31. Ma, Y.; Olendzki, B.C.; Merriam, P.A.; Chiriboga, D.E.; Culver, A.L.; Li, W.; Pagoto, S.L. A randomized clinical trial comparing low-glycemic index versus ADA dietary education among individuals with type 2 diabetes. *Nutrition* **2008**, *24*, 45–56. [CrossRef] [PubMed]

32. Gonçalves Reis, C.E.; Dullius, J. Glycemic acute changes in type 2 diabetics caused by low and high glycemic index diets. *Nutr. Hosp.* **2011**, *26*, 546–552. [PubMed]

33. Stenvers, D.J.; Schouten, L.J.; Jurgens, J.; Endert, E.; Kalsbeek, A.; Fliers, E.; Bisschop, P.H. Breakfast replacement with a low-glycaemic response liquid formula in patients with type 2 diabetes: A randomised clinical trial. *Br. J. Nutr.* **2014**, *112*, 504–512. [CrossRef] [PubMed]

34. Visek, J.; Lacigova, S.; Cechurova, D.; Rusavy, Z. *Comparison of a Low-Glycemic Index vs. Standard Diabetic Diet*; Biomedical Papers of the Medical Faculty of The University Palacky; The University Palacky: Olomouc, Czechoslovakia, 2014; Volume 158, pp. 112–116.

35. Wolever, T.; Gibbs, A.; Mehling, C.; Chiasson, J.; Connelly, P.; Josse, R.; Ryan, E. The Canadian Trial of Carbohydrates in Diabetes (CCD), a 1-y controlled trial of low-glycemic-index dietary carbohydrate in type 2 diabetes: No effect on glycated hemoglobin but reduction in C-reactive protein. *Am. J. Clin. Nutr.* **2008**, *87*, 114–125. [CrossRef] [PubMed]

36. Yusof, B.M.; Talib, R.A.; Kamaruddin, N.A.; Karim, N.A.; Chinna, K.; Gilbertson, H. A low-GI diet is associated with a short-term improvement of glycaemic control in Asian patients with type 2 diabetes. *Diabetes Obes. Metab.* **2009**, *11*, 387–396. [CrossRef] [PubMed]

37. Miller, C.K.; Headings, A.; Peyrot, M.; Nagaraja, H. A behavioural intervention incorporating specific glycaemic index goals improves dietary quality, weight control and glycaemic control in adults with type 2 diabetes. *Public Health Nutr.* **2011**, *14*, 1303–1311. [CrossRef] [PubMed]

38. American Diabetes Association. Life style management: Standards of Medical Care in Diabetes–2018. *Diabetes Care* **2018**, *41* (Suppl. 1), S38–S50.

39. Ojo, O.; Brooke, J. Evaluation of the role of enteral nutrition in managing patients with diabetes: A systematic review. *Nutrients* **2014**, *6*, 5142–5152. [CrossRef] [PubMed]

40. Widanagamage, R.D.; Ekanayake, S.; Welihinda, J. Carbohydrate-rich foods: Glycaemic indices and the effect of constituent macronutrients. *Int. J. Food Sci. Nutr.* **2009**, *60*, 215–223. [CrossRef] [PubMed]

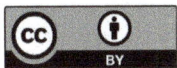

nutrients

MDPI

Article

Effects of Different Dietary and Lifestyle Modification Therapies on Metabolic Syndrome in Prediabetic Arab Patients: A 12-Month Longitudinal Study

Hanan A. Alfawaz [1,2], Kaiser Wani [1,3], Abdullah M. Alnaami [1,3], Yousef Al-Saleh [4], Naji J. Aljohani [5], Omar S. Al-Attas [1,3], Majed S. Alokail [1,3], Sudhesh Kumar [6] and Nasser M. Al-Daghri [1,3,*]

[1] Prince Mutaib Chair for Biomarkers of Osteoporosis, Biochemistry Department, College of Science, King Saud University, Riyadh 11451, Saudi Arabia; halfawaz@ksu.edu.sa (H.A.A.); wani.kaiser@gmail.com (K.W.); aalnaami@yahoo.com (A.M.A.); omrattas@ksu.edu.sa (O.S.A.-A.); msa85@yahoo.co.uk (M.S.A.)

[2] Department of Food Science and Nutrition, College of Food Science & Agriculture, King Saud University, Riyadh 11451, Saudi Arabia

[3] Biomarkers Research Program, Biochemistry Department, College of Science, King Saud University, Riyadh 11451, Saudi Arabia

[4] College of Medicine, King Saud bin Abdulaziz University for Health Sciences, Riyadh 11461, Saudi Arabia; alaslawi@hotmail.com

[5] Specialized Diabetes and Endocrine Center, King Fahad Medical City, Faculty of Medicine, King Saud bin Abdulaziz University for Health Sciences, Riyadh 11525, Saudi Arabia; najijohani@gmail.com

[6] Division of Metabolic and Vascular Health, Clinical Sciences Research Institute, University Hospitals Coventry and Warwickshire Trust, Walsgrave, Coventry CV2 2DX, UK; Sudhesh.Kumar@warwick.ac.uk

* Correspondence: aldaghri2011@gmail.com; Tel.: +966-11-467-5939

Received: 12 February 2018; Accepted: 15 March 2018; Published: 20 March 2018

Abstract: This three-arm, randomized, controlled study aimed to determine the differences in the effects of general advice (GA) on lifestyle change, intensive lifestyle modification programme (ILMP) and GA + metformin (GA + Met) in reducing the prevalence of full metabolic syndrome (MetS) in subjects with prediabetes; 294 Saudis with prediabetes (fasting glucose 5.6–6.9 mmol/L) were initially randomized, 263 completed 6 months and 237 completed 12 months. They were allocated into three groups: GA group which received a standard lifestyle change education; ILMP which followed a rigorous lifestyle modification support on diet and physical activity; and a GA + Met group. Anthropometric and biochemical estimations were measured. Full MetS (primary endpoint) and its components (secondary endpoint) were screened at baseline, 6 and 12 months. Full MetS in the ILMP group decreased by 26% ($p < 0.001$); in GA + Met group by 22.4% ($p = 0.01$) and in GA group by 8.2% ($p = 0.28$). The number of MetS components decreased significantly in the ILMP and GA + Met groups (mean change 0.81, $p < 0.001$ and 0.35, $p = 0.05$, respectively). Between-group comparison revealed a clinically significant decrease in MetS components in favor of the ILMP group (-0.58 (-0.88–0.28), $p < 0.001$). This study highlights the clinical potency of ILMP versus other diabetes prevention options in reducing MetS in Saudi adults with elevated fasting glucose.

Keywords: impaired glucose regulation; lifestyle modifications; metabolic syndrome; type 2 diabetes; metformin

1. Introduction

Type 2 diabetes mellitus (T2DM) has a huge impact on the health status of patients and the overall health care cost of the country. One big opportunity to reduce such an impact is to reduce the incidence of the disease by focusing on high-risk people such as those with impaired glucose regulation. This condition is characterized either by impaired fasting glucose (IFG) (fasting glucose levels 5.6–6.9 mmol/L) or impaired glucose tolerance (IGT) (2-h oral glucose tolerance test (OGTT) 7.8–11 mmol/L) [1]. Every year, about 5–10% of people with IGT progress to T2DM [2]. Fortunately, landmark clinical trials like the Diabetes Prevention Programme (DPP) [3] and others [4,5] have revealed the effectiveness of lifestyle modifications in reducing the incidence of T2DM. The major focus of these interventions were weight loss and physical activity. However, a recent meta-analysis [6,7] concluded that when translated into routine clinical settings, these expensive programmes have more effect on weight reduction and less effect on diabetes risk reduction. Clearly, such intervention studies need to be done, not only to add to the literature to better predict the outcomes on a global health-care perspective but also to devise large-scale effective and low cost intervention programmes on a regional level such as in Saudi Arabia, where data are limited.

Identification of individual risk factors associated with the increased effectiveness of lifestyle intervention programmes may help in devising them in a more economical and practical way. Metabolic Syndrome (MetS), an amalgam of cardiovascular risk factors, is a major health problem globally. It is defined by the National Cholesterol Education Program Adult Treatment Panel III (NCEP ATP III) as the presence of at least three out of five risk factors (central obesity, hyperglycemia, low HDL-cholesterol, hypertriglyceridemia and elevated blood pressure) [8]. The prevalence of MetS is increasing rapidly worldwide, including Saudi Arabia, as a result of rapid economic growth and Westernization of diet [9,10].

The risk of developing incident T2DM in patients with MetS is manifold compared to those without this condition [11]. Also, all components of MetS are independent risk factors for developing T2DM [12]. Prevention of T2DM in subjects with impaired glucose regulation through lifestyle modifications in diet, physical activity or by giving drugs like metformin have been studied in the past, however, the applicability of these treatments in prevention or reversal of MetS is largely unknown, particularly in a population like Saudi Arabia where the prevalence of both T2DM and MetS is high [13,14]. We hypothesize that lifestyle modifications in diet and physical activity have a role in preventing or reversal of Mets in subjects with impaired glucose regulation. Hence, this study aimed to investigate the differences in the effectiveness of lifestyle modifications (diet and physical activity) and drug therapy (metformin), in an adult Saudi population with impaired glucose regulation, in preventing or reversing full MetS and its individual components.

2. Materials and Methods

This is a 12 months, 2-center, 3-arm randomized controlled (1:1:1), lifestyle intervention study conducted from April 2013 until March of 2017. This lifestyle intervention programme was approved by the Ethics Committee of the College of Science, King Saud University; Riyadh, Saudi Arabia (Reference# 8/25/220355) and funded by the National Plan for Science and Technology; Riyadh, Saudi Arabia (Grant# 12-MED2881-02). All procedures followed were in accordance with the ethical standards of the responsible committee on human experimentation (institutional and national) and with the Helsinki Declaration of 1975, as revised in 2008. Written informed consent was obtained from each participant prior to inclusion in this 12-month interventional study.

2.1. Study Population

A total of 294 Saudi males and females (age range 25–60) attending King Khalid University Hospital and King Salman Hospital in Riyadh, Saudi Arabia, agreed to take part in this lifestyle intervention Programme. The criteria for selection was a fasting glucose level of 5.6 to 6.9 mmol/L, identified as one of the five components of MetS (NCEP ATP III criteria) [15]. Interested participants were referred to the concerned physician who used the guidelines stated under section "prevention or delay of type 2 diabetes" in "standards for medical care in diabetes" [16] to screen the candidates. Subjects who were already on anti-hyperglycemic treatment; pregnant or lactating women; with known renal, hepatic, pulmonary, cardiac, etc., complications were excluded.

A computer-generated serial number, randomly assigned to one of the three intervention groups (GA, ILMP, and GA + Met), was given blindly to each participant. All participants were allocated (1:1:1) to receive one of the three interventions. True allocation concealment was done since the research personnel involved cannot adjust randomization. The total duration of this lifestyle intervention programme was 12 months. Fasting blood samples and anthropometric data was collected at recruitment, at 6-month and at the end of the programme. Out of the 294 initially recruited, the data for 217 was used in this study. A flow chart summarizing the programme is provided in Figure 1.

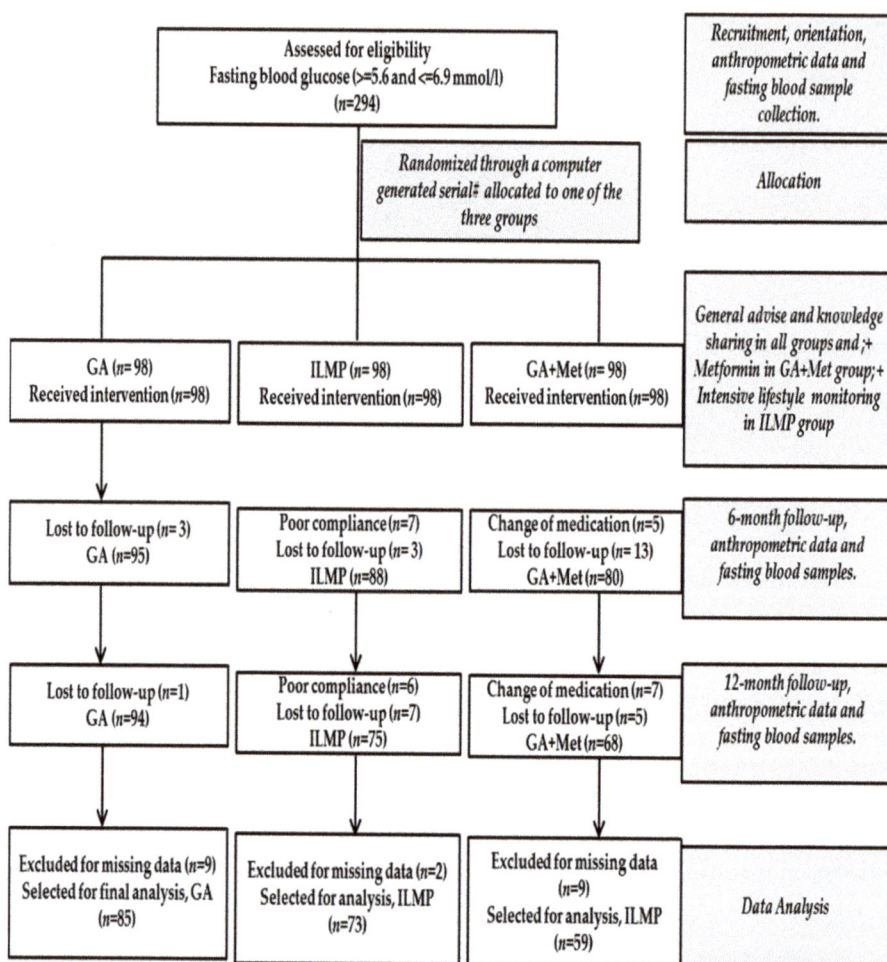

Figure 1. Flow chart detailing the participation of subjects and their allocation to treatment groups.

2.2. Intervention

All participants had an orientation session with concerned physician and a dietician where they were educated about risk of developing T2DM and the current scenario of diabetes worldwide and Saudi Arabia. They were advised to adopt lifestyle modifications in their dietary habits; weight reduction; exercise; increased physical activity etc. This knowledge sharing included distributing pamphlets and booklets with information related to lifestyle modifications in earlier programmes, done elsewhere [17,18]. In addition to this, every four months, seminars were conducted at the auditorium of the respective hospitals in which the investigators of the current study educated the participants about lifestyle modifications to prevent T2DM. This intervention process was unified across the two study centers.

The participants in the general advice (GA) group received the usual instructions to lifestyle change as described above. In addition to this the participants in intensive lifestyle modification programme (ILMP) group were followed with a rigorous lifestyle modification support published earlier [19,20], which included:

(a) Individual consultation with the dietician was done to assess the participant's food intake. Special dietary charts were supplied to participants explaining how to reduce the total fat intake to less than 30% of energy consume and increase the fiber intake to 15 g/1000 Kcal.

(b) Guidelines for physical activity were supplied as pamphlets to each participant. Also, each participant was given a pedometer (081564483, Patterson Medical) and recommended at least 5000 steps per day to gradually increase as tolerance develops.

(c) Individual consultation with an expert on vitamin D to educate about the benefits of optimal levels of vitamin D for good health. They were recommended to expose to sunlight for at least 30 min either before 10 a.m. and/or after 3 p.m. twice a week.

The intervention in ILMP group was monitored regularly which were scheduled every three months during the course of the programme.

The third intervention group (GA + Met) was provided with the same general advice and were given 500 mg of metformin hydrochloride, twice a day. The participants in ILMP and GA + Met groups were regularly contacted by research assistants to reinforce instructions through phone calls.

2.3. Anthropometric and Biochemical Measurements

Anthropometrics were collected at recruitment (baseline), 6-month and 12-month. The anthropometrics included height (cm), weight (kg), waist and hip circumferences (cm), systolic and diastolic blood pressure by standard methods. Fasting blood samples, taken at each time point, were sent immediately to Prince Mutaib Chair for biomarkers in Osteoporosis (PMCO), King Saud University (KSU), Riyadh where they were processed, aliquoted and stored at recommended temperature for further analysis.

Fasting blood glucose and lipid profile was quantified using routine biochemical tests in an automated biochemistry analyzer (Konelab 20, Thermo-Fischer scientific, Helsinki, Finland). The reagents were supplied ready to use by Thermo Fischer (catalog# 981379 for glucose; 981812 for total cholesterol; 981823 for HDL-cholesterol and 981301 for triglyceride). The imprecision, calculated as the total CV, was $\leq$5%, $\leq$3.5%, $\leq$4% and $\leq$4% for these tests respectively. 25(OH)vitamin D was quantified using COBAS e-411 autoanalyzer (Roche Diagnostics, Indianapolis, IN, USA). Glycated haemoglobin (HbA1c) was quantified in DCA vantage analyzer (Siemens, Munich, Germany). The imprecision of the HbA1c assay was $\leq$3.6% in the important clinical ranges. The standards and controls used for these biochemical assays were routinely tested by Quality assurance department of KSU, for highly reproducible research data.

2.4. Outcome Variables

For the purpose of this study, the status of MetS and its five components were evaluated at follow up (6-month and 12-month) versus baseline. MetS was defined by the criteria set in "The National

Cholesterol Education Programme Adult Treatment Panel III" (NCEP ATP III) as having atleast three of the five components [15]:

(a) Central obesity-waist circumference of >101.6 cm in males and >88.9 cm in females.
(b) Hyperglycemia-fasting glucose > 5.6 mmol/L.
(c) Low HDL-Cholesterol < 1.03 mmol/L in males and <1.30 mmol/L in females.
(d) Hypertriglyceridemia-fasting triglycerides > 1.7 mmol/L.
(e) Hypertension-systolic blood pressure > 130 mmHg and/or diastolic blood pressure > 85 mmHg.

Two other variables were tested in this study for the intervention effects between groups. One was the total number of MetS components (taken as a continuous variable) and the other was the MetS risk-score. The MetS risk-score was constructed for the evaluation of continuous MetS status, calculated using the formula with cut-off values employed to define each component of MetS, with consideration to age and gender as follows:

MetS risk-score = ((waist/101.6 for males or 88.9 for males) + (fasting glucose/5.6) − (HDL-Cholesterol/1.03 for males or 1.30 for females) + (triglyceride/1.7) + (systolic BP/130) + (diastolic BP/85)) × (Age/45 for males or 50 for females).

The Receiver Operating Characteristic (ROC) analysis was employed to test this score for predicting MetS in our data, with full MetS positive (≥3 MetS components) versus full MetS negative (<3 MetS components). The ROC revealed an area under the curve (AOC) of 0.890 with 95% confidence interval of 0.86 and 0.92 and a *p*-value of <0.001. The cut-off of MetS risk-score for predicting MetS, obtained in ROC analysis, was 3.85 (Supplementary Figure S1, Table S1–S2).

2.5. Data Analysis

As expected with longitudinal studies, the data in this study had random missing values which are a limitation for utilizing any test on repeated measure data. Hence, the missing data (<5% of the total data points in any variable) was dealt with the last observation carried forward (LOCF) method. However, as much as possible, the LOCF was minimized by removing the data of the subjects lost to follow up at 6-month or 12-month and also by removing ones with >5% missing data in any variable (Figure 1). The remaining data (*n* = 217) was analyzed using SPSS 21. Continuous normally distributed variables were summarized as mean ± standard deviation while median (25th percentile, 75th percentile) was used for continuous non-normal variables. Simple One-way ANOVA and Kruskal-Wallis one-way ANOVA were used to test the differences between the three treatment groups at baseline. The status of MetS and its five components were evaluated as present/absent at all three time-points, which were presented as frequency (% of the present in the respective group) and chi-square test (McNemar 2 × 2 contingency table) was used to calculate the *p*-value of the difference in percentages. The intervention effect within each group was shown as Odds ratio (95% confidence interval) and respective *p*-value representing odds of having MetS and its components independently at follow-up compared to baseline and this data was generated by Generalized Estimating Equation (GEE) in SPSS for repeated measures of nominal data. Finally, the intervention effect between the groups was shown as mean Change (95% confidence interval), *p*-value for the total number of MetS components (taking MetS components as scalar quantity) and MetS risk-score by mixed repeated measures ANCOVA. *p*-Values were considered significant at <0.05.

3. Results

A total of 294 (98 in each group) Saudi adults with impaired fasting glucose were initially randomized and 237 (94 in GA, 75 in ILMP and 68 in GA + Met) completed the entire 12 months of this intervention. The most common reasons for drop out included loss to follow-up and poor compliance. After excluding persons with missing data >5% in any parameter, the data for 217 subjects (85 in GA, 73 in ILMP and 59 in GA + Met) were used for analysis (Figure 1).

3.1. Anthropometric and Biochemical Characteristics at Baseline and over Time

Table 1 shows the anthropometric, glycemic, and lipid characteristics of the study participants at baseline, 6-month, and 12-month, according to treatment groups. The mean change in fasting glucose from baseline to end of study for ILMP and GA + Met groups decreased significantly (-0.39 mmol/L, $p = 0.003$ and -0.81 mmol/L, $p < 0.001$ respectively). This was not observed in the GA group (-0.005 mmol/L, $p = 0.65$). Weight was significantly reduced in the GA + Met group from baseline to 12 months (mean change of -4.15 kg, $p < 0.001$). ILMP group also showed a significant reduction in weight (mean change $= -1.86$ kg, $p = 0.015$) while the average weight for GA group increased from baseline to the end of the study by 0.49 kg. Waist, systolic blood pressure and triglycerides significantly reduced from baseline to 12 months in the ILMP group (-1.61 cm, $p = 0.004$; -2.59 mmHg, $p = 0.049$ and -0.23 mmol/L, $p = 0.03$ respectively). At baseline, the three treatment groups were significantly different in waist ($p < 0.01$), systolic blood pressure ($p = 0.01$), diastolic blood pressure ($p = 0.02$), fasting glucose ($p < 0.01$), HbA1c ($p < 0.01$) and vitamin D levels ($p = 0.03$).

Table 1. Anthropometric and biochemical characteristics at baseline and follow-up.

Treatment (*n*) Female/Male	GA (85) 64/21	ILMP (73) 51/22	GA+Met (59) 42/17	*p* [B]
Anthropometrics				
Age (years)	42.3 ± 11.2	43.4 ± 7.8	42.6 ± 6.9	0.74
Weight (Kg)				
Baseline	81.7 ± 13.9	79.6 ± 15.9	80.4 ± 14.9	
6-month	82.3 ± 13.9	78.7 ± 15.9	77.6 ±13.9	
12-month	82.2 ±13.4	77.7 ± 16.2	76.3 ±14.1	0.67
Change at 6 months	0.61	−0.93	−2.86 **	
Change at 12 months	0.49	−1.86 *	−4.15 **	
BMI (kg/m^2)				
Baseline	32.6 ± 5.8	31.3 ± 6.4	32.1 ± 5.7	
6-month	32.8 ± 5.9	31.0 ± 6.7	31.0 ± 5.4	
12-month	32.8 ± 5.7	30.6 ± 6.6	30.4 ± 5.3	0.18
Change at 6 months	0.26	−0.32	−1.14 **	
Change at 12 months	0.21	−0.71 *	−1.68 **	
Waist (cm)				
Baseline	95.6 ± 6.8	97.9 ± 13	103.6 ± 12.5	
6-month	95.7 ± 6.7	97.7 ± 13.5	102.6 ± 12.8	
12-month	95.5 ± 6.2	96.3 ± 13	102.6 ± 12.3	<0.01
Change at 6 months	0.12	−0.25	−0.95	
Change at 12 months	−0.09	−1.61 **	−0.96	
Hips (cm)				
Baseline	110.2 ± 7.9	111. 9 ± 12	111.0 ± 12	
6-month	110.5 ± 7.9	111.0 ± 11.6	109.5 ± 10.9	
12-month	110.6 ± 7.6	109.9 ± 12.2	109.6 ± 10.9	0.60
Change at 6 months	0.26	−0.86 *	−1.48 **	
Change at 12 months	0.44	−1.98 **	−1.39 *	
Systolic BP (mmHG)				
Baseline	120.0 ± 12.1	122.1 ± 15.8	127.4 ± 11.6	
6-month	117.8 ± 14.4	120.0 ± 18.5	129.2 ± 11.1	
12-month	119.2 ± 15.8	119.5 ± 16.6	129.3 ± 10.7	0.01
Change at 6 months	−2.25	−2.12	1.86	
Change at 12 months	−0.86	−2.59 *	1.97	
Diastolic BP (mmHG)				
Baseline	76.4 ± 9.7	76.0 ± 11.9	80.6 ± 9.0	
6-month	76.4 ± 12.1	76.0 ± 12.1	81.2 ± 11.1	
12-month	77.1 ± 13.7	74.6 ± 12.8	83.3 ± 9.2	0.02
Change at 6 months	0.06	0.14	0.68	
Change at 12 months	0.71	−1.38	2.73	

Table 1. *Cont.*

Treatment (n) Female/Male	GA (85) 64/21	ILMP (73) 51/22	GA+Met (59) 42/17	p^B
Glycemic Profile				
Fasting Glucose (mmol/L)				
Baseline	6.0 ± 0.4	6.1 ± 0.4	6.6 ± 0.5	
6-month	6.1 ± 0.7	5.7 ± 0.8	6.0 ± 1.3	
12-month	5.9 ± 0.9	5.7 ± 0.8	5.8 ± 1.7	<0.01
Change at 6 months	0.09	−0.40 **	−0.56 **	
Change at 12 months	−0.05	−0.39 **	−0.81 **	
HbA1c				
Baseline	5.6 ± 0.5	5.8 ± 0.4	5.6 ± 0.5	
6-month	5.7 ± 1.6	5.6 ± 0.4	5.1 ± 1.5	
12-month	5.6 ± 1.5	5.5 ± 1.0	5.0 ± 1.7	<0.01
Change at 6 months	0.06	−0.22	−0.47 **	
Change at 12 months	−0.06	−0.30	−0.53 **	
Lipid Profile				
Total Cholesterol (mmol/l)				
Baseline	4.8 ± 1.0	5.2 ± 1.3	4.8 ± 1.2	
6-month	4.8 ± 1.2	5.0 ± 1.1	4.9 ± 1.0	
12-month	4.6 ± 1.1	5.0 ± 1.0	4.9 ± 1.2	0.06
Change at 6 months	−0.05	−0.19	0.04	
Change at 12 months	−0.22	−0.24	0.06	
HDL-Cholesterol (mmol/l)				
Baseline	1.1 ± 0.3	1.2 ± 0.4	1.2 ± 0.4	
6-month	0.93 ± 0.4	1.2 ± 0.4	1.1 ± 0.4	
12-month	0.96 ± 0.4	1.2 ± 0.4	1.2 ± 0.3	0.49
Change at 6 months	−0.16	0.02	−0.02	
Change at 12 months	−0.13	0.03	0.01	
Triglycerides (mmol/l)				
Baseline	1.4 (1.1, 2.1)	1.5 (1.1, 1.8)	1.6 (1.2, 2.0)	
6-month	1.5 (1.1, 2.1)	1.3 (1.1, 1.8)	1.6 (1.3, 2.2)	
12-month	1.4 (1.1, 2.0)	1.2 (1.0, 1.7)	1.6 (1.3, 2.0)	0.75
Change at 6 months	0.11	−0.12	0.03	
Change at 12 months	−0.03	−0.23 *	0.00	
25(OH) vitamin D (nmol/l)				
Baseline	41.7 (24.0, 73.0)	47.3 (30, 67.2)	57.0 (38, 96)	
6-month	45.0 (28.5, 72.6)	54.1 (40, 68)	62.4 (41, 95)	
12-month	48.3 (28.3, 74.7)	56.1 (40, 72.2)	62.4 (42, 96)	0.03
Change at 6 months	0.66	3.78	0.98	
Change at 12 months	2.49	5.82	3.79	

Note: Data presented as Mean ± SD for continuous normal variables and medians (25th–75th percentile) for continuous non-normal variables; * and ** represent significant mean change at $p < 0.05$ and $p <0.01$ respectively. p^B represents difference between treatment groups at baseline. GA is "general advice group", ILMP is "intensive lifestyle monitoring programme group", GA + Met is "Metformin group", BMI is "body mass index", BP is "blood pressure", HbA1c is "glycated haemoglobin", HDL is "high density lipoprotein". $p < 0.05$ is considered significant.

3.2. Prevalence of MetS and Its Components at Baseline and Overtime

Table 2 shows the percentage of subjects having different components of MetS and full MetS in the three treatment groups at baseline, follow-up and percentage of subjects in which there was a change in status over time. MetS and its components were evaluated as binomial variables. Component 1 (central obesity) and component 4 (hypertriglyceridemia) showed the lowest changes at follow-up in all the three groups (−1.2%, −1.4% and −1.7% in central obesity; and +3.5%, −4.1% and 0% in hypertriglyceridemia for groups GA, ILMP and GA + Met respectively). Component 3 (Low HDL-Cholesterol) increased by 7.1% (n = 6) in GA group at end of the study compared to baseline while it decreased by 6.8% (n = 5) and 3.4% (n = 2), respectively, in ILMP and GA + Met groups. Component 5 (Hypertension) increased by 2.4% (n = 2) and by 8.5% (n = 5, p = 0.035) in GA and GA + Met groups, respectively, while it decreased by 1.4% ($n = 1$) in the ILMP group. The highest change was seen in component 2 (hyperglycemia) where from baseline to end of the study, hyperglycemia was reduced by 22.4% ($n = 19$), 38.4% ($n = 28$) and 39% ($n = 23$), respectively, in GA, ILMP, and GA+ILMP groups respectively. Full MetS was also significantly reduced by 8.2% ($n = 7$), 26% ($n = 19$, $p < 0.001$), and 22.4% ($n = 13$, $p = 0.013$), respectively, in GA, ILMP, and GA + Met groups.

Table 2. Prevalence of MetS and its 5 components at baseline and follow-up.

		Central Obesity	Hyperglycemia	Hyper Triglyceridemia	Low HDL-Cholesterol	Hypertension	MetS
GA (85)	Baseline	63 (74.1)	85 (100)	64 (75.3)	36 (42.4)	14 (16.5)	62 (72.9)
	6-month	61 (71.8)	76 (89.4)	71 (83.5)	36 (42.4)	19 (22.4)	63 (74.1)
	12-month	62 (72.9)	66 (77.6)	70 (82.4)	33 (38.8)	16 (18.8)	55 (64.7)
	% change-6	−2.3	−10.6	8.2	0.0	5.9	1.2
	% change-12	−1.2	−22.4	7.1	−3.5	2.4	−8.2
ILMP (73)	Baseline	45 (61.6)	73 (100)	47 (64.4)	23 (31.5)	22 (30.1)	45 (61.6)
	6-month	46 (63.0)	56 (76.7)	43 (58.9)	21 (28.8)	22 (30.1)	36 (49.3)
	12-month	44 (60.3)	45 (61.6)	42 (57.5)	20 (27.4)	21 (28.8)	26 (35.6)
	% change-6	1.4	−23.3	−5.5	−2.7	0.0	−12.3
	% change-12	−1.4	−38.4	−6.8	−4.1	−1.4	−26.0 **
GA + Met (59)	Baseline	47 (79.7)	59 (100)	39 (66.1)	25 (42.4)	22 (37.3)	49 (83.1)
	6-month	46 (78.0)	43 (72.9)	42 (71.2)	24 (40.7)	29 (49.2)	42 (71.2)
	12-month	46 (78.0)	36 (61.0)	37 (62.7)	25 (42.4)	27 (45.8)	38 (64.4)
	% change-6	−1.7	−27.1	5.1	−1.7	11.9 *	−11.9
	% change-12	−1.7	−39.0	−3.4	0.0	8.5 *	−22.4 *

Note: Data presented as n (%). % change (6 for 6-month and 12 for 12-month) represents the overall percentage change in respective treatment groups; * and ** represents significant change at $p < 0.05$ and $p < 0.01$ respectively.

3.3. Odds of Having MetS and Its Components at Follow-Up Compared to Baseline

Table 3 shows the odds of having MetS and its individual components at follow-up compared to baseline in each group. Supplementary Table S3 shows the odds of having MetS for these covariates, independent of each other.

Table 3. Odds ratio representing the risk of having MetS and its individual components at follow-up compared to baseline in respective groups.

		Baseline	6-Month		12-Month	
		Reference	O.R. (95% C.I.)	p	O.R. (95% C.I.)	p
Central Obesity						
GA	Model a	1.00	0.89 (0.8, 1.0)	0.15	0.94 (0.7, 1.2)	0.65
	Model b	1.00	0.73 (0.5, 1.1)	0.13	0.85 (0.4, 1.7)	0.65
	Model c	1.00	0.71 (0.5, 1.1)	0.12	0.84 (0.4, 1.8)	0.65
ILMP	Model a	1.00	1.06 (0.8, 1.4)	0.65	0.94 (0.7, 1.2)	0.65
	Model b	1.00	1.08 (0.8, 1.5)	0.65	0.92 (0.7, 1.3)	0.654
	Model c	1.00	1.25 (0.5, 3.2)	0.64	0.80 (0.3, 2.2)	0.67
GA + Met	Model a	1.00	0.90 (0.6, 1.3)	0.56	0.90 (0.5, 1.5)	0.71
	Model b	1.00	0.88 (0.6, 1.4)	0.56	0.88 (0.4, 1.7)	0.70
	Model c	1.00	0.74 (0.3, 2.1)	0.56	0.74 (0.2, 3.5)	0.71
Low HDL-Cholesterol						
GA	Model a	1.00	1.66 (0.9, 3.2)	0.13	1.53 (0.8, 2.8)	0.18
	Model b	1.00	1.80 (0.8, 3.8)	0.13	1.64 (0.8, 3.4)	0.18
	Model c	1.00	1.83 (0.8, 4.0)	0.13	1.66 (0.8, 3.5)	0.18
ILMP	Model a	1.00	0.75 (0.4, 1.3)	0.34	0.79 (0.4, 1.4)	0.43
	Model b	1.00	0.75 (0.4, 1.4)	0.34	0.79 (0.4, 1.4)	0.43
	Model c	1.00	0.74 (0.4, 1.4)	0.34	0.79 (0.4, 1.4)	0.43
GA + Met	Model a	1.00	1.27 (0.7, 2.4)	0.47	0.86 (0.4, 1.7)	0.67
	Model b	1.00	1.27 (0.6, 2.4)	0.47	0.86 (0.4, 1.7)	0.67
	Model c	1.00	1.27 (0.7, 2.4)	0.47	0.86 (0.4, 1.7)	0.67

Table 3. *Cont.*

		Baseline	6-Month		12-Month	
		Reference	O.R. (95% C.I.)	*p*	O.R. (95% C.I.)	*p*
			Hypertriglyceridemia			
	Model a	1.00	1.00 (0.7, 1.5)	1.00	0.86 (0.6, 1.3)	0.49
GA	Model b	1.00	1.00 (0.6, 1.5)	1.00	0.86 (0.6, 1.3)	0.49
	Model c	1.00	1.00 (0.6, 1.6)	1.00	0.86 (0.5, 1.3)	0.49
	Model a	1.00	0.88 (0.5, 1.5)	0.62	0.82 (0.5, 1.4)	0.44
ILMP	Model b	1.00	0.87 (0.5, 1.5)	0.62	0.80 (0.5, 1.4)	0.44
	Model c	1.00	0.86 (0.5, 1.5)	0.62	0.80 (0.5, 1.4)	0.44
	Model a	1.00	0.93 (0.6, 1.5)	0.78	1.00 (0.6, 1.7)	1.00
GA + Met	Model b	1.00	0.93 (0.5, 1.6)	0.78	1.00 (0.6, 1.7)	1.00
	Model c	1.00	0.92 (0.5, 1.6)	0.78	1.00 (0.6, 1.8)	1.00
			Hypertension			
	Model a	1.00	1.46 (0.8, 2.6)	0.19	1.18 (0.6, 2.1)	0.59
GA	Model b	1.00	1.48 (0.8, 2.7)	0.19	1.18 (0.6, 2.2)	0.59
	Model c	1.00	1.80 (0.8, 4.2)	0.18	1.28 (0.5, 3.1)	0.59
	Model a	1.00	1.00 (0.7, 1.5)	1.00	0.94 (0.6, 1.4)	0.76
ILMP	Model b	1.00	1.00 (0.6, 1.6)	1.00	0.93 (0.6, 1.5)	0.76
	Model c	1.00	1.00 (0.5, 2.2)	1.00	0.88 (0.4, 2.1)	0.76
	Model a	1.00	**2.13 (1.1, 4.0)**	**0.019**	**1.86 (1.1, 3.1)**	**0.016**
GA + Met	Model b	1.00	**2.25 (1.1, 4.5)**	**0.020**	**1.95 (1.1, 3.4)**	**0.017**
	Model c	1.00	**2.85 (1.2, 6.7)**	**0.017**	**2.36 (1.2, 4.6)**	**0.012**
			MetS			
	Model a	1.00	1.06 (0.6, 1.8)	0.83	0.68 (0.4, 1.2)	0.21
GA	Model b	1.00	1.07 (0.6, 2.0)	0.83	0.64 (0.3, 1.3)	0.21
	Model c	1.00	1.08 (0.6, 2.1)	0.83	0.62 (0.3, 1.3)	0.21
	Model a	1.00	**0.61 (0.4, 0.9)**	**0.035**	**0.34 (0.2, 0.5)**	**<0.001**
ILMP	Model b	1.00	**0.56 (0.3, 0.9)**	**0.033**	**0.29 (0.2, 0.5)**	**<0.001**
	Model c	1.00	**0.52 (0.3, 0.9)**	**0.033**	**0.25 (0.1, 0.4)**	**<0.001**
	Model a	1.00	**0.50 (0.3, 0.9)**	**0.049**	**0.37 (0.2, 0.8)**	**0.006**
GA + Met	Model b	1.00	**0.49 (0.2, 0.9)**	**0.047**	**0.36 (0.2, 0.7)**	**0.006**
	Model c	1.00	**0.46 (0.2, 0.9)**	**0.043**	**0.32 (0.1, 0.7)**	**0.005**

Note: Data presented as O.R. (95% C.I.) for Odds ratio (95% confidence interval). Model "a" is univariate. Model "b" is adjusted at age, sex and BMI at baseline. Model "c" is adjusted with additional covariates like waist, systolic and diastolic BP, fasting glucose, HbA1c, and vitamin D (baseline). Hyperglycemia as a component of MetS is excluded in this analysis as this component is present in all subjects at reference (baseline).

The odds of central obesity and hypertriglyceridemia showed marginal changes in all groups, with odds ratio (95% confidence interval (C.I.)) of 0.84 (0.4, 1.8) and 0.86 (0.5, 1.3), respectively, in GA group; 0.80 (0.3, 2.2) and 0.80 (0.5, 1.4) in ILMP group and 0.74 (0.2, 3.5) and 1.0 (0.6, 1.8) in GA + Met group. The odds of low HDL-cholesterol increased (1.66 (0.8, 3.5)) in GA group, but was reduced both in ILMP (0.79 (0.4, 1.4)) and GA + Met (0.86 (0.4, 1.7)) groups. The odds of hypertension increased in GA + Met group (2.36 (1.2, 4.6), *p*-value = 0.012) and GA group (1.28 (0.5, 3.1)) but was modestly decreased in ILMP group (0.88 (0.4, 2.1)). The odds of full MetS was significantly reduced both in ILMP (0.25 (0.1, 0.4), *p*-value < 0.001) and GA + Met (0.32 (0.1, 0.7), *p*-value = 0.005) groups only.

Figure 2 shows the odds ratio of MetS and its components at the end of the study compared to baseline for different treatment groups. The odds for MetS were significantly reduced in ILMP group followed by GA + Met group.

3.4. Intervention Effects in Total Number of MetS Components and MetS Risk Factor

Table 4 shows the intervention effects in the total number of MetS components and the MetS risk-score. The number of MetS components significantly decreased from baseline to the end of the study in the ILMP group (mean change (standard error)) of 0.81 (0.13), *p*-value < 0.001. Similarly, it decreased in GA + Met group by 0.35 (0.18), *p*-value = 0.05. Between-group comparison revealed that the decrease in the number of MetS components in ILMP was statistically more significant than GA (*p* < 0.001). Between (GA + Met) and GA groups, this decrease was not significant. Intervention effects between groups for MetS risk score showed the same trend between ILMP vs. GA group (0.31 (−0.53, −0.09); *p* = 0.003).

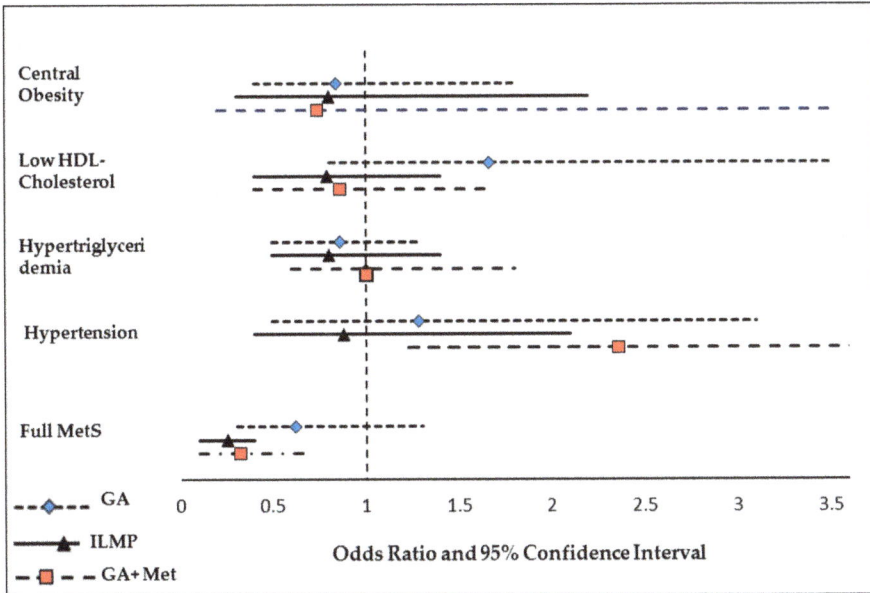

Figure 2. Odds ratio (OR) of MetS and its components for three treatment groups. The model is adjusted for age, sex, BMI and baseline covariates: waist, systolic and diastolic BP, fasting glucose, HbA1c, and vitamin D.

Table 4. Intervention effects in number of MetS components and the MetS risk-score.

	Treatment Groups			Intervention Effects: Mean Change (95% C.I.), *p*	
	GA	ILMP	GA + Met	ILMP-GA	(GA + Met)-GA
	No. of MetS Components				
Baseline	3.15 (0.10)	2.91 (0.11)	3.11 (0.15)		
6-month	3.14 (0.11)	2.41 (0.12)	2.93 (0.16)		
12-month	2.88 (0.11)	2.10 (0.12)	2.77 (0.16)	−0.58 (−0.88, −0.28), <0.001	−0.12 (−0.53, 0.27), 1.0
6 M	−0.02 (0.12)	−0.49 (0.13) **	−0.18 (0.17)		
12 M	−0.28 (0.12)	−0.81 (0.13) **	−0.35 (0.18) *		
	MetS Risk-score				
Baseline	4.22 (0.08)	4.13 (0.09)	4.28 (0.10)		
6-month	4.25 (0.07)	3.82 (0.08)	4.22 (0.09)		
12-month	4.12 (0.07)	3.72 (0.08)	4.16 (0.10)	−0.31 (−0.53, −0.09), 0.003	−0.11 (−0.42, 0.19), 1.0
6 M	0.04 (0.07)	−0.31 (0.07) *	−0.06 (0.09)		
12 M	−0.09 (0.07)	−0.41 (0.08) **	−0.12 (0.10)		

Note: Data presented as Mean (Standard error) for baseline, 6 months and 12 months. Changes at time-intervals are presented as mean change (standard error), where 6 M (6-month minus baseline) and 12 M (12-month minus baseline). Overall change in ILMP and GA + Met groups versus GA group are reported as Mean Change (95% confidence interval). Values were adjusted for baseline covariates age, sex and BMI, systolic and diastolic BP, waist, fasting glucose, HbA1c, and vitamin D (baseline values). * represents *p*-value < 0.05 and ** represents *p*-value < 0.01. *p* < 0.05 considered significant.

Figure 3 shows the intervention effects of the three treatment strategies on MetS, represented by bar graphs showing changes in total number of MetS components and MetS risk-score overtime.

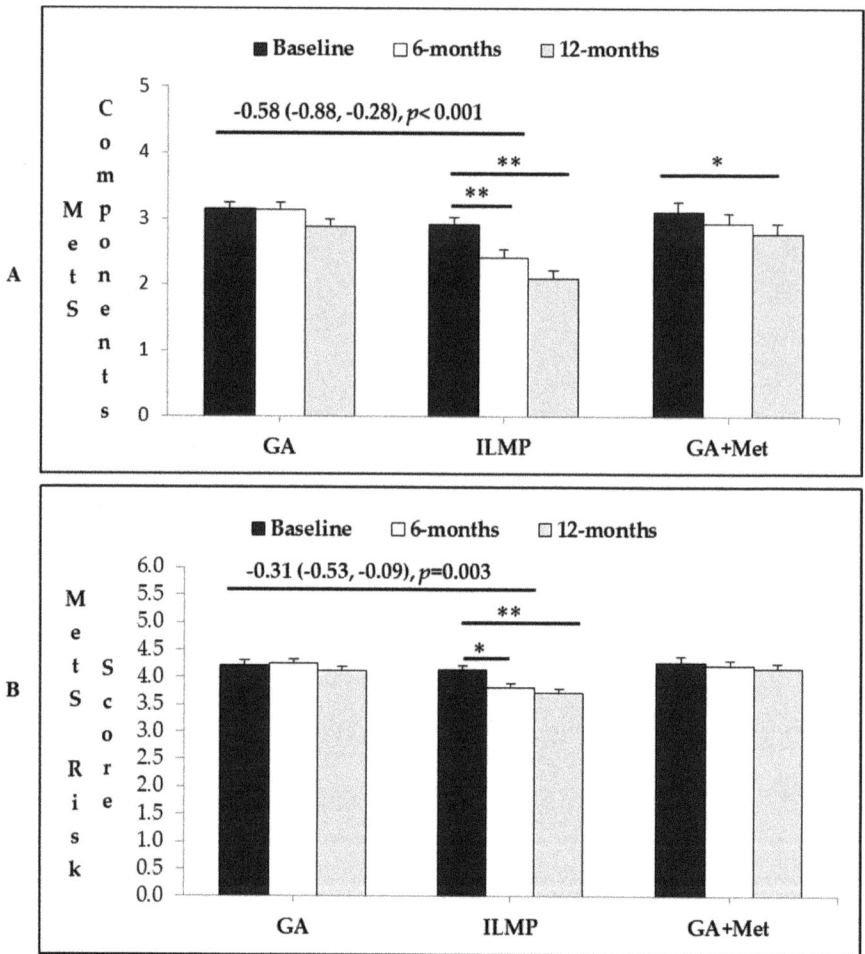

Figure 3. Intervention effects in total number of MetS components (**A**) and MetS risk-score (**B**) for three treatment strategies calculated at baseline and follow-up. Data is adjusted for age, sex and BMI, systolic and diastolic BP, waist, fasting glucose, HbA1c, and vitamin D (all baseline values). The overall change in ILMP and GA + Met groups versus GA group reported as Mean Change (95% confidence interval). Within group intervention effect is shown as * for $p < 0.05$ or ** for $p < 0.01$.

4. Discussion

In this study, Saudi adults with impaired glucose regulation were given treatment based on lifestyle modifications in diet and exercise or low doses of metformin to assess the status of MetS and its individual components over time. Changing lifestyle and reducing the burden of chronic diseases in this population is of great public health importance, however, the impact of such programmes on full MetS and components of MetS in the pre-diabetic Saudi population has not been studied. It is notable that, for the past two decades since these lifestyle intervention studies started, the study outcome variables in most of them has been the incidence of diabetes. In this study, we chose a broader set of outcome measures and focused on the status of MetS and its components together, as well as those independently considered as risk factors for the incidence of T2DM. To the best of our knowledge, this is the first such study in Saudi Arabia which emphasizes the changes in the status of MetS and its components through lifestyle modifications. A similar study was done by the Diabetes Prevention Program (DPP) research group in 2005 [21] and focused on lifestyle intervention and metformin-based therapies for MetS.

Mean fasting glucose was significantly reduced in the ILMP and GA + Met groups while in the GA group this reduction was modest. Similarly, the prevalence of hyperglycemia was reduced significantly by 38.4% and 39% in the ILMP and GA + Met groups, respectively. This improvement in mean fasting glucose is similar to previous studies done in USA [22], Italy [23], and Iran [24] where, on an average, fasting glucose was reduced by 6 mg/dl from baseline to the end of the study in the dietary intervention group. Lifestyle modifications, including replacing high-glycemic index diet with low-glycemic index diet like vegetables, dairies, and whole grains, etc. might have played a role in the reduction in mean fasting glucose [25]. However, as expected, the mean reduction in fasting glucose in the ILMP group is lesser than that found in the GA + Met group. Though the molecular mechanism of the action of metformin remains debated, a consensus is on the direct action of metformin on hepatic glucose production and improving insulin sensitivity in muscle and fat cells [26]. Furthermore, metformin's action is not limited to glucose reduction and insulin sensitivity, it is also an effective weight loss drug due to its effect on appetite and its regulation of fat oxidation, storage in liver and adipose tissue [27]. In our study, the mean weight loss from baseline to the end of the study was 4.15 kg in GA + Met group and this was higher than the ILMP group (1.86 kg).

The ILMP group showed modest improvements in all of the other components of MetS, namely, central obesity, low HDL-cholesterol, hypertriglyceridemia and hypertension. Waist circumference also decreased from baseline to the end of study in the ILMP group by an average of 1.86 cm. This change in waist circumference is close to a mean decrease of 2.7 cm found in a meta-analysis of six interventions [28]. The odds for low HDL-cholesterol was 1.66 (95% confidence interval 0.8 to 3.5) in the GA group, indicating a higher risk in the absence of an intensive lifestyle change program. Similarly, the odds for hypertriglyceridemia at the end of the study versus baseline in the metformin group was 1.0 (0.6, 1.8), which together with the odds obtained for low HDL-cholesterol indicated that GA + Met induce less effects on lipid levels than the ILMP. This was in agreement with studies like [29] which reported significantly larger improvement in lipid indexes in the ILMP group than in the GA + Met group.

The prevalence of hypertension was significantly higher at the end of the study compared to baseline in the GA + Met group (O.R. 2.36 (1.2, 4.6), *p*-value 0.012). The literature on the effect of metformin on hypertension has yielded conflicting results. While some [30] suggest metformin has no intrinsic effect on blood pressure, others, like a recent meta-analysis from 26 studies [31], suggested that metformin could effectively lower systolic blood pressure especially in those with IGT. There are also reports on the role of metformin in reversing pulmonary hypertension through inhibition of aromatase synthesis [32]. In any case, the findings in this study related to hypertension in the GA + Met group should be looked at keeping in mind that most of the study participants (72.3% of all subjects and 71.2% of GA + Met group) are females. Women normally tend to have lower blood pressure than men, related to sex differences in concentrations of angiotensin II and sodium reabsorption in distal nephron [33].

The decrease in the prevalence of full MetS at the end of the study compared to baseline was greater in ILMP (−26%, *p*< 0.001) and GA + Met groups (−22.4%, *p* = 0.013) than the GA group (−8.2%, *p* = 0.281). Furthermore, the analysis of the number of MetS components as well as MetS risk-score suggests that although ILMP was superior to GA + Met, both are more effective compared to GA. The biological mechanism whereby ILMP or metformin exerts its protective effect from MetS is complex and unclear; however, greater intakes of dietary fibers, low-glycemic index foods, vitamins, more physical activity, etc. in ILMP all contribute to the reduction in low-grade inflammation, normally associated with MetS [34,35].

The MetS risk-score, employed in testing the hypothesis of the study regarding MetS reversal/reduction with three different treatments, had high discriminative power for presence/absence of MetS (AOC of 0.890, 95% C.I. of 0.86 to 0.92 and a p-value of <0.001, Supplementary Figure S1, Tables S1–S2). A continuous risk-score for predicting MetS has been developed by approaches such as taking standardized residuals (z-scores) or scores from principal component analysis of risk factors [36,37]. These scores, although precise, are complex and require specialized statistical software. While the authors attempted an easy-to-calculate continuous MetS risk-score, it should be used with caution as the values apply to the population and local laboratory reference values.

The authors acknowledge certain limitations of the study. Firstly, the study was done on subjects with IGT and, hence, the results may not hold true for those with normal glucose regulation but having full MetS manifestations. Such intensive lifestyle change programmes should be conducted in these categories to have a better understanding of the benefits. Secondly, the study does not give details about the actual changes in lifestyle that each participant in this programme carried out in terms of variables related to diet or physical activity, measured before intervention and follow up. Despite the study being based on self-monitoring; it showed a significant reversal in MetS in the ILMP group which suggests that, if guided properly, people are willing to change from a sedentary to a healthy lifestyle. The study also offered a unique statistical approach in assessing MetS and its components and by evaluating the change in the total number of MetS components as an outcome variable. Also, the MetS risk-score devised in this study, if further researched, may provide a simplistic estimate for assessing MetS in an individual.

5. Conclusions

Intensive lifestyle modifications or low dose metformin for a period of 12 months significantly reduces MetS manifestation in individuals with prediabetes, with lifestyle modifications being superior to metformin, as the latter's potency is limited to weight loss and reduction of hyperglycemia, while the former improves all the components of MetS together as well as independently.

Supplementary Materials: The following are available online at http://www.mdpi.com/2072-6643/10/3/383/s1, Figure S1: ROC curve depicting power of MetS_risk factor (RS) for predicting full metabolic syndrome; Table S1: Data showing area under the curve (AUC); Table S2: Data showing coordinates of the ROC curve; Table S3: Odds ratio representing the risk of having metabolic syndrome and its individual components in all samples.

Acknowledgments: The authors thank Deanship of Scientific Research, KSU and Prince Mutaib Bin Abdullah Chair for Biomarkers of Osteoporosis (PMCO) for its continuous support. We also acknowledge Hamza Saber for his efforts in maintaining/providing good quality samples for analysis during this study. The authors are also thankful to Malak Nawaz Khan Kattak and Syed Danish for critical comments on data analysis. This work was supported by the National Plan for Science and Technology (NPST), Riyadh, Saudi Arabia (grant# 12-MED2881-02).

Author Contributions: Study conception and design: N.M.A.-D., H.A.A.; Study execution: H.A.A., N.J.A., Y.A.S., O.S.A.-A., M.S.A.; Sample analysis: K.W., A.M.A.; Manuscript writing: K.W.; Statistical analysis: K.W.; Manuscript review: H.A.A., N.M.A., S.K.

Conflicts of Interest: The authors declare no conflict of interest.

References

1. American Diabetes Association. Diagnosis and classification of diabetes mellitus. *Diabetes Care* **2014**, *37*, S81–S90.

2. Prediabetes and the Potential to Prevent Diabetes. *Lancet* **2012**, *379*. Available online: http://www.thelancet.com/journals/lancet/article/PIIS0140-6736%2812%2960960-X/fulltext (accessed on 15 March 2018).

3. Bray, G.A.; Ehrmann, D.A.; Goldberg, R.B.; Diabetes Prevention Program Research Group. Reduction in the incidence of type 2 diabetes with lifestyle intervention or metformin. *N. Engl. J. Med.* **2002**, *346*, 393–403.

4. Pan, X.R.; Li, G.W.; Hu, Y.H.; Wang, J.X.; Yang, W.Y.; An, Z.X.; Hu, Z.X.; Xiao, J.Z.; Cao, H.B.; Liu, P.A. Effects of diet and exercise in preventing NIDDM in people with impaired glucose tolerance: The Da Qing IGT and Diabetes Study. *Diabetes Care* **1997**, *20*, 537–544. [CrossRef] [PubMed]

5. Ramachandran, A.; Snehalatha, C.; Mary, S.; Mukesh, B.; Bhaskar, A.; Vijay, V. The Indian Diabetes Prevention Programme shows that lifestyle modification and metformin prevent type 2 diabetes in Asian Indian subjects with impaired glucose tolerance (IDPP-1). *Diabetologia* **2006**, *49*, 289–297. [CrossRef] [PubMed]

6. Cardona-Morrell, M.; Rychetnik, L.; Morrell, S.L.; Espinel, P.T.; Bauman, A. Reduction of diabetes risk in routine clinical practice: Are physical activity and nutrition interventions feasible and are the outcomes from reference trials replicable? A systematic review and meta-analysis. *BMC Public Health* **2010**, *10*, 653. [CrossRef] [PubMed]

7. Johnson, M.; Jones, R.; Freeman, C.; Woods, H.B.; Gillett, M.; Goyder, E.; Payne, N. Can diabetes prevention programmes be translated effectively into real-world settings and still deliver improved outcomes? A synthesis of evidence. *Diabet. Med.* **2013**, *30*, 3–15. [CrossRef] [PubMed]

8. Expert Panel on Detection, Evaluation. Executive summary of the Third Report of the National Cholesterol Education Program (NCEP) expert panel on detection, evaluation, and treatment of high blood cholesterol in adults (Adult Treatment Panel III). *JAMA* **2001**, *285*, 2486–2497.

9. Al-Qahtani, D.A.; Imtiaz, M.L. Prevalence of metabolic syndrome in Saudi adult soldiers. *Saudi Med. J.* **2005**, *26*, 1360–1366. [PubMed]

10. Al-Nozha, M.; Al-Khadra, A.; Arafah, M.R.; Al-Maatouq, M.A.; Khalil, M.Z.; Khan, N.B.; Al-Mazrou, Y.Y.; Al-Marzouki, K.; Al-Harthi, S.S.; Abdullah, M.; et al. Metabolic syndrome in Saudi Arabia. *Saudi Med. J.* **2005**, *26*, 1918–1925. [PubMed]

11. Wilson, P.W.; D'Agostino, R.B.; Parise, H.; Sullivan, L.; Meigs, J.B. Metabolic syndrome as a precursor of cardiovascular disease and type 2 diabetes mellitus. *Circulation* **2005**, *112*, 3066–3072. [CrossRef] [PubMed]

12. Hanson, R.L.; Imperatore, G.; Bennett, P.H.; Knowler, W.C. Components of the "metabolic syndrome" and incidence of type 2 diabetes. *Diabetes* **2002**, *51*, 3120–3127. [CrossRef] [PubMed]

13. Al-Daghri, N.M.; Al-Attas, O.S.; Alokail, M.S.; Alkharfy, K.M.; Yousef, M.; Sabico, S.L.; Chrousos, G.P. Diabetes mellitus type 2 and other chronic non-communicable diseases in the central region, Saudi Arabia (Riyadh cohort 2): A decade of an epidemic. *BMC Med.* **2011**, *9*, 76. [CrossRef] [PubMed]

14. Aljohani, N.J. Metabolic syndrome: Risk factors among adults in Kingdom of Saudi Arabia. *J. Fam. Community Med.* **2014**, *21*, 170–175. [CrossRef] [PubMed]

15. Huang, P.L. A comprehensive definition for metabolic syndrome. *Dis. Models Mech.* **2009**, *2*, 231–237. [CrossRef] [PubMed]

16. American Diabetes Association. Standards of Medical Care in Diabetes. *Diabetes Care* **2017**, *40*. Available online: http://care.diabetesjournals.org/content/diacare/suppl/2016/12/15/40.Supplement_1.DC1/DC_40_S1_final.pdf (accessed on 2 February 2018).

17. Tuomilehto, J.; Lindström, J.; Eriksson, J.G.; Valle, T.T.; Hämäläinen, H.; Ilanne-Parikka, P.; Keinänen-Kiukaanniemi, S.; Laakso, M.; Louheranta, A.; Rastas, M. Prevention of type 2 diabetes mellitus by changes in lifestyle among subjects with impaired glucose tolerance. *N. Engl. J. Med.* **2001**, *344*, 1343–1350. [CrossRef] [PubMed]

18. Kosaka, K.; Noda, M.; Kuzuya, T. Prevention of type 2 diabetes by lifestyle intervention: A Japanese trial in IGT males. *Diabetes Res. Clin. Pract.* **2005**, *67*, 152–162. [CrossRef] [PubMed]

19. Al-Daghri, N.M.; Alfawaz, H.; Aljohani, N.J.; Al-Saleh, Y.; Wani, K.; Alnaami, A.M.; Alharbi, M.; Kumar, S. A 6-month "self-monitoring" lifestyle modification with increased sunlight exposure modestly improves vitamin D status, lipid profile and glycemic status in overweight and obese Saudi adults with varying glycemic levels. *Lipids Health Dis.* **2014**, *13*, 87. [CrossRef] [PubMed]

20. Al-Daghri, N.M.; Alfawaz, H.; Aljohani, N.J.; Wani, K.; Alharbi, M.; Al-Saleh, Y.; Al-Attas, O.S.; Alokail, M.S. Age-specific improvements in impaired fasting glucose and vitamin D status using a lifestyle intervention programme in overweight and obese Saudi subjects. *Int. J. Clin. Exp. Med.* **2016**, *9*, 19850–19857.

21. Orchard, T.J.; Temprosa, M.; Goldberg, R.; Haffner, S.; Ratner, R.; Marcovina, S.; Fowler, S. The effect of metformin and intensive lifestyle intervention on the metabolic syndrome: The Diabetes Prevention Program randomized trial. *Ann. Intern. Med.* **2005**, *142*, 611–619. [CrossRef] [PubMed]

22. Watkins, L.L.; Sherwood, A.; Feinglos, M.; Hinderliter, A.; Babyak, M.; Gullette, E.; Waugh, R.; Blumenthal, J.A. Effects of exercise and weight loss on cardiac risk factors associated with syndrome X. *Arch. Intern. Med.* **2003**, *163*, 1889–1895. [CrossRef] [PubMed]

23. Esposito, K.; Marfella, R.; Ciotola, M.; Di Palo, C.; Giugliano, F.; Giugliano, G.; D'armiento, M.; D'andrea, F.; Giugliano, D. Effect of a Mediterranean-style diet on endothelial dysfunction and markers of vascular inflammation in the metabolic syndrome: A randomized trial. *JAMA* **2004**, *292*, 1440–1446. [CrossRef] [PubMed]

24. Azadbakht, L.; Mirmiran, P.; Esmaillzadeh, A.; Azizi, T.; Azizi, F. Beneficial effects of a Dietary Approaches to Stop Hypertension eating plan on features of the metabolic syndrome. *Diabetes Care* **2005**, *28*, 2823–2831. [CrossRef] [PubMed]

25. Brand-Miller, J.; Hayne, S.; Petocz, P.; Colagiuri, S. Low–glycemic index diets in the management of diabetes. *Diabetes Care* **2003**, *26*, 2261–2267. [CrossRef] [PubMed]

26. Rena, G.; Hardie, D.G.; Pearson, E.R. The mechanisms of action of metformin. *Diabetologia* **2017**, *60*, 1577–1585. [CrossRef] [PubMed]

27. Malin, S.K.; Kashyap, S.R. Effects of metformin on weight loss: Potential mechanisms. *Curr. Opin. Endocrinol. Diabetes Obes.* **2014**, *21*, 323–329. [CrossRef] [PubMed]

28. Yamaoka, K.; Tango, T. Effects of lifestyle modification on metabolic syndrome: A systematic review and meta-analysis. *BMC Med.* **2012**, *10*, 138. [CrossRef] [PubMed]

29. American Diabetes Association. Impact of intensive lifestyle and metformin therapy on cardiovascular disease risk factors in the diabetes prevention program. *Diabetes Care* **2005**, *28*, 888–894.

30. Wulffelé, E.M.; Kooy, A.; Zeeuw, D.D.; Stehouwer, C.; Gansevoort, R. The effect of metformin on blood pressure, plasma cholesterol and triglycerides in type 2 diabetes mellitus: A systematic review. *J. Intern. Med.* **2004**, *256*, 1–14. [CrossRef] [PubMed]

31. Zhou, L.; Liu, H.; Wen, X.; Peng, Y.; Tian, Y.; Zhao, L. Effects of metformin on blood pressure in nondiabetic patients: A meta-analysis of randomized controlled trials. *J. Hypertens.* **2017**, *35*, 18–26. [CrossRef] [PubMed]

32. Dean, A.; Nilsen, M.; Loughlin, L.; Salt, I.P.; MacLean, M.R. Metformin reverses development of pulmonary hypertension via aromatase inhibition. *Hypertension* **2016**, *68*, 446–454. [CrossRef] [PubMed]

33. Kagan, A.; Faibel, H.; Ben-Arie, G.; Granevitze, Z.; Rapoport, J. Gender differences in ambulatory blood pressure monitoring profile in obese, overweight and normal subjects. *J. Hum. Hypertens.* **2007**, *21*, 128–134. [CrossRef] [PubMed]

34. Gleeson, M.; Bishop, N.C.; Stensel, D.J.; Lindley, M.R.; Mastana, S.S.; Nimmo, M.A. The anti-inflammatory effects of exercise: Mechanisms and implications for the prevention and treatment of disease. *Nat. Rev. Immunol.* **2011**, *11*, 607–615. [CrossRef] [PubMed]

35. Messier, S.P.; Mihalko, S.L.; Legault, C.; Miller, G.D.; Nicklas, B.J.; DeVita, P.; Beavers, D.P.; Hunter, D.J.; Lyles, M.F.; Eckstein, F. Effects of intensive diet and exercise on knee joint loads, inflammation, and clinical outcomes among overweight and obese adults with knee osteoarthritis: The IDEA randomized clinical trial. *JAMA* **2013**, *310*, 1263–1273. [CrossRef] [PubMed]

36. Andersen, L.B.; Harro, M.; Sardinha, L.B.; Froberg, K.; Ekelund, U.; Brage, S.; Anderssen, S.A. Physical activity and clustered cardiovascular risk in children: A cross-sectional study (The European Youth Heart Study). *Lancet* **2006**, *368*, 299–304. [CrossRef]

37. Katzmarzyk, P.T.; Perusse, L.; Malina, R.M.; Bergeron, J.; Despres, J.; Bouchard, C. Stability of indicators of the metabolic syndrome from childhood and adolescence to young adulthood: The Quebec Family Study. *J. Clin. Epidemiol.* **2001**, *54*, 190–195. [CrossRef]

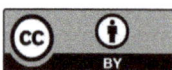

nutrients

MDPI

Article

Dietary Inflammatory Index and Type 2 Diabetes Mellitus in Adults: The Diabetes Mellitus Survey of Mexico City

Edgar Denova-Gutiérrez [1], Paloma Muñoz-Aguirre [2], Nitin Shivappa [3,4,5], James R. Hébert [3,4,5], Lizbeth Tolentino-Mayo [1], Carolina Batis [6] and Simón Barquera [1,*]

[1] Nutrition and Health Research Center, National Institute of Public Health, Cuernavaca 62100, Mexico; edgar.denova@insp.mx (E.D.-G.); mltolentino@insp.mx (L.T.-M.)
[2] Center for Research on Population Health , National Institute of Public Health, Cuernavaca 62100, Mexico; pmz.aguirre@gmail.com
[3] Cancer Prevention and Control Program, University of South Carolina, Columbia, SC 29208, USA; shivappa@email.sc.edu (N.S.); JHEBERT@mailbox.sc.edu (J.R.H.)
[4] Department of Epidemiology and Biostatistics, Arnold School of Public Health, University of South Carolina, Columbia, SC 29208, USA
[5] Connecting Health Innovations LLC, Columbia, SC 29250, USA
[6] CONACYT-Nutrition and Health Research Center, National Institute of Public Health, Cuernavaca 62100, Mexico; Carolina.batis@insp.mx
* Correspondence: sbarquera@insp.mx; Tel.: +52-(777)-329-3017 or +52-(777)-311-2219

Received: 23 February 2018; Accepted: 19 March 2018; Published: 21 March 2018

Abstract: Diet and inflammation are both associated with type 2 diabetes mellitus (T2DM). In the present study, we aimed to assess the relation between the dietary inflammatory index (DII) and the presence of T2DM in Mexican adults participating in the Diabetes Mellitus Survey administered in Mexico City (DMS-MC). The study involved 1174 subjects (48.5% men) between 20–69 years of age. A validated semi-quantitative food frequency questionnaire was employed to evaluate dietary intake and to compute DII. The DII is based on scientific evidence about the association between dietary compounds and six established inflammatory biomarkers. Multivariate logistic regression models were used to estimate the odds ratios (ORs) and 95% confidence intervals (95% CIs) of DII in relation to T2DM. Our results suggest that subjects in the highest quintile of the DII had higher odds of T2DM (OR = 3.02; 95% CI: 1.39, 6.58; $p = 0.005$) compared to subjects in the lowest quintile of DII scores. Assessing possible effect modification, an association with T2DM was evident when comparing DII quintile 5 to quintile 1 for participants aged ≥ 55 years (OR = 9.77; 95% CI: 3.78, 25.50; $p = 0.001$). These results suggest that a pro-inflammatory diet is associated with significantly higher odds of T2DM among adult Mexicans.

Keywords: type 2 diabetes mellitus; dietary inflammatory index; obesity; Mexican population; survey

1. Introduction

Low-grade, systemic inflammation, which provides the substrate for many chronic diseases, is characterized by elevated pro-inflammatory markers, including interleukin-6 (IL-6), and tumor necrosis factor-alpha (TNF-α) [1]. Chronic systemic inflammation has been linked to non-communicable diseases such as cancer, cardiovascular disease, and diabetes [2]. Globally, type 2 diabetes mellitus (T2DM) has become a serious public health problem, affecting 382 million people in 2013 [3] and had led to a loss of approximately 64 million disability adjusted life-years (DALYs) in 2015 [4]. Currently, 80% of people with T2DM live in low-income and middle-income countries [5]. In Mexico, T2DM prevalence has reached 14.7% of the population and two million DALYs lost in 2013 [5,6].

Recent evidence indicates that risk factors can induce chronic inflammation, which are also related with T2DM such as adiposity [7], a sedentary lifestyle [8], and diet [9]. In the past several decades, certain individual dietary factors have been widely investigated regarding their association with diabetes risk and inflammation, including high intake of saturated fatty acids, sugar-sweetened beverages, and starchy food, combined with low consumption of fruits, vegetables, and whole grains [10]. More recently, alternative approaches have been used in order to capture the complicated nutrient interactions and cumulative effects in the food matrix [11]. Based on evidence linking diet with inflammation and chronic conditions such as T2DM, we used a literature-derived, population-based dietary inflammatory index (DII) [12] to evaluate the potential inflammatory properties of diet. The DII has been validated with different inflammatory biomarkers [13,14]. Furthermore, it has been associated with components of metabolic syndrome [15], as well as a variety of chronic disease outcomes [16,17].

To the best of our knowledge, no study has yet explored the relation between the DII and T2DM in a Mexican population. Thus, we aimed to explore the association between DII and the prevalence of T2DM in adults participating in the Diabetes Mellitus Survey in Mexico City 2015 (DMS-MC 2015).

2. Materials and Methods

2.1. Study Design

The present analysis was conducted with data from the DMS-MC 2015, a cross-sectional probabilistic population-based survey, designed and implemented by our group at the National Institute of Public Health (INSP by its Spanish acronym), representative of adults aged 20–69 years living in Mexico City. The DMS-MC 2015 sample was randomly stratified into clusters according to city district. In the first stage, 16 primary sampling units were selected and by means of a probabilistic and systematic sampling, six secondary sampling units were designated. Then, six houses per secondary sampling unit were included. Finally, per household, we evaluated up to two adults between 20–69 years of age. Fasting venous blood samples were collected in a subsample of participants randomly selected based on estimations of the Mexican National Health and Nutrition Survey 2012 [18].

For the present analysis, we excluded participants with >10% blank items on their food frequency questionnaires, and who did not consume between 600 kcal and 5500 kcal daily (*n* = 10), determined with the standard deviation method suggested by Rosner [19]. Additionally, we excluded participants with incomplete biomarkers data or with missing information on other important covariates (*n* = 142). Finally, we excluded those subjects with more than 12 months past their T2DM diagnosis date (*n* = 90). A total of 1174 individuals were included in our final sample.

This study was managed according to the Declaration of Helsinki guidelines. The Research, Ethics and Biosecurity Committee at INSP reviewed and approved the study protocol (No. 1658) and informed consent forms (No. B04). Written informed consent was obtained from each participant.

2.2. Dietary Assessment

To assess dietary intake, a previously validated semi-quantitative food frequency questionnaire (SFFQ) [20] was used. The instrument describes the consumption of 140 foods over the past seven days prior to the interview. For each food, a commonly used portion size was specified on the SFFQ. Frequency of food consumption was characterized by set categories ranging from never to six. First, frequency was expressed as times per day, but then was converted into portion size per day. To compute the energy (kcal/day) and daily nutrient intake, we multiplied the frequency of consumption of each food by the estimated nutrient content with a comprehensive database of food contents, compiled by the INSP [21]. The SFFQ was administered by interviewers and were collected by personnel trained using standardized data collection and entry procedures.

2.3. Dietary Inflammatory Index (DII) Assessment

SFFQ-derived dietary data was used to calculate DII scores for each participant. A complete description of the DII is available elsewhere [12]. Briefly, the body of literature on DII consists of all qualifying publications between 1950 and 2010 reporting one or more associations between dietary components and the following inflammatory markers: IL-1β, IL-4, IL-6, IL-10, TNF-α and C-reactive protein [12]. A total of 45 different food parameters were identified as being related to the six inflammatory biomarkers in the literature review. Each was assigned a "food parameter-specific inflammatory effect score" through a process of counting the number of studies reporting a pro-inflammatory, anti-inflammatory, and no inflammatory effect on one or more of the six inflammatory markers, and weighing the scores by study design and size of the literature for each food parameter/inflammatory marker relation. In previous analyses, the DII was positively correlated with circulating level of high-sensitivity C-reactive protein (hs-CRP) [13,22].

To calculate DII scores for the participants of this study, the dietary data was first linked to the world database that provided estimates of a mean intake and standard deviation for each food parameter [12]. These then became the multipliers to express an individual's exposure relative to the "standard global mean" as a z-score. This was achieved by subtracting the "standard global mean" from the amount reported and dividing this value by the standard deviation. Since data was skewed to the right (a common occurrence with dietary data), we converted this value into a centered percentile score. The centered percentile score from every individual was multiplied by the food parameter-specific inflammatory effect score in order to obtain a food parameter-specific DII score for an individual. All of the food parameter-specific DII scores were then summed to create the overall DII score for every participant in the study [12]. DII scores for individuals in the DMS-MC 2015 were calculated using the 27 food items and nutrients (out of the 45 possible items) for which we had intake data available from the SFFQ: carbohydrate, protein, fat, alcohol, fiber, cholesterol, saturated fatty acids, mono-unsaturated fatty acids, poly-unsaturated fatty acids, omega 3 fat, omega 6 fat, trans fat, niacin, thiamin, riboflavin, vitamin B12, vitamin B6, iron, magnesium, zinc, vitamin A, vitamin C, vitamin E, folic acid, beta carotene, garlic, and onion. Since the DII was calculated per 1000 calories of food consumed we used the energy-standardized version of the world database to control for the effect of total energy intake.

2.4. Biomarkers Assessment

A fasting venous blood sample (fasting time was ≥8 h) from an antecubital vein was collected from each participant. Serum aliquots were stored in cryovials and transported to a laboratory, where the aliquots were stored at −70 °C until they were used for analysis.

Plasma triglycerides were measured with a colorimetric method following enzymatic hydrolysis performed with the lipase technique. Total cholesterol, high-density lipoprotein-cholesterol (HDL-c), and low-density lipoprotein-cholesterol (LDL-c) were measured using the colorimetric method following enzymatic assay. Additionally, plasma glucose was measured with the enzymatic colorimetric methods by using glucose oxidize. Finally, the proportion of hemoglobin A1c (HbA1c) was determined using the immunocolorimetric method [23].

2.5. Type 2 Diabetes Mellitus Definition

For the present study, subjects who declared to have a previous T2DM physician-diagnosis independent of their survey glucose concentration were called "previously diagnosed". Of these, respondents who were diagnosed with T2DM less than 11 months prior to administration of the SFFQ, had fasting glucose concentrations ≥126 mg/dL (at the moment of the survey) and poor glycemic control (HbA1c (%) ≥ 6.5) [24]. These subjects were considered participants with T2DM. Furthermore, subjects whose glucose concentration in the fasting blood sample taken during the survey was ≥ 126 mg/dL and had levels of (HbA1c (%) ≥ 6.5) were defined as displaying fasting glucose and/or HbA1c values consistent with T2DM diagnostic criteria and were also defined as participants with T2DM.

2.6. Anthropometric and Blood Pressure Assessment

Participants' height and weight were measured by trained personal using standardized procedures. Height was measured by using a conventional stadiometer (SECA 213, Medical Measuring Systems and Scales, Hamburg, Germany) to the nearest 0.1 cm and body weight was measured with a previously calibrated electronic (SECA 874, Medical Measuring Systems and Scales, Hamburg, Germany) scale with a precision of 0.1 kg. Body mass index (BMI = weight (kg)/height (m^2)) was calculated based on measured weight and height. We defined overweight/obesity as BMI $\geq$25 kg/m^2. Waist circumference was measured to the nearest 0.1 cm at the high point of the iliac crest at the end of normal expiration, with a measuring tape, which was placed below any clothing, directly touching the participant's skin. Abdominal obesity was defined as a waist circumference of $\geq$90 cm in men and $\geq$80 cm in women [25].

Subjects' blood pressure was measured twice by a trained personal using an automatic medical grade monitor (OMROM HEM-907, OMROM Mexico, Mexico City, Mexico). The first measurement was taken after five minutes of rest, while participants were sitting with the dominant arm supported at heart level. The second measurement was taken in the same way, five minutes after the first.

2.7. Physical Activity Assessment

Physical activity was evaluated with a previously used and validated [26] short version of the international physical activity questionnaire (s-IPAQ). The questionnaire includes 9 items that assesses time spent performing moderate-intense physical activity for at least 10 min for each activity over seven days. The s-IPAQ data was analyzed in agreement with IPAQ protocol [27], as follows: first, physical activity interval duration gathered in hours was converted into minutes; second, data which was described as a weekly frequency was transformed into an average daily time; and third, subjects whose responses were "do not know", or "refused", or had "missing data" for time duration or frequency were removed from the present analysis. Based on the reported time spent performing moderate to intense physical activity, participants were classified as inactive (<150 min/week), physically active (150–299 min/week), or highly active ($\geq$300 min/week) according to the World Health Organization (WHO) physical activity guidelines [28].

2.8. Socioeconomic Status and Education Assessment

Socioeconomic status (SES) was constructed by combining eight variables that assessed household characteristics, goods, and available services including: construction materials of the floor, ceiling, and walls; household goods (stove, microwave, washing machine, refrigerator and boiler); and electrical goods (television, computer, radio and telephone). The index was divided into tertiles and used as a proxy for low, medium, and high SES. Education level was stratified into three groups according to the highest level of education obtained: primary or less, secondary/high school, and/or higher education.

2.9. Other Participant Characteristics

Participants completed two self-administered questionnaires (home and individual level) and delivered detailed information regarding their demographic characteristics (e.g., age, sex, education, marital status), self-perception of body weight, past medical history, current medication use, lifestyle information (e.g., diet, physical activity, smoking status, alcohol consumption, etc.), depression symptoms, sleep quantity, and information on reproductive history (for females).

2.10. Statistical Analysis

We conducted descriptive analyses of the main characteristics of interest to assess adherence to model assumptions. One-way analysis of variance (ANOVA) was used to test for differences for general characteristics across quintiles of DII, while, chi-square tests were used to evaluate the distribution of qualitative variables across DII quintiles. To evaluate the magnitude of the association between specific DII and diabetes, we estimated multivariable adjusted odds ratios (OR) 95% CI using logistic regression models. In all multivariate models, the first quintile of the DII score was considered the reference. The Mantel–Haenszel extension chi-square test was used to assess the overall trend of OR across increasing quintile of DII scores.

Additionally, to assess possible effect modification, we conducted a stratified analysis by age groups (<55 years vs. ≥55 years), sex, BMI (<25.0 kg/m^2 vs. ≥25.0 kg/m^2), and physical activity (inactive vs. active or highly active). We tested the significance using a likelihood ratio test by comparing a model with the main effects of each intake and the stratified variable and the reduced model interaction terms with only the main effects.

All *p*-values presented are two-tailed, $p < 0.05$ was considered significant. All analyses were performed using STATA software (College Station, StataCorp LP, TX, USA), version 13.0.

3. Results

Participants' baseline characteristics are shown in Table 1. A total of 1174 subjects (48.5% men) between 20–69 years were included in the present analysis. The overall prevalence of T2DM was 13.6%; of these, 10.1% were previously diagnosed individuals, whereas 3.5% were individuals with glucose and/or HbA1c values consistent with T2DM definition at the time of the survey. The mean age among participants with T2DM was 52.3 years. Subjects with T2DM had a significantly higher prevalence of obesity, abdominal obesity, had lower levels of physical activity and intake of cereal fiber, and also, as expected, levels of total cholesterol, triglycerides, and glycated hemoglobin were all significantly higher in participants with T2DM.

Table 1. Characteristics of the study population: The Diabetes Mellitus Survey of Mexico City, 2015.

Variables	Overall Study (*n* = 1174)	Non-T2DM Subjects (*n* = 973)	T2DM Subjects (*n* = 201)	*p*-Value [a]
Sex, %				
Men	48.5	48.4	48.7	0.17
Women	51.5	51.6	51.3	
Age (years) [b]	39.9 (0.48)	38.0 (0.46)	52.3 (0.83)	<0.001
Socioeconomic status, %				
Low	21.9	20.2	33.5	
Medium	36.4	36.1	37.4	<0.001
High	41.7	43.7	29.1	
Education, %				
Elementary and secondary education	19.3	16.5	37.4	
High school	27.2	26.5	32.0	<0.001
Bachelor's degree or higher	53.5	57.0	30.6	
Smoking status, %				
Current	45.6	45.2	48.8	
Past	11.6	12.1	7.8	0.41
Never	42.8	42.7	43.4	
Physical activity, %				
Inactive	23.0	22.8	24.4	
Active/highly active	77.0	77.2	75.6	0.17
Family history of DM2, %	41.9	38.2	66.5	<0.001
Hypertension, (%)	15.9	11.5	44.1	<0.001
Body mass index (kg/m^2) [b]	28.8 (0.22)	28.2 (0.23)	31.2 (0.48)	<0.001

Table 1. *Cont.*

Variables	Overall Study (*n* = 1174)	Non-T2DM Subjects (*n* = 973)	T2DM Subjects (*n* = 201)	*p*-Value [a]
Body mass index, %				
Normal (<25.0 kg/m^2)	25.5	28.2	9.1	
Overweight (≥25.0 to <30.0 kg/m^2)	40.2	39.9	41.8	<0.001
Obesity (≥30.0 kg/m^2)	34.3	31.9	49.1	
Abdominal obesity, %	43.1	38.9	70.2	<0.001
Glucose (mg/dL) [b]	107.7 (2.0)	91.3 (0.53)	213.8 (7.7)	<0.001
Glycated hemoglobin (HbA1c %) [b]	5.9 (0.07)	5.3 (0.02)	9.8 (0.23)	<0.001
Triglycerides (mg/dL) [b]	205.6 (6.3)	189.8 (6.3)	307.3 (15.1)	<0.001
Total cholesterol (mg/dL) [b]	189.1 (1.5)	186.2 (1.5)	207.8 (4.0)	<0.001
High density lipoprotein (mg/dL) [b]	42.3 (0.41)	42.8 (0.49)	39.9 (0.68)	0.39
Low density lipoprotein (mg/dL) [b]	84.0 (2.1)	80.9 (2.0)	87.6 (4.9)	<0.001
Dietary variables				
Energy intake (kcal/day) [c]	2224 (2106–2342)	2329 (2196–2462)	1801 (1673–1927)	<0.001
Carbohydrates (% energy) [c]	55.4 (54.7–56.1)	55.1 (54.3–55.9)	56.8 (55.4–58.1)	0.06
Total fats (% energy) [c]	31.1 (30.5–31.7)	31.3 (30.6–31.9)	30.2 (29.3–31.2)	0.03
Saturated fats (% energy) [c]	11.6 (11.3–11.9)	11.8 (11.5–12.0)	11.2 (10.7–11.6)	0.001
Monounsaturated fatty acids (% energy) [c]	10.9 (10.7–11.1)	11.0 (10.7–11.2)	10.4 (10.0–10.8)	0.03
Polyunsaturated fatty acids (% energy) [c]	7.0 (6.8–7.2)	7.0 (6.8–7.2)	7.0 (6.8–7.3)	0.61
Fiber (g/day) [c]	27.7 (25.9–29.6)	28.3 (26.3–30.3)	25.6 (23.8–27.4)	<0.001
Alcohol intake (g/day) [c]	9.4 (7.4–11.3)	10.4 (8.2–12.6)	5.0 (2.5–7.5)	0.003
Magnesium (mg/day) [c]	409.7 (386.5–432.9)	417.7 (392.3–443.1)	377.3 (351.4–403.2)	<0.001

[a] $p < 0.05$, difference in mean and proportion between diabetic and non-diabetic subjects. Values were determined using a student's *t*-test for continuous variables and Chi-square test for categorical variables. [b] Mean and (standard error); [c] Mean and 95% confidence intervals (95% CI). T2DM, type 2 diabetes mellitus; HbA1c, hemoglobin A1c.

According to DII score quintiles, subjects with the most pro-inflammatory diet were significantly older, less educated, had lower SES, smoked less, had a higher prevalence of obesity, abdominal obesity, and T2DM (Table 2). The most pro-inflammatory diet was characterized by a higher consumption of carbohydrates (56.1%; (95% CI: 54.3, 57.8) vs. 53.8% (52.6, 55.1)), red meat and processed meat (78.3 g/day (66.3, 90.2) vs. 40.1 g/day (33.7, 46.5)), refined cereals (173.9 g/day (147.1, 200.6) vs. 109.2 g/day (96.0, 122.5)), and soft drinks (401.7 mL/day (343.3, 460.1) vs. 69.5 mL/day (51.6, 87.4)) compared to the most anti-inflammatory diet. All of these differences were statistically significant. Also, significantly decreasing trends were observed for the anti-inflammatory nutrients: fiber, vitamin C, vitamin D, and magnesium (Table 3).

After adjusting for age and sex, the odds of having T2DM, across all DII score quintiles were 1.00, 1.63, 1.80, 1.84, and 2.29 (95% CI: 1.11, 4.75; $p = 0.01$). Finally, after additional adjustment for co-variables, we observed that subjects with the most pro-inflammatory diet had approximately three times greater odds of having T2DM (OR: 3.02, 95% CI: 1.39, 6.58; $p = 0.005$), compared to individuals in the lowest DII quintile (Table 4).

Additionally, a sensitivity analysis included individuals with glucose and/or HbA1c values consistent with T2DM definition at the time of the survey. In this case, we observed that subjects with the most pro-inflammatory diet had greater odds of having T2DM (OR = 3.56; 95% CI: 1.13, 9.11) (data not shown).

In addition, we evaluated the effect-modifying role of age; we observed a greater association with T2DM contrasting DII extreme quintiles (Q_5 vs. Q_1) for participants aged ≥ 55 years (OR = 9.77; 95% CI: 3.78, 25.50; $p = 0.001$) (Figure 1).

Table 2. Characteristics of participants according to quintiles of the dietary inflammatory index: The Diabetes Mellitus Survey of Mexico City, 2015.

	Dietary Inflammatory Index					p-Value [a]
	Quintile 1: Most Anti-Inflammatory	Quintile 2	Quintile 3	Quintile 4	Quintile 5: Most Pro-Inflammatory	
	(n = 235)	(n = 235)	(n = 235)	(n = 235)	(n = 234)	
Mean DII-density	−3.05	−1.85	−0.81	0.24	1.79	<0.001
Sex, %						
Men	24.7	37.5	38.9	40.1	48.9	<0.001
Women	75.3	62.5	61.1	59.9	51.1	
Age (years) [b]	39.9 (0.91)	42.9 (1.2)	45.5 (1.11)	46.2 (1.08)	48.5 (1.05)	0.001
Socioeconomic status, %						
Low	21.5	22.8	21.5	22.3	34.8	<0.001
Medium	32.2	39.0	38.5	41.0	34.3	
High	46.3	38.2	40.0	36.7	30.9	
Education, %						
Elementary and secondary education	10.6	26.1	27.3	27.6	34.4	<0.001
High school	24.5	21.3	27.2	29.8	31.7	
Bachelor's degree or higher	59.9	52.6	45.5	42.6	33.9	
Smoking status, %						
Current	52.9	51.8	47.8	39.5	31.7	<0.001
Past	10.5	6.1	10.0	17.9	15.2	
Never	36.6	42.1	42.2	42.6	53.1	
Physical activity, %						
Inactive	25.7	27.8	29.5	26.5	23.8	0.14
Active/highly active	74.3	72.2	70.5	73.5	76.2	
Body mass index (kg/m^2) [b]	28.1 (0.38)	28.3 (0.40)	28.7 (0.47)	28.9 (0.45)	29.8 (0.48)	0.007
Body mass index, %						
Normal (<25.0 kg/m^2)	29.2	25.3	23.5	25.4	20.8	0.005
Overweight (≥25.0 to <30.0 kg/m^2) [b]	38.5	38.8	41.4	38.6	36.2	
Obesity (≥30.0 kg/m^2)	32.3	35.8	35.1	36.0	43.0	

Table 2. *Cont.*

	Dietary Inflammatory Index					
	Quintile 1: Most Anti-Inflammatory	Quintile 2	Quintile 3	Quintile 4	Quintile 5: Most Pro-Inflammatory	p-Value [a]
	(n = 235)	(n = 235)	(n = 235)	(n = 235)	(n = 234)	
Abdominal obesity, %						
Yes	39.3	47.2	48.3	50.3	54.2	<0.001
Glucose (mg/dL) [b]	100.9 (3.6)	103.8 (2.8)	108.8 (3.6)	112.4 (3.9)	117.2 (4.7)	<0.001
Glycated hemoglobin (HbA1c %) [b]	5.7 (0.10)	5.8 (0.12)	6.2 (0.14)	6.2 (0.13)	6.7 (0.11)	0.006
Triglycerides (mg/dL) [b]	200.6 (10.8)	188.3 (12.3)	217.9 (13.0)	203.1 (11.6)	216.7 (13.1)	0.96
Total cholesterol (mg/dL) [b]	187.7 (3.1)	181.6 (3.0)	192.4 (3.5)	190.9 (3.2)	196.4 (3.3)	0.02
High density lipoprotein (mg/dL) [b]	42.8 (1.03)	41.2 (0.81)	42.1 (0.75)	42.1 (0.76)	41.7 (0.71)	0.17
Low density lipoprotein (mg/dL) [b]	81.2 (4.4)	85.2 (3.4)	80.2 (4.7)	88.7 (4.4)	88.9 (4.8)	0.79
Type 2 Diabetes Mellitus, %						
Yes	6.4	11.1	13.3	16.2	22.8	<0.001

[a] *p*-values were determined using analysis of variance (ANOVA) test for continuous variables and Chi-square test for categorical variables. [b] Data are given as means, with standard error (SE) in parentheses, unless otherwise specified.

Table 3. Nutrient and food consumption according to quintiles of the dietary inflammatory index: in the Diabetes Mellitus Survey of Mexico City, 2015.

| | Dietary Inflammatory Index | | | | | | | | | | |
| Variables | Quintile 1: Most Anti-Inflammatory | | Quintile 2 | | Quintile 3 | | Quintile 4 | | Quintile 5: Most Pro-Inflammatory | | p-Value [a] |
	Mean	(95% CI)	Mean	(95% CI)	Mean	(95% CI)	Mean	(95% CI)	Mean	(95% CI)	
Carbohydrates intake (% energy) [b]	53.8	(52.6, 55.1)	55.0	(53.7, 56.4)	56.0	(55.2, 58.4)	56.1	(54.7, 57.5)	56.1	(54.3, 57.8)	<0.001
Protein intake (% energy)	14.4	(13.9, 14.8)	13.9	(13.4, 14.6)	13.7	(13.1, 14.0)	13.0	(12.6, 13.5)	12.6	(11.7, 13.7)	<0.001
Total fat intake (% energy)	31.8	(30.9, 32.9)	30.8	(29.8, 31.6)	30.3	(29.2, 31.3)	31.2	(30.1, 32.3)	31.3	(29.9, 32.7)	0.08
Saturated fats (% energy)	11.4	(10.9, 11.9)	11.7	(11.2, 12.2)	11.3	(10.9, 11.8)	11.3	(10.8, 11.8)	12.3	(11.5, 13.2)	0.51
Monounsaturated fats (% energy)	11.2	(10.8, 11.6)	10.8	(10.4, 11.2)	10.6	(10.1, 11.1)	10.9	(10.4, 11.4)	10.9	(10.3, 11.4)	0.20
Polyunsaturated fats (% energy)	7.6	(7.3, 7.9)	7.2	(6.9, 7.5)	6.9	(6.6, 7.2)	6.8	(6.5, 7.1)	6.7	(6.5, 7.0)	<0.001
Fiber (g/day)	42.7	(40.0, 45.4)	31.5	(27.8, 35.2)	24.7	(23.5, 25.9)	24.2	(22.6, 25.9)	13.3	(12.7, 14.0)	<0.001
Alcohol consumption (g/day)	15.2	(9.4, 21.0)	11.8	(7.2, 16.4)	6.6	(2.2, 11.0)	6.6	(1.2, 13.2)	2.5	(1.2, 3.9)	<0.001
Magnesium (mg/day)	600.3	(568.8, 631.8)	453.5	(402.1, 504.8)	365.5	(350.3, 380.7)	355.9	(333.7, 388.2)	219.5	(208.6, 230.5)	<0.001
Vitamin C (mg/day)	374.4	(344.5, 404.2)	288.0	(258.2, 317.8)	194.5	(181.0, 208.2)	160.6	(141.4, 179.7)	82.0	(72.9, 91.2)	<0.001
Vitamin A (µg/day)	1900.2	(1666.1, 2134.2)	1219.9	(1071.6, 1368.2)	830.1	(772.7, 887.6)	701.5	(635.1, 767.9)	396.3	(360.0, 432.6)	<0.001
Vitamin E (mg/day)	13.0	(12.3, 13.6)	8.9	(7.6, 10.1)	6.5	(6.2, 6.8)	6.5	(6.2, 7.3)	3.4	(3.4, 3.9)	<0.001
Vitamin D (µg/day)	7.7	(7.1, 8.3)	5.1	(4.4, 5.7)	4.4	(3.9, 4.9)	3.8	(3.4, 4.2)	2.5	(2.5, 3.1)	<0.001
Vegetables (g/day)	370.0	(321.2, 418.8)	245.5	(212.8, 278.4)	139.4	(121.3, 157.5)	112.2	(95.9, 128.5)	69.3	(60.0, 78.6)	<0.001
Fruits (g/day)	327.6	(293.3, 362.0)	259.9	(225.9, 294.0)	178.8	(162.2, 195.5)	134.5	(114.3, 154.6)	74.2	(64.4, 84.0)	<0.001
Legumes (g/day)	67.4	(49.5, 85.3)	51.0	(29.2, 72.6)	31.6	(26.0, 37.2)	33.7	(26.6, 40.8)	21.2	(16.2, 26.1)	<0.001
Fish and seafood (g/day)	24.1	(15.0, 33.1)	13.9	(4.7, 23.0)	10.8	(5.9, 15.7)	10.4	(5.1, 15.7)	3.2	(1.5, 4.9)	<0.001
Dairy products (g/day)	242.5	(209.9, 275.1)	225.8	(188.9, 262.6)	177.9	(142.3, 213.5)	172.5	(134.3, 210.8)	139.2	(109.3, 169.1)	<0.001
Red meat and processed meat (g/day)	40.1	(33.7, 46.5)	46.9	(41.3, 52.6)	55.0	(44.4, 65.5)	55.3	(41.8, 68.7)	78.3	(66.3, 90.2)	<0.001
Eggs (g/day)	28.9	(23.8, 33.9)	30.8	(25.1, 36.5)	32.2	(25.2, 39.2)	35.5	(28.4, 42.6)	34.3	(26.6, 41.9)	<0.001
Refined cereals (g/day)	109.2	(96.0, 122.5)	145.0	(129.8, 160.3)	145.4	(125.5, 165.3)	158.2	(122.7, 193.6)	173.9	(147.1, 200.6)	<0.001
Potatoes (g/day)	9.7	(5.2, 14.2)	11.8	(7.7, 15.8)	11.5	(7.8, 15.3)	8.3	(4.9, 11.7)	7.1	(5.1, 9.2)	0.87
Soft drinks (mL/day)	69.5	(51.6, 87.4)	146.9	(109.6, 184.1)	219.5	(175.7, 263.3)	262.4	(202.2, 322.6)	401.7	(343.3, 460.1)	<0.001

[a] p-values were determined using ANOVA test. [b] Data are given as means, with 95% CI in parentheses.

Table 4. Odds ratio (OR) and 95% confidence intervals (CI) for the relation between the dietary inflammatory index and T2DM in the Diabetes Mellitus Survey of Mexico City, 2015.

	Dietary Inflammatory Index									
	Quintile 1: Most Anti-Inflammatory	Quintile 2		Quintile 3		Quintile 4		Quintile 5: Most Pro-Inflammatory		*p*-Value
	OR	OR	(95% CI)	OR	(95% CI)	OR	(95% CI)	OR	(95% CI)	
Model I	1.0	1.55	(0.86, 2.78)	1.80	(0.90, 3.56)	1.78	(0.93, 3.53)	2.29	(1.11, 4.75)	0.01
Model II	1.0	1.73	(0.94, 3.20)	1.88	(0.91, 3.89)	1.97	(1.06, 3.64)	3.00	(1.38, 6.55)	0.005
Model III	1.0	1.80	(0.95, 3.38)	2.01	(0.97, 4.13)	2.10	(1.07, 3.78)	3.02	(1.39, 6.58)	0.005

Model I: Adjusted by age and sex. Model II: Model I plus physical activity (inactive vs. active/highly active); hours of television watching; tobacco use (current, past, and never); socioeconomic status (low, medium, and high); education (elementary and secondary education, high school, and Bachelor's degree or higher); family history of diabetes mellitus (yes vs. no); persona history of hypertension (yes vs. no), medication use (yes vs. no), multivitamin use (yes vs. no), and alcohol intake (gr/day). Model III: Model II plus body mass index (<25.0 vs. ≥25.0 kg/m^2).

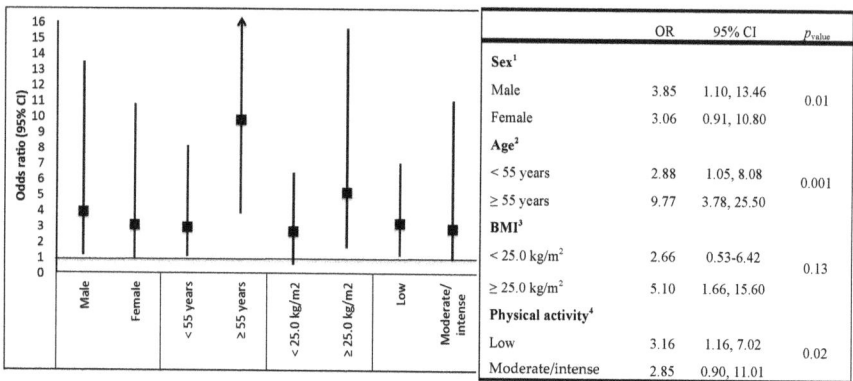

	OR	95% CI	p_{value}
Sex[1]			
Male	3.85	1.10, 13.46	0.01
Female	3.06	0.91, 10.80	
Age[2]			
< 55 years	2.88	1.05, 8.08	0.001
≥ 55 years	9.77	3.78, 25.50	
BMI[3]			
< 25.0 kg/m^2	2.66	0.53-6.42	0.13
≥ 25.0 kg/m^2	5.10	1.66, 15.60	
Physical activity[4]			
Low	3.16	1.16, 7.02	0.02
Moderate/intense	2.85	0.90, 11.01	

Figure 1. Subgroup analysis. Odds ratios (95% CI) for the association between extreme quintiles of the dietary inflammatory index (DII) and type 2 diabetes mellitus (T2DM). [1] Adjusted for age (years), physical activity (inactive vs. active/highly active), hours of television watching; tobacco use (current, past, and never), socioeconomic status (low, medium, and high), education (elementary and secondary education, high school, and Bachelor's degree or higher), family history of diabetes mellitus (yes vs. no), personal history of hypertension (yes vs. no), medication use (yes vs. no), multivitamin use (yes vs. no), alcohol intake (gr/day), body mass index (<25.0 vs. ≥25.0 kg/m^2). [2] Adjusted for sex, physical activity (inactive vs. active/highly active), hours of television watching; tobacco use (current, past, and never), socioeconomic status (low, medium, and high); education (elementary and secondary education, high school, and Bachelor's degree or higher), family history of diabetes mellitus (yes vs. no), personal history of hypertension (yes vs. no), medication use (yes vs. no), multivitamin use (yes vs. no), alcohol intake (gr/day vs. ≥25.0 kg/m^2). [3] Adjusted for age (years), sex, physical activity (inactive vs. active/highly active), hours of television watching, tobacco use (current, past, and never), socioeconomic status (low, medium, and high); education (elementary and secondary education, high school, and Bachelor's degree or higher), family history of diabetes mellitus (yes vs. no), personal history of hypertension (yes vs. no), medication use (yes vs. no), multivitamin use (yes vs. no), alcohol intake (gr/day). [4] Adjusted for age (years), sex, hours of television watching, tobacco use (current, past, and never); socioeconomic status (low, medium, and high); education (elementary and secondary education, high school, and Bachelor's degree or higher), family history of diabetes mellitus (yes vs. no), personal history of hypertension (yes vs. no), medication use (yes vs. no), multivitamin use (yes vs. no), alcohol intake (gr/day), body mass index (<25.0 vs. ≥25.0 kg/m^2).

4. Discussion

In the Mexico City Diabetes Mellitus Survey, we observed that participants in the DII score highest quintile, representing the most pro-inflammatory diet, had higher odds of T2DM (independent of other diabetes risk factors) compared with participants in the DII score lowest quintile (maximum anti-inflammatory potential). When we stratified by age (<55 years vs. ≥55 years), we observed positive associations between DII and T2DM, with larger magnitude of association among participants ≥55 years of age.

In the present study, we used a previously derived and validated DII score [13] to appraise the capacity of a pro-inflammatory diet on T2DM. The DII scores computed from a Mexican population included 27 food parameters, ranged from −5.49 to +4.12 with a mean of −0.68. This result is consistent with prior publications conducted in Italy, France, and Spain [16,17,29,30]. For example, Ramallal and colleagues at the University of Navarra cohort study reported a DII score ranging from −5.14 to +3.97 [30].

We also evaluated associations between food groups and nutrient intake and the DII, and found that subjects in the highest DII quintile (most pro-inflammatory diet) consumed more red and processed meat, eggs, refined cereals, and soft drinks, and had a lower intakes of vegetables, fruits, fish, and seafood. Similar to these results, the "PREvención con DIeta MEDiterránea" (PREDIMED) study found that consumption of vegetables and fruit was less frequent among men and women in the highest DII quintile [29].

Regarding nutrient intake, we observed that subjects with the most pro-inflammatory diet had lower intakes of polyunsaturated fatty acids, fiber, magnesium, and some vitamins. Similar to our results, the PREDIMED study found that subjects in the highest DII quintile consumed fewer polyunsaturated fatty acids, vitamins, and fiber. Moreover, other studies using the dietary pattern or dietary score approach, have observed an inverse association between healthy diets or patterns (mainly characterized by fruits, vegetables, whole grains and fiber) and inflammation and T2DM, as well as a positive association with Western patterns or unhealthy diet scores [9,10,30,31].

In the present analysis, we studied the association between DII and T2DM. We observed that subjects in the highest DII quintile had approximately three times greater odds of T2DM compared with subjects in the lowest DII quintile. The findings in our analysis agree with prior studies that evaluate the relation between diet and T2DM. For example, in the Insulin Resistance Atherosclerosis Cohort study, including subjects with a diet high in red meat, low-fiber cereals, fried potatoes, eggs, cheese, and low in wine had approximately 4.5 times greater risk of T2DM comparing extreme quartiles of the dietary pattern [31]. Similar results were observed in the Nurses' Health Study [32], where a pattern higher in sugar-sweetened soft drinks, refined grains, and processed meat but low in vegetables was associated with an increased risk of T2DM (OR = 3.09; 95% CI: 1.99, 4.79; compared to diet characterized by lower consumption of these dietary components). On the other hand, multiple prospective studies have reported an inverse association between the adherence to Mediterranean diet (with anti-inflammatory effects) [33] and the risk of T2DM [34]. Furthermore, a recent study [35] that evaluated the relation between DII and the risk of prediabetes found that subjects in the highest DII tertile had higher odds of prediabetes (OR = 18.88; 95% CI: 7.02, 50.82) compared to those who consumed a more anti-inflammatory diet. Additionally, most of the highly consumed food groups in the most pro-inflammatory DII quintile (red and processed meat, refined cereals, and soft drinks) have been associated with T2DM and with inflammatory markers [10]. For example, soft drinks have been linked to T2DM and inflammatory biomarkers due to their significant contribution to the glycemic load [36]. Whereas, low intakes of whole grains, fruits, and vegetables in the highest DII quintile have been related with reduced diabetes risk, probably mediated by a reduction of CRP, and certain interleukins, and by an improvement in the endothelial function [37].

Other results in the present study indicate that a pro-inflammatory effect of diet on T2DM could be particularly unfavorable among older (≥55 years) or inactive individuals (<150 min/week). Although not statistically significant, there was a suggestion of an interaction between DII and overweight/obesity in relation to T2DM. Despite the lack of significance, this result could be biologically important. Similar results were obtained in the Multiethnic Cohort (MEC) Study. In this study, the stratified analysis suggests that, among men, the risk for T2DM increased with higher consumption of fat and meat patterns among overweight (Hazard ratio = 1.49; 95% CI: 1.23, 1.81) and obese (HR = 1.57; 95% CI: 1.16, 2.12) individuals [38]. In women, similar results were observed, although these results were not statistically significant. In our case, this finding should be interpreted with caution; it is difficult to determine, with our study design, the role of BMI in the causal sequence (i.e., whether it is a confounder or an effect modifier). The relation between DII and T2DM remained strong after adjustment for BMI, indicating that the DII may be associated with diabetes in all individuals, but especially among obese subjects.

The connection between DII and T2DM could be explained through the effect of a pro-inflammatory diet on insulin resistance that has been linked to the inflammatory process [39]. In this sense, prior studies suggest a positive relationship between markers of chronic inflammation, including CRP, IL-1β, IL-6, and TNF-α, and insulin resistance [39]. Furthermore, it has been established that insulin resistance increases levels of these adhesion molecules in diabetic and nondiabetics individuals [40]. On the other hand, the functional effects of food or food groups and nutrients like meat, processed meat, refined cereals, and soft drinks, which corresponded with high DII scores in our study, have been also shown to influence systemic inflammation [32].

Strengths of our study include: (1) the random stratified cluster design of the DMS-MC; (2) the use of previously validated questionnaires; (3) the inclusion of many potential demographic, behavioral, and other factors as potential effect modifiers or confounders in the multivariate analysis; and (4) the use of a validated DII score specially constructed to assess the inflammatory potential of any diet [12,13]. As reported in other studies [17,29], the DII can be adapted for use in different populations including the Mexican population providing results that can be compared to those from studies based in diverse populations in many parts of the world.

Some potential weaknesses of our study need to be highlighted. Because of its cross-sectional design, this study cannot infer causality. Therefore, these results need to be further investigated in future longitudinal studies. Although the SFFQ used in this study had been previously validated [20], other possible limitations are related to information bias. In this regard, it is important to note that dietary factors used to calculate the DII were evaluated from a single measurement of SFFQ, which is subject to random error that would tend to underestimate the true association between DII and T2DM in our study. As observed in previous studies [29], some dietary components such as saffron, thyme, turmeric, and others were not available to compute the DII in the present analysis; however, as they are not habitually consumed in large quantities or common in Mexican diet, they may not have an important impact on the DII score. Another probable weakness could be related to the T2DM definition; nevertheless, we provided appropriate allowance for the prevalent ascertainment in the present analysis. In other words, prevalent cases of T2DM (previously diagnosed) were included only if they were recently diagnosed (less than 11 months), had fasting glucose concentrations ≥126 mg/dL, and had poor glycemic control (HbA1c ≥ 6.5) at the time of the survey. Additionally, we conducted a sensitivity analysis including only subjects diagnosed at the time of the survey and we observed similar results (OR = 3.56; 95% CI: 1.13, 9.11). We adjusted for many potentially confounding factors, however, residual confounding due to measurement error, mainly in assessing some self-reported lifestyle variables or due to insufficient control in statistical models, might have produced some degree of bias in our results. However, it is improbable that such a bias would explain the consistently robust association observed between DII and T2DM.

5. Conclusions

Our data suggest that a higher DII score (revealing a more pro-inflammatory diet) was associated with increased odds of T2DM compared with DII scores in the lowest quintile of the DII (indicative of an anti-inflammatory diet) among participants from the DMS-MC. In addition, we observed that the magnitude of the association appeared to be more pronounced among overweight/obesity subjects, older individuals, and those with low levels of physical activity. Further longitudinal investigations evaluating this relationship are needed to determine causality. Finally, the DII may be an important tool to characterize the diet of the Mexican population and further explore associations with non-communicable diseases.

Acknowledgments: This study was possible thanks to an unrestricted research grant obtained by SB from Novo Nordisk (number Project: 1295. Cities Changing Diabetes: Mexico City Representative Diabetes survey) and a NIH-Fogarty grant (NIH-Fogarty RO3 TW009061) to the National Institute of Public Health. Shivappa and Hébert were supported by grant number R44DK103377 from the United States National Institute of Diabetes and Digestive and Kidney Diseases.

Author Contributions: S.B. and E.D.-G. designed the study; E.D.-G., S.B., L.T.-M. conducted the research; E.D.-G., P.M.-A. and N.S. performed the statistical analyses; E.D.-G. wrote the first draft of the manuscript; E.D.-G., P.M.-A., N.S., J.R.H., L.T.-M., C.B., and S.B. critically reviewed and commented on the manuscript. All authors read and approved the final version of the manuscript.

Conflicts of Interest: E. Denova-Gutiérrez, P. Muñoz-Aguirre, L. Tolentino-Mayo, C. Batis, S. Barquera, declare no conflict of interest. James R. Hébert owns controlling interest in Connecting Health Innovations LLC (CHI), a company planning to license the right to his invention of the dietary inflammatory index (DII^{TM}) from the University of South Carolina in order to develop computer and smart phone applications for patient counseling and dietary intervention in clinical settings. Dr. Nitin Shivappa is an employee of CHI.

References

1. Calder, P.C.; Albers, R.; Antoine, J.M.; Blum, S.; Bourdet-Sicard, R.; Ferns, G.A.; Folkerts, G.; Friedmann, P.S.; Frost, G.S.; Guarner, F.; et al. Inflammatory disease processes and interactions with nutrition. *Br. J. Nutr.* **2009**, *101*, S1–S45. [CrossRef] [PubMed]

2. Fung, T.T.; McCullough, M.L.; Newby, P.K.; Manson, J.E.; Meigs, J.B.; Rifai, N.; Willett, W.C.; Hu, F.B. Diet-quality scores and plasma concentrations of markers of inflammation and endotelial dysfunction. *Am. J. Clin. Nutr.* **2005**, *82*, 163–173. [CrossRef] [PubMed]

3. Zimmet, P.Z.; Magliano, D.J.; Herman, W.H.; Shaw, J.E. Diabetes: A 21st century challenge. *Lancet Diabetes Endocrinol.* **2014**, *2*, 56–64. [CrossRef]

4. Kassebaum, N.J.; DALYs and GBD collaborators, 2015. Global, regional, and national disability-adjusted life-years (DALYs) for 315 diseases and injuries and healthy life expectancy (HALE), 1990–2015: A systematic analysis for the Global Burden of Disease Study 2015. *Lancet* **2016**, *388*, 1603–1658. [CrossRef]

5. Guariguata, L.; Whiting, D.R.; Hambleton, I.; Beagley, J.; Linnenkamp, U.; Shaw, J.E. Global estimates of diabetes prevalence for 2013 and projections for 2035. *Diabetes Res. Clin. Pract.* **2014**, *103*, 137–149. [CrossRef] [PubMed]

6. Gómez-Dantés, H.; Fullman, N.; Lamadrid-Figueroa, H.; Cahuana-Hurtado, L.; Darney, B.; Avila-Burgos, L.; Correa-Rotter, R.; Rivera, J.A.; Barquera, S.; González-Pier, E.; et al. Dissonant health transition in the states of Mexico, 1990–2013: A systematic analysis for the Global Burden of Disease Study 2013. *Lancet* **2016**, *388*, 2386–2402. [CrossRef]

7. Visser, M.; Bouter, L.M.; McQuillan, G.M.; Wener, M.H.; Harris, T.B. Elevated C-reactive protein levels in overweight and obese adults. *JAMA* **1999**, *282*, 2131–2135. [CrossRef] [PubMed]

8. Petersen, A.M.; Pedersen, B.K. The anti-inflammatory effect of exercise. *J. Appl. Physiol.* **2005**, *98*, 1154–1162. [CrossRef] [PubMed]

9. Calder, P.C.; Ahluwalia, N.; Brouns, F.; Buetler, T.; Clement, K.; Cunningham, K.; Esposito, K.; Jönsson, L.S.; Kolb, H.; Lansink, M.; et al. Dietary factors and low-grade inflammation in relation to overweight and obesity. *Br. J. Nutr.* **2011**, *106*, S5–S78. [CrossRef] [PubMed]

10. Schulze, M.B.; Hu, F.B. Primary prevention of diabetes: What can we done and how much can be prevented? *Annu. Rev. Public Health* **2005**, *26*, 445–467. [CrossRef] [PubMed]

11. Fung, T.T.; Schulze, M.; Manson, J.E.; Willett, W.C.; Hu, F.B. Dietary patterns, meat intake, and the risk of type 2 diabetes in women. *Arch. Intern. Med.* **2004**, *164*, 2235–2240. [CrossRef] [PubMed]

12. Shivappa, N.; Steck, S.E.; Hurley, T.G.; Hussey, J.R.; Hébert, J.R. Designing and developing a literature-derived, population-based dietary inflammatory index. *Public Health Nutr.* **2014**, *17*, 1689–1696. [CrossRef] [PubMed]

13. Shivappa, N.; Steck, S.E.; Hurley, T.G.; Hussey, J.R.; Ma, Y.; Ockene, I.S.; Tabung, F.; Hébert, J.R. A population based dietary inflammatory index predicts levels of C-reactive protein in the seasonal variation of blood cholesterol study (SEASONS). *Public Health Nutr.* **2014**, *17*, 1825–1833. [CrossRef] [PubMed]

14. Shivappa, N.; Hébert, J.R.; Rietzschel, E.R.; De Buyzere, M.L.; Langlois, M.; Debruyne, E.; Marcos, A.; Huybrechts, I. Associations between dietary inflammatory index and inflammatory markers in the Asklepios Study. *Br. J. Nutr.* **2015**, *113*, 665–671. [CrossRef] [PubMed]

15. Alkerwi, A.; Shivappa, N.; Crichton, G.; Hébert, J.R. No significant independent relationships with cardiometabolic biomarkers were detected in the Observation of Cardiovascular Risk Factors in Luxemburgo Study population. *Nutr. Res.* **2014**, *34*, 1058–1065. [CrossRef] [PubMed]

16. Shivappa, N.; Zucchetto, A.; Montella, M.; Serraino, D.; Steck, S.E.; La Vecchia, C.; Hébert, J.R. Inflammatory potential of diet and risk of colorectal cancer: A case-control study from Italy. *Br. J. Nutr.* **2015**, *114*, 152–158. [CrossRef] [PubMed]

17. Neufcourt, L.; Assmann, K.E.; Fezeu, L.K.; Touvier, M.; Graffouillère, L.; Shivappa, N.; Hébert, J.R.; Wirth, M.D.; Hercberg, S.; Galan, P.; et al. Prospective association between the dietary inflammatory index and cardiovascular diseases in the SUpplémentation en VItamines et Minéraux AntiOXydants (SU.VI.MAX) cohort. *J. Am. Heart Assoc.* **2016**, *5*, e002735. [CrossRef] [PubMed]

18. Romero-Martínez, M.; Shamah-Levy, T.; Franco-Nuñez, A.; Villalpando, S.; Cuevas-Nasu, L.; Gutiérrez, J.P.; Rivera-Dommarco, J.Á. National Health and Nutrition Survey 2012: Design and coverage. *Salud Publica Mex.* **2013**, *55*, S332–S340. [CrossRef] [PubMed]

19. Rosner, B.; Willett, W.C. Interval estimates for correlation coefficients corrected for within-person variation: Implications for study design and hypothesis testing. *Am. J. Epidemiol.* **1988**, *127*, 377–386. [CrossRef] [PubMed]

20. Denova-Gutiérrez, E.; Ramírez-Silva, I.; Rodríguez-Ramírez, S.; Jiménez-Aguilar, A.; Shamah-Levy, T.; Rivera-Dommarco, J.A. Validity of a food frequency questionnaire to assess food intake in Mexican adolescent and adult population. *Salud Publica Mex.* **2016**, *58*, 617–628. [CrossRef] [PubMed]

21. Hernández-Ávila, J.E.; González-Avilés, L.; Rosales-Mendoza, E. *Manual de Usuario. SNUT Sistema de Evaluación de Hábitos Nutricionales y Consumo de Nutrimentos*; Instituto Nacional de Salud Pública: Cuernavaca, México, 2003. (In Spanish)

22. Hebert, J.R.; Ockene, I.S.; Hurley, T.G.; Luippold, R.; Well, A.D.; Harmatz, M.G. Development and testing of a seven-day dietary recall. *J. Clin. Epidemiol.* **1997**, *50*, 925–937. [CrossRef]

23. Twetz, N. *Textbook of Clinical Chemistry*; WB Saunders: Philadelphia, PA, USA, 1999.

24. American Diabetes Association. Standards of medical care in diabetes-2014. *Diabetes Care* **2014**, *37*, S14–S80. [CrossRef]

25. Alberti, K.G.; Zimmet, P.; Shaw, J. The metabolic syndrome: A new worldwide definition. *Lancet* **2005**, *366*, 1059–1062. [CrossRef]

26. Martinez, S.M.; Ainsworth, B.E.; Elder, J.P. A review of physical activity measures used among US Latinos: Guidelines for developing culturally appropriate measures. *Ann. Behav. Med.* **2008**, *36*, 195–207. [CrossRef] [PubMed]

27. International Physical Activity Questionnaire. Guidelines for Data Processing and Analysis of the International Physical Activity Questionnaire (IPAQ)-Short and Long Forms. Available online: http://www.ipaq.ki.se/scoring.pdf (accessed on 30 May 2016).

28. World Health Organization. Global Recommendations on Physical Activity for Health. Available online: http://whqlibdoc.who.int/publications/2010/9789243599977_spa.pdf (accessed on 29 May 2016).

29. Ruiz-Canela, M.; Zazpe, I.; Shivappa, N.; Hébert, J.R.; Sánchez-Tainta, A.; Corella, D.; Salas-Salvadó, J.; Fitó, M.; Lamuela-Raventós, R.M.; Rekondo, J.; et al. Dietary inflammatory index and anthropometric measures of obesity in a population sample at high cardiovascular risk from the PREDIMED (PREvención con DIeta MEDiterránea) trial. *Br. J. Nutr.* **2015**, *113*, 984–995. [CrossRef] [PubMed]

30. Ramallal, R.; Toledo, E.; Martínez-González, M.A.; Hernández-Hernández, A.; García-Arellano, A.; Shivappa, N.; Hébert, J.R.; Ruiz-Canela, M. Dietary inflammatory index and incidence of cardiovascular disease in the SUN Cohort. *PLoS ONE* **2015**, *10*, e0135221. [CrossRef] [PubMed]

31. Liese, A.D.; Weis, K.E.; Schulz, M.; Tooze, J.A. Food intake patterns associated with incident type 2 diabetes. *Diabetes Care* **2009**, *32*, 263–268. [CrossRef] [PubMed]

32. Schulze, M.B.; Hoffmann, K.; Manson, J.E.; Willett, W.C.; Meigs, J.B.; Weikert, C.; Heidemann, C.; Colditz, G.A.; Hu, F.B. Dietary pattern, inflammation, and incidence of type 2 diabetes in women. *Am. J. Clin. Nutr.* **2005**, *82*, 675–684. [CrossRef] [PubMed]

33. Casas, R.; Sacanella, E.; Urpí-Sardà, M.; Chiva-Blanch, G.; Ros, E.; Martínez-González, M.A.; Covas, M.I.; Lamuela-Raventos, R.M.; Salas-Salvadó, J.; Fiol, M.; et al. The effects of the Mediterranean diet on biomarkers of vascular wall inflammation and plaque vulnerability in subjects with high risk for cardiovascular disease. A randomize trial. *PLoS ONE* **2014**, *9*, e100084. [CrossRef] [PubMed]

34. Mozaffarian, D.; Marfisi, R.; Levantesi, G.; Silletta, M.G.; Tavazzi, L.; Tognoni, G.; Valagussa, F.; Marchioli, R. Incidence of new-onset diabetes and impaired fasting glucose in patients with recent myocardial infarction and the effect of clinical and lifestyle risk factors. *Lancet* **2007**, *370*, 667–675. [CrossRef]

35. Vahid, F.; Shivappa, N.; Karamati, M.; Naeini, A.J.; Hebert, J.R.; Davoodi, S.H. Association between Dietary Inflammatory Index (DII) and risk of prediabetes: A case-control study. *Appl. Physiol. Nutr. Metab.* **2017**, *42*, 399–404. [CrossRef] [PubMed]

36. Schulze, M.B.; Manson, J.E.; Ludwig, D.S.; Colditz, G.A.; Stampfer, M.J.; Willett, W.C.; Hu, F.B. Sugar-sweetend beverages, weight gain, and incidence of type 2 diabetes in young and middle-aged women. *JAMA* **2004**, *292*, 927–934. [CrossRef] [PubMed]

37. Whincup, P.H.; Donin, A.S. Cereal fibre and type 2 diabetes: Time now for randomised control trials? *Diabetologia* **2015**, *58*, 1383–1385. [CrossRef] [PubMed]

38. Erber, E.; Hopping, B.N.; Grandinetti, A.; Park, S.Y.; Kolonel, L.N.; Maskarinec, G. Dietary pattern and risk for diabetes. The multiethnic cohort. *Diabetes Care* **2010**, *33*, 532–538. [CrossRef] [PubMed]

39. Festa, A.; D'Agostino, R., Jr.; Howard, G.; Mykkänen, L.; Tracy, R.P.; Haffner, S.M. Chronic subclinical inflammation as part of the insulin resistance syndrome: The Insulin ResistanceAtherosclerosis Study (IRAS). *Circulation* **2000**, *102*, 42–47. [CrossRef] [PubMed]

40. Gearing, A.J.; Newman, W. Circulating adhesion molecules in disease. *Immunol. Today* **1993**, *14*, 506–512. [CrossRef]

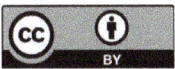

nutrients

MDPI

Article

Effects of Virgin Olive Oils Differing in Their Bioactive Compound Contents on Metabolic Syndrome and Endothelial Functional Risk Biomarkers in Healthy Adults: A Randomized Double-Blind Controlled Trial

Estefania Sanchez-Rodriguez [1], Elena Lima-Cabello [2], Sara Biel-Glesson [3], Jose R. Fernandez-Navarro [3], Miguel A. Calleja [3], Maria Roca [4], Juan A. Espejo-Calvo [5], Blas Gil-Extremera [6], Maria Soria-Florido [7], Rafael de la Torre [8], Montserrat Fito [7,9], Maria-Isabel Covas [9,10], Juan de Dios Alche [2], Emilio Martinez de Victoria [11], Angel Gil [1,9,*] and Maria D. Mesa [1]

[1] Department of Biochemistry and Molecular Biology II, Institute of Nutrition and Food Technology "José Mataix", Biomedical Research Center, University of Granada, Parque Tecnológico de la Salud, Avenida del Conocimiento s/n, 18100 Armilla, Granada, Spain; estefaniasr@outlook.com (E.S.-R.); mdmesa@ugr.es (M.D.M.)

[2] Department of Biochemistry, Cell and Molecular Biology of Plants, Estación Experimental del Zaidín (CSIC), Profesor Albareda 1, 18008 Granada, Spain; elimacabello@gmail.com (E.L.-C.); juandedios.alche@eez.csic.es (J.d.D.A.)

[3] Fundación Pública Andaluza para la Investigación Biosanitaria de Andalucía Oriental "Alejandro Otero" (FIBAO), Avenida de Madrid 15, 18012 Granada, Spain; sbiel@fibao.es (S.B.-G.); estrategia@innofood.es (J.R.F.-N.); mangel.calleja.sspa@juntadeandalucia.es (M.A.C.)

[4] Food Phytochemistry Department, Instituto de la Grasa, Consejo Superior de Investigaciones Científicas (CSIC), University Campus Pablo de Olavide, 41013 Sevilla, Spain; mroca@ig.csic.es

[5] Instituto para la Calidad y Seguridad Alimentaria (ICSA), Avenida de la Hispanidad 17, 18320 Santa Fe, Granada, Spain; jaespejo@hotmail.com

[6] Department of Medicine, University of Granada, Avenida de la Investigación 11, 18071 Granada, Spain; blasgil@ugr.es

[7] Cardiovascular Risk and Nutrition Research Group, Hospital del Mar Medical Research Institute (IMIM), Dr. Aiguader 88, 08003 Barcelona, Spain; mariat.soria@gmail.com (M.S.-F.); mfito@imim.es (M.F.)

[8] Integrative Pharmacology and Systems Neuroscience Research Group, IMIM (Hospital del Mar Research Institute), Universitat Pompeu Fabra (CEXS-UPF), Dr. Aiguader 88, 08003 Barcelona, Spain; rtorre@imim.es

[9] Spanish Biomedical Research Networking Centre, Physiopathology of Obesity and Nutrition (CIBEROBN), Instituto de Salud Carlos III, Monforte de Lemos 3-5, 28029 Madrid, Spain; maria.nuproas@gmail.com

[10] NUPROAS Handelsbolag, Nackã, Sweden, NUPROAS HB, Apartado de Correos 93, 17242 Girona, Spain

[11] Department of Physiology, Institute of Nutrition and Food Technology "José Mataix", Biomedical Research Center, University of Granada, Parque Tecnológico de la Salud, Avenida del Conocimiento s/n, 18100 Armilla, Granada, Spain; emiliom@ugr.es

* Correspondence: agil@ugr.es; Tel.: +34-958-246-187

Received: 10 April 2018; Accepted: 14 May 2018; Published: 16 May 2018

Abstract: The aim of this study was to evaluate the effect of virgin olive oils (VOOs) enriched with phenolic compounds and triterpenes on metabolic syndrome and endothelial function biomarkers in healthy adults. The trial was a three-week randomized, crossover, controlled, double-blind, intervention study involving 58 subjects supplemented with a daily dose (30 mL) of three oils: (1) a VOO (124 ppm of phenolic compounds and 86 ppm of triterpenes); (2) an optimized VOO (OVOO) (490 ppm of phenolic compounds and 86 ppm of triterpenes); and (3) a functional olive oil (FOO) high in phenolic compounds (487 ppm) and enriched with triterpenes (389 ppm). Metabolic syndrome and endothelial function biomarkers were determined in vivo and ex vivo. Plasma high density lipoprotein cholesterol (HDLc) increased after the OVOO intake. Plasma endothelin-1 levels decreased after the intake of the three olive oils, and in blood cell cultures challenged. Daily intake of VOO enriched in phenolic compounds improved plasma HDLc, although no differences were found at the end of the three interventions, while VOO with at least 124 ppm of phenolic compounds, regardless of the triterpenes content improved the systemic endothelin-1 levels in vivo and ex vivo. No effect of triterpenes was observed after three weeks of interventions. Results need to be confirmed in subjects with metabolic syndrome and impaired endothelial function (Clinical Trials number NCT02520739).

Keywords: olive oil; virgin olive oil; olive oil polyphenols; maslinic acid; oleanolic acid; cardiovascular diseases; endothelial function; phenolic compounds; triterpenes; metabolic syndrome

---

1. Introduction

Metabolic syndrome (MS) is a cluster of associated metabolic and clinical disturbances that tend to occur together [1]. This syndrome is commonly represented by the combination of obesity (particularly abdominal), hyperglycemia, dyslipidemia, and hypertension [2]. MS is associated with an increased risk of cardiovascular disease (CVD), which is the main cause of disability and mortality in industrialized countries, and is associated with a chronic inflammatory response characterized by abnormal cytokine production leading to endothelial dysfunction [3].

There is consolidated clinical evidence that the Mediterranean diet (MD) is associated with a lower risk of CVDs, including myocardial infarction, stroke and cardiovascular death [4]. Mayneris-Perxachs et al. [5] proposed the MD as a successful tool for the prevention and treatment of MS and related comorbidities. A large study in a high cardiovascular risk population has found that the MD supplemented with virgin olive oil (VOO) protects people from vascular disease, suggesting a key role of olive oil [6]. A recent systematic review and meta-analysis provided evidence that olive oil might exert beneficial effects on endothelial function and biomarkers of inflammation, thus representing a key ingredient contributing to the MD cardiovascular-protective effects [7]. Olive oil is not only a source of monounsaturated fatty acids (MUFAs) but also an important source of bioactive compounds, such as phenols and triterpenes [8,9]. Previous studies suggested a protective effect of olive oil phenolic compounds on endothelial dysfunction [10], whereas olive oil triterpenes could be useful for the prevention of multiple diseases related to cell oxidative damage [11]. Maslinic and oleanolic acids are the principal triterpenes found in VOO. The potential of these olive oil triterpenic acids for use as a therapeutic strategy to improve vascular function and treating CVD has been recently reviewed [12]. However, to our best knowledge, no clinical trial has been performed to provide evidence of their benefits in healthy adults, according to EFSA requirement [13]. The present study which acronyms is NUTRAOLEUM, aimed to evaluate the effect of VOO enriched with bioactive compounds, such as phenolic compounds and triterpenes, on MS and endothelial function biomarkers in healthy adults. We reported that daily intake of VOO enriched in phenolic compounds during three weeks improved plasma high density lipoprotein cholesterol levels (HDLc), one of the features of metabolic syndrome, although no differences were found at the end of the three interventions. In addition, VOO with at least 124 ppm of phenolic compounds, regardless of the triterpenes content, improved the systemic endothelin-1 levels in vivo and ex vivo, while no additional effect of triterpenes was observed.

2. Materials and Methods

2.1. Subjects

Information about subjects, sample size and their eligibility and dietary control have been referenced in detail elsewhere [14]. In brief, fifty-eight intention-to-treat subjects were eligible.

The inclusion criteria were as follows: people in good health on the basis of a physical examination and basic biochemical and hematological analyses, and willingness to provide written informed consent. The exclusion criteria were as follows: smoking, intake of antioxidant supplements, aspirin or any other drug with established antioxidant properties, hyperlipidemia, obesity (body mass index (BMI) >30 kg/m^2), diabetes, hypertension, celiac or other intestinal disease, any condition limiting mobility, life-threatening diseases, or any other disease or condition that would impair compliance. Five subjects declined to participate for personal reasons before olive oil type allocation. Fifty-three subjects (27 men and 26 women) aged from 20 to 50 years from the general population of Granada were enrolled in the study from February 2014 to July 2014 and were assigned into groups. Two subjects did not complete the study. After the first intervention, one subject refused to continue for personal reasons, and the other did not follow the protocol correctly. At the end of the experimental period, 51 subjects remained in the study (Figure 1) [14]. All subjects provided written informed consent according to the principles of the Declaration of Helsinki, and the local institutional review board, the Ethics Committee Research Centre of Granada, approved the protocol (13/11 C38).

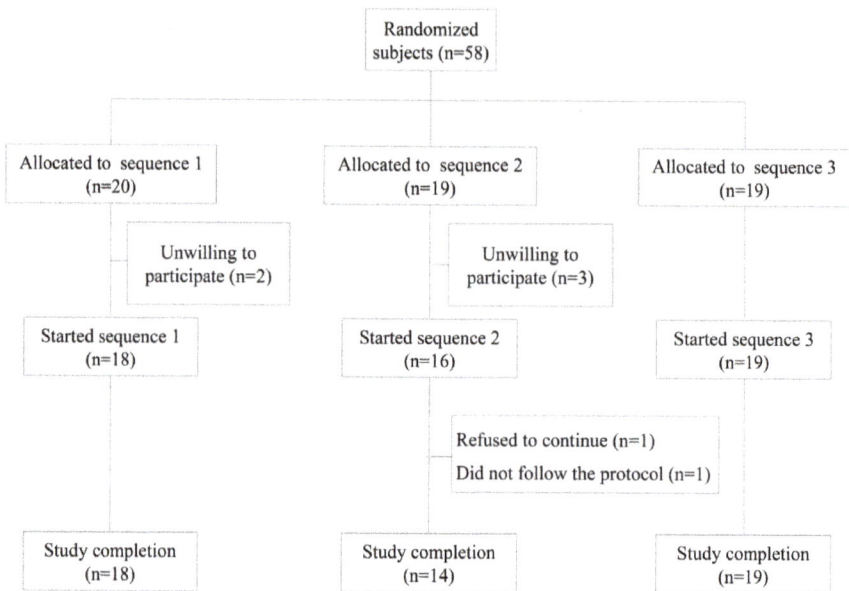

Figure 1. CONSORT Based Flow Diagram of the recruitment, enrollment and randomization process.

2.2. Study Design

The NUTRAOLEUM study has been designed to evaluate the effects of VOO high in phenolic compounds and enriched with triterpenes, maslinic and oleanolic acids, from olive exocarp, on MS features and endothelial function risk biomarkers in comparison with a standard VOO. The characteristics of the olive oils used in the study, the design of the study, and the detailed study procedures of the sustained consumption study have been previously published [14]. In brief, the trial was a randomized, crossover, controlled and double-blind clinical trial involving three oils: (1) an optimized VOO high in phenolic compounds (OVOO) (490 ppm of phenolic compounds and 86 ppm of triterpenes) produced from Picual olives (Andalucía, Spain); (2) a functional olive oil (FOO), that was the same OVOO high in phenolic compounds (487 ppm) and enriched with triterpenes (389 ppm) from olive exocarp; and (3) a VOO obtained from the OVOO after washing to eliminate the majority of phenolic compounds (124 ppm of phenolic compounds and 86 ppm of triterpenes).

San Francisco de Asís Cooperative (Montefrío (Granada), Spain) provided the olive oils used in the present study. Daily doses of 30 mL of the three types of raw olive oils, as recommended by the US Food and Drug Administration [15], were distributed over three meals. Olive oils were blindly prepared in special containers; the three types of olive oil were labeled "A","B", and "C". Containers with the corresponding 30 mL olive oil daily dose and enough amount of the same oil for cooking during each intervention period were delivered to the subjects at the beginning of each intervention period. The subjects were randomly assigned to three orders of administration of olive oil, paired by gender and age, using the block-randomization method of a software program for sequence generation [14]. The randomization lists were concealed in a lightproof sealed envelope. The sealed envelopes were kept by the independent statistician during the study, avoiding the breaking of the seal. Thus, the subjects, investigators, and outcome assessors were blinded and could not foresee the treatment allocation throughout the study. Hence, blinding of outcome assessment was also ensured. According to previous published studies, olive oils were sequentially administered over three periods of 3 weeks [16] preceded by two weeks of washout periods [17] during which the subjects were requested to avoid olives and olive oil consumption. A nutritionist personally advised subjects on replacing all types of habitually consumed raw fats using only the assigned oil. The advantage of using a crossover design is that each subject served as his or her own control. Olive oils were specially prepared for the trial and differed only in phenolic compound and triterpenes contents (Table 1). The oils were prepared in dark, sealed containers and were similar in appearance and color, thus ensuring blinding of the subjects and study personnel. The trial has been registered at ClinicalTrials.gov ID: NCT02520739.

Table 1. Characteristics of the administered olive oils.

	VOO	OVOO	FOO
Fatty Acid Profile (%)			
C18:0	2.3	2.2	2.1
C18:1n9	78.9	78.2	78.4
C18:2n6	6.6	6.8	6.9
C18:3n3	0.6	0.7	0.7
C20:0	0.4	0.4	0.4
C20:1	0.3	0.4	0.4
C22:0	0.1	0.1	0.1
C24:0	<0.1	<0.1	<0.1
Total phenolic compounds (ppm)	124	490	487
Hydroxytyrosol and derivates	105	424.0	423.0
Lignanes	18.2	61.3	59.2
Flavonoids	0.7	3.4	3.2
Simple phenols	0.0	0.9	0.9
Total triterpenes (mg/kg)	86.5	86.3	388.8
Maslinic acid	47.3	47.3	217.7
Oleanolic acid	39.2	39.1	171.1
Ursolic acid	<10	<10	<10
α-tocopherol (ppm)	174	183	176
Squalene (mg/100 g)	529.2	536.2	545.5
Total pigments (ppm)	15.73	17.59	16.78
Total carotenoid pigments (ppm)	7.08	6.79	6.97
Total sterols (ppm)	1437	1396	1460

FOO, functional olive oil; OVOO, optimized virgin olive oil; VOO, virgin olive oil.

2.3. Evaluation of Dietary Intake

Subjects completed a 3-day dietary record at baseline and during each intervention period [18]. Energy consumption and dietary intakes of macro- and micronutrients data were processed using CSG software (General ASDE) and the Spanish Food Composition Database (BEDCA) for the subjects who completed the intervention [19].

2.4. Blood Sample Collection

Fasting venous blood samples were collected at the beginning of the study (baseline) and before (pre-intervention, after the washout period) and at the end (post-intervention) of each olive oil intervention period using EDTA-coated tubes. Three-milliliter aliquots were stored at 4 °C for the ex vivo experiments. The rest of the blood samples were centrifuged (4 °C, 10 min at $1750\times g$), and plasma aliquots were immediately frozen and stored at -80 °C until analysis.

2.5. Ex-Vivo Whole Blood Cultures

An aliquot of blood samples (as indicated above) were collected using lithium–heparin tubes (BD Vacutainer System, Heidelberg, Germany) from a subsample of 36 subjects. Blood was diluted 1:3 with Dulbecco's modified Eagle's medium and agitated gently in 3-mL tubes (Greiner Bio-one, Solingen, Germany) within 3 h after collection. One-milliliter aliquots were seeded in each well of 24-well plates (Nunc, VWR International GmbH, Langenfeld, Germany) and cultured for 24 h at 37 °C under an atmosphere of 5% CO_2. From each blood drawing, we performed triplicate incubations in parallel with positive and negative controls, separate cultures that included phytohaemagglutinin (PHA, 10 µg/mL), *E. coli* lipopolysaccharide (LPS, 1 µg/mL) and phorbol 12-myristate 13-acetate plus ionomycin (PMA, 25 ng/mL + IO, 1 µg). The same lots of PHA, LPS, PMA + IO and phosphate buffered saline were used in all experiments. Blood cultures were removed from each well and centrifuged at $700\times g$ for 5 min at 20 °C. The resulting supernatants (plasma) were aliquoted and pooled from eight subjects from each of the three assigned orders of administration of olive oil and stored at -20 °C until further analysis of endothelin-1 [20,21].

2.6. Measurement of Metabolic Syndrome Biomarkers

In the fasting state, anthropometric measurements (weight, height and waist circumference) were determined at baseline and before and after each intervention period by the same member of the professional staff. For all measurements, the subjects did not wear shoes. MS biomarkers were determined as primary outcomes. BMI was calculated as weight (kg) divided by height squared (m²). Total cholesterol, triacylglycerols and serum glucose were determined by standard enzymatic methods using a PENTRA-400 autoanalyzer (ABX-Horiba Diagnostics, Montpellier, France). Plasma HDLc was measured as soluble HDLc as determined using an accelerator selective detergent method (ABX-Horiba Diagnostics). Plasma low density lipoprotein cholesterol (LDLc) concentrations were calculated using the Friedewald formula. Systolic (SBP) and diastolic (DBP) blood pressures were measured with a mercury sphygmomanometer after a minimum of 10 min resting in the seated position; the average of two measurements was recorded. The pulse pressure was calculated as the difference between SBP and DBP. Total cholesterol, triacylglycerols, serum glucose, HDLc and LDLc could only be measured for 46 subjects.

2.7. Measurement of Selected Plasma Hormones and Endothelial Function Biomarkers

A Milliplex Map Kit, human monoclonal antibody kits (EMD Millipore Corporation, Billerica, MA, USA) were used according to the manufacturer's instructions in conjunction with a Luminex® 200 system with the XMap technology (Luminex Corporation, Austin, TX, USA) to determine the concentrations of the following biomarkers as secondary outcomes: adiponectin (coefficient of variation

(CV): 10.3%), resistin (CV: 7.7%), soluble intercellular adhesion molecule (sICAM-1) (CV: 6.1%) and soluble vascular adhesion molecule (sVCAM-1) (CV: 5.4%), (Cat. #HADK1MAG-61K).

Endothelin-1 was determined as a secondary outcome by ELISA (CV): 7.2%) (R&D Systems, Minneapolis, MN, USA; Cat. DET100) in both plasma and whole blood culture supernatants.

2.8. Measurements of Triterpenes and Phenolic Compounds in Urine

To ensure the subjects' compliance with the assigned intervention, triterpenes (maslinic and oleanolic acid) derivatized with 2-picolylamine (see Appendix A) and olive oil phenolic compounds (hydroxytyrosol and metabolites) were analyzed in 24-h urine from 12 random subjects by liquid chromatography coupled to a mass spectrometer [22].

2.9. Statistical Analysis

Baseline data are presented as the mean values ± standard error of the mean (SEMs) unless otherwise indicated. The normality of variables was assessed using Q-Q graphs. The χ^2 test was used for categorical variables to determine differences in the baseline. One-factor ANOVA or Kruskal-Wallis tests were used (depending on whether the normality assumption was met) for continuous variables to determine differences among the three olive oil interventions, in terms of baseline characteristics, nutrient intake and for the ex vivo endothelin-1 experiment.

Biochemical parameters are presented as adjusted mean values ± SEMs and were analyzed using a linear mixed-effects model (LMM). The normality of the residues was evaluated using Q-Q graphs. Missing data were imputed using appropriate methods. The outliers for each intervention were removed if kurtosis > 1 and asymmetry > 1 in the distribution of the responses. In all cases, more than 80% of the data were analyzed.

Variables with a skewed distribution were logarithm-transformed for analysis (nutritional variables and resistin). A LMM was used to compare variables before and after each intervention (pre- vs. post-interventions, intra-treatment effect) and to compare the results between the groups after the 3-week intervention (inter-treatment effect), adjusting for age, gender, pre-intervention and period as fixed effects and for subjects and hospital as random effects. The same model was also used to compare changes of the variables (post-intervention minus pre-intervention) without adjusting for pre-intervention. Carryover effects were assessed as the interaction between period and intervention [23]. The multiple comparison post hoc is given by the estimated means in the model (adjusted by Sidak). This statistical model (LMM) takes into account all the possible confounders (covariates) which are included on it. In addition, the baselines are used as outcomes but without effect, so they can act as a control and take into account a possible carryover effect [24]. Within the LMMs, the factor treatment, time and the random effect considered by participant are taken into account in the structure of the data.

In addition, an interaction term was checked for differences on the effect part intervention by gender. Model goodness-of-fit was tested using residual plots. The Bayesian Information Criterion was used to assess model reduction and the selection of variables and interactions. We performed all analysis on an intention-to-treat basis. A $p < 0.05$ value was considered significant. Statistical Package for the Social Sciences version 20 software was used to perform the statistical analysis (SPSS Inc., Chicago, IL, USA).

3. Results

3.1. Baseline Characteristics

Tables 2 and 3 show the clinical and biochemical characteristics, and the average daily nutritional intakes, respectively, of the subjects grouped according to the sequence of olive oil administration at the beginning of the study. No differences were observed among the three groups of subjects at baseline.

Table 2. Clinical and biochemical characteristics of subjects at baseline according to olive oil administration sequence.

Characteristics	Sequence 1	Sequence 2	Sequence 3
Age, years	32 ± 2	29 ± 2	28 ± 2
Gender, male n (%)	12 (60)	10 (53)	8 (42)
BMI, kg/m^2	24 ± 1	24 ± 1	24 ± 1
Waist circumference, cm	80 ± 2	78 ± 3	77 ± 2
Males	80 ± 3	82 ± 4	82 ± 2
Females	81 ± 5	73 ± 3	73 ± 2
HDLc, mg/dL	58 ± 2	58 ± 3	59 ± 2
Males	55 ± 3	51 ± 3	52 ± 3
Females	64 ± 2	65 ± 5	64 ± 3
LDLc, mg/dL	117 ± 9	107 ± 7	102 ± 5
Total cholesterol, mg/dL	192 ± 10	180 ± 7	175 ± 7
Triacylglycerols, mg/dL	87 ± 7	81 ± 13	67 ± 5
Glucose, mg/dL	90 ± 2	92 ± 2	87 ± 2
Adiponectin, mg/L	11.40 ± 1.38	12.49 ± 1.69	17.20 ± 2.78
Resistin, µg/L	16.38 ± 1.88	16.57 ± 1.82	15.26 ± 1.69
SBP, mmHg	121 ± 2	120 ± 3	118 ± 3
DBP, mmHg	77 ± 2	74 ± 2	71 ± 2
Pulse pressure, mmHg	44 ± 2	46 ± 3	47 ± 2
Endothelin-1, pg/mL	1.35 ± 0.08	1.36 ± 0.10	1.38 ± 0.12
sICAM, ng/mL	74.48 ± 4.50	62.26 ± 3.16	66.10 ± 4.63
sVCAM, ng/mL	459 ± 21	459 ± 30	443 ± 25

Values are expressed as the means $\pm$ SEMs. ANOVA and χ^2 tests were used to compare results between groups. Sequence 1: OVOO, VOO and FOO olive oil, n = 20; Sequence 2: VOO, FOO and OVOO olive oil, n = 19; Sequence 3: FOO, OVOO and VOO olive oil, n = 19. BMI, body mass index; DBP, diastolic blood pressure; FOO, functional olive oil; HDLc, high density lipoprotein cholesterol; LDLc, low density lipoprotein cholesterol; n, number of observations; OVOO, optimized virgin olive oil; SBP, systolic blood pressure; SEM, standard error of the mean; sICAM-1, soluble intercellular adhesion molecule; sVCAM-1, soluble vascular cell adhesion molecule; VOO, virgin olive oil.

Table 3. Average daily energy and selected nutrient intake of subjects at baseline according to olive oil administration sequence.

Nutritional Characteristics	Sequence 1	Sequence 2	Sequence 3
Energy, kcal	1976 ± 90	2151 ± 138	2074 ± 109
Total carbohydrates, g	200 ± 10	213 ± 16	214 ± 13
Proteins, g	80 (16–222)	96 (37–258)	93 (21–215)
Total fat, g	86 ± 4	102 ± 10	89 ± 6
MUFA, g	31 (12–80)	33 (6–85)	33(6–89)
PUFA, g	13 (3–43)	11 (1–44)	14 (2–49)
SFA, g	21 (6–64)	27 (11–80)	26 (4–66)
Vitamin A, µg retinol equivalents	440 (111–1552)	512 (109–158)	539 (7–1669)
Vitamin C, mg ascorbic acid	70 (4–400)	88 (11–428)	81 (3–335)
Vitamin D, µg	2 (0–41)	2 (0–40)	2 (0–34)
Vitamin E, mg α-tocopherol equivalents	9 (2–29)	9 (1–67)	11 (1–39)
Cholesterol, mg	284 ± 26	354 ± 31	287 ± 24
Alcohol, g	0 (0–52)	0 (0–48)	0 (0–84)
Selenium, µg	31 (5–130)	34 (1–114)	36 (3–117)

Values are expressed as the means $\pm$ SEMs or as medians (range). ANOVA was used to compare results between groups for those variables that followed normality, and the Kruskal Wallis test was used for those that did not. Data of 51 subjects were obtained from the 3-day dietary record at baseline. Sequence 1: OVOO, VOO and FOO olive oil, n = 54; Sequence 2: VOO, FOO and OVOO olive oil, n = 42; Sequence 3: FOO, OVOO and VOO olive oil, n = 57. FOO, functional olive oil; MUFA, monounsaturated fatty acids; n, number of observations; OVOO, optimized virgin olive oil; PUFA, polyunsaturated fatty acids; SEM, standard error of the mean; SFA, saturated fatty acids; VOO, virgin olive oil.

3.2. Nutritional Analysis

Table 4 shows the average daily energy and selected nutrient intakes after the three olive oil interventions. No differences were observed among the three interventions (Table 4).

Table 4. Average daily energy and selected nutrient intake of subjects after the three olive oil interventions.

Nutritional Characteristics	VOO	OVOO	FOO
Energy, kcal	1983 (873–4342)	2006 (697–4561)	1914 (780–3457)
Total carbohydrates, g	199 (47–408)	203 (30–531)	175 (38–533)
Proteins, g	77 (24–180)	80 (17–200)	73 (25–207)
Total fat, g	89 (27–244)	94 (24–257)	91 (20–227)
MUFA, g	44 (8–119)	44 (8–113)	45 (9–123)
PUFA, g	11 (4–37)	12 (4–36)	13 (3–41)
SFA, g	25 (7–74)	27 (6–82)	24 (5–69)
Vitamin A, μg retinol equivalents	433 (34–1477)	427 (26–1504)	452 (39–1515)
Vitamin C, mg ascorbic acid	48 (0–280)	60 (0–255)	55 (1–305)
Vitamin D, μg	1.5 (0–32)	1.2 (0–82)	1.2 (0–81)
Vitamin E, mg α-tocopherol equivalents	10 (2–30)	11 (3–32)	11 (2–32)
Cholesterol, mg	285 (11–981)	253 (28–853)	272 (15–1011)
Alcohol, g ethanol	0 (0–97)	0 (0–54)	0 (0–78)
Selenium, μg	30 (0–260)	31 (0–198)	31 (1–160)

Values are expressed as median (range). ANOVA was used to compare intakes between interventions. Data for 51 subjects were obtained from the 3-day dietary record at baseline. Data for 51 subjects were obtained from the 3-day dietary record at baseline. FOO, functional olive oil; MUFA, monounsaturated fatty acids; *n*, number of observations; OVOO, optimized virgin olive oil; PUFA, polyunsaturated fatty acids; SFA, saturated fatty acids; VOO, virgin olive oil.

3.3. Plasma Metabolic Syndrome and Endothelial Function Biomarkers

Table 5 shows MS and endothelial function biomarker data before and after the three interventions. All clinical and biochemical MS biomarkers were within normal values at the beginning and at the end of the study. BMI, waist circumference, pulse pressure, and fasting plasma glucose, adiponectin and resistin concentrations were unchanged during the study.

When comparing pre- vs. post-intervention data (intra-treatment effect), HDLc levels significantly increased only after the OVOO intervention ($p = 0.041$), and only in females ($p = 0.005$). However, no differences were observed between the three interventions. Total cholesterol increased after the FOO intervention ($p = 0.021$). LDLc was unaffected. Fasting plasma triacylglycerol concentrations increased after the VOO and OVOO interventions ($p = 0.037$ and $p = 0.002$, respectively) but not after the FOO intervention. However, plasma triacylglycerols were low at the beginning of the study (78 ± 5 mg/dL). On the other hand, SBP decreased after the VOO intervention ($p = 0.019$) and increased after the FOO intervention ($p = 0.004$), while DBP and pulse pressure were unchanged after the three interventions. Plasma endothelin-1 concentrations decreased after the VOO, OVOO, and FOO interventions ($p = 0.006$, $p = 0.006$ and $p = 0.014$, respectively), and the plasma concentrations of sICAM-1 and sVCAM-1 were unchanged after the three interventions.

When analyzing the inter-treatment effects, LDLc levels were higher after the FOO intervention compared with the OVOO intervention ($p = 0.033$), and SBP was higher after the FOO intervention compared with the VOO intervention ($p = 0.001$).

The changes in metabolic clinical variables and endothelial function biomarkers (Supplementary Table S1) were similar in all the subjects after the three interventions except SBP, which increased up to 118 mmHg after the FOO but decreased after the VOO and OVOO interventions (up to 115 and 116 mmHg, respectively) ($p < 0.001$). The results show differences by gender for all interventions. However, no interactions were observed between gender and intervention.

Table 5. Metabolic syndrome and endothelial function biomarkers before and after each olive oil intervention in healthy adults.

Characteristics	VOO		OVOO		FOO	
	Pre-Intervention	Post-Intervention	Pre-Intervention	Post-Intervention	Pre-Intervention	Post-Intervention
BMI, kg/m^2	23.9 ± 0.1	24 ± 0.1	23.9 ± 0.1	24 ± 0.1	24 ± 0.1	24 ± 0.1
Waist circumference, cm	77.4 ± 0.7	77.2 ± 0.7	77.2 ± 0.7	76.8 ± 0.7	77.4 ± 0.7	76.9 ± 0.7
HDLc, mg/dL	58 ± 2	59 ± 2	57 ± 2	60 ± 2 *	58 ± 2	60 ± 2
Males	52 ± 2	53 ± 2	52 ± 2	52 ± 2	52 ± 2	54 ± 2
Females	64 ± 2	65 ± 2	63 ± 2	67 ± 2 *	65 ± 2	66 ± 2
LDLc, mg/dL	105 ± 4	108 ± 4 [a,b]	104 ± 4	106 ± 4 [a]	104 ± 4	111 ± 4 [b]
Total cholesterol, mg/dL	179 ± 5	182 ± 5	177 ± 5	183 ± 5	178 ± 5	186 ± 5 *
Triacylglycerols, mg/dL	72 ± 7	75 ± 7 *	74 ± 7	81 ± 7 *	75 ± 7	75 ± 7
Glucose, mg/dL	91 ± 2	91 ± 2	91 ± 2	91 ± 2	90 ± 2	91 ± 2
Adiponectin, mg/L	13.74 ± 1.7	12.8 ± 1.7	12.48 ± 1.7	13.6 ± 1.71	12.62 ± 1.71	13.74 ± 1.71
Resistin, µg/L	14.1 ± 1.1	14.1 ± 1.1	14.5 ± 1.1	13.8 ± 1.1	13.8 ± 1.1	14.1 ± 1.1
SBP, mmHg	117 ± 3	115 ± 3 *,[a]	119 ± 3	116 ± 3 [a,b]	114 ± 3	118 ± 3 *,[b]
DBP, mmHg	72 ± 2	72 ± 2	75 ± 2	73 ± 2	72 ± 2	74 ± 2
Pulse pressure, mmHg	45 ± 1	43 ± 1	44 ± 1	42 ± 1	42 ± 1	45 ± 1
Endothelin-1, pg/mL	1.53 ± 0.15	1.38 ± 0.15 *	1.58 ± 0.15	1.41 ± 0.15 *	1.49 ± 0.15	1.35 ± 0.15 *
sICAM-1, ng/mL	68.09 ± 3.19	67.11 ± 3.19	65.17 ± 3.20	67.73 ± 3.19	65.1 ± 3.20	66.7 ± 3.21
sVCAM-1, ng/mL	451 ± 22	443 ± 23	435 ± 22	451 ± 22	431 ± 22	442 ± 23

Values are expressed as the adjusted means ± SEMs. LMM was used to compare pre-intervention vs. post-interventions with each oil data, and data after the three interventions (post-interventions). * Significant differences between pre-intervention vs. post-intervention data within each intervention with the three olive oils. Different superscript letters indicate significant differences between post-intervention results ([a,b]), $p < 0.05$ was considered significant. DBP, diastolic blood pressure; FOO, functional olive oil; HDLc, high density lipoprotein cholesterol; LDLc, low density lipoprotein cholesterol; OVOO, optimized virgin olive oil; SBP, systolic blood pressure; SEM, standard error of the mean; sICAM-1, soluble intercellular adhesion molecule; sVCAM-1, soluble vascular cell adhesion molecule; VOO, virgin olive oil.

3.4. Plasma Endothelin-1 Ex Vivo Experiments

Before the three interventions, pooled blood cultures challenging with PHA, LPS, or PMA + IO induced a potent increase in the supernatant concentrations of endothelin-1 in whole blood cultures.

Figure 2 shows that the supernatant endothelin-1 concentration changes (post-intervention minus pre-intervention data) in whole blood cultures from the subjects were similar after the VOO and OVOO interventions and were significantly lower after the FOO intervention: -26.7 ± 15.3 pg/mL, -41.0 ± 12.9 pg/mL, and -119.5 ± 28.5 pg/mL for the VOO, OVOO and FOO interventions, respectively ($p = 0.035$), when stimulating with PHA; -30.3 ± 6.5 pg/mL, -58.2 ± 10.1 pg/mL and -109.6 ± 9.7 pg/mL for the VOO, OVOO, and FOO interventions, respectively, when stimulating with LPS ($p = 0.002$); and -38.9 ± 3.4 pg/mL, -50.8 ± 8.5 pg/mL and -87.0 ± 11.1 pg/mL for the VOO, OVOO, and FOO interventions, respectively, when stimulating with PMA+IO ($p = 0.015$).

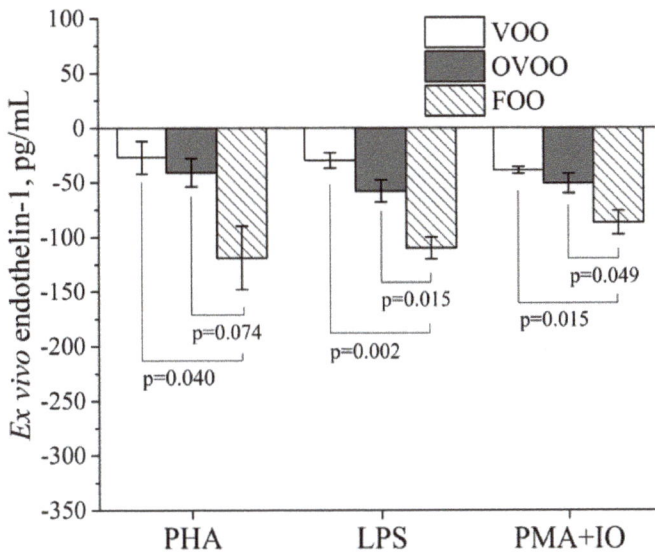

Figure 2. Plasma endothelin-1 ex vivo changes (post-intervention minus pre-intervention data) when stimulated with PHA, LPS or PMA + IO in whole blood cultures from healthy adults. Values are expressed as the means ± SEMs. ANOVA was used to compare differences between interventions and induction treatments. The Tukey post-hoc test was used for multiple comparisons among groups. $p < 0.05$ was considered significant. FOO, functional olive oil; IO, ionomycin; OVOO, optimized virgin olive oil; PHA, phytohemagglutinin; PMA, phorbol 12-myristate 13-acetate; VOO, virgin olive oil.

Supplemental Figure S1 shows the supernatant endothelin-1 concentrations that were induced ex vivo with PHA, LPS, and PMA + IO in whole blood cultures from the subjects before and after the three interventions. After the VOO, OVOO, and FOO interventions, challenging with LPS or PMA + IO induced a significantly lower increase of endothelin-1 secretion in whole blood cultures, while challenging with PHA induced a significantly lower increase of endothelin-1 secretion only after the OVOO and FOO interventions.

3.5. Biomarkers of Intervention Compliance

Recoveries of triterpenes in urine were consistent with the olive oils consumed in each intervention. Figure 3 shows urinary triterpenes changes (post-intervention minus pre-intervention data) for each olive oil intervention. The amounts of both triterpenic acids in urine after the FOO intervention were about four times higher than those recovered after the VOO and OVOO interventions ($p = 0.004$ and $p < 0.001$, respectively, for maslinic acid, and $p = 0.026$ and $p < 0.001$, respectively, for oleanolic acid). Urine concentrations of total hydroxytyrosol (the sum of hydroxytyrosol and its glucuronide and sulfate conjugates) were higher after the OVOO (2444 mM, $p = 0.003$) and FOO (2876 mM, $p = 0.002$) interventions than after the VOO (115 mM, $p = 0.011$) intervention.

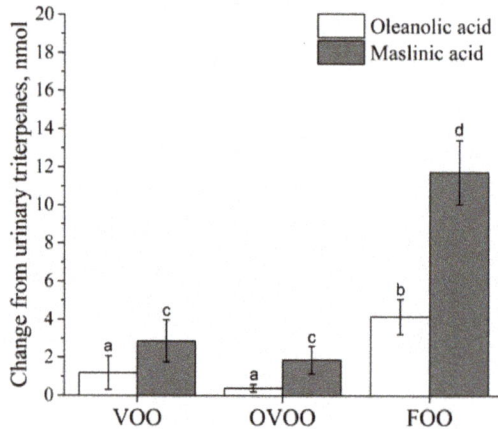

Figure 3. In vivo urinary triterpenes changes (post-intervention minus pre-intervention data) for each olive oil intervention in healthy adults. Values are expressed as the means ± SEMs. ANOVA was used to compare differences between the three interventions. Different superscript letters indicate significant differences between the interventions for oleanolic acid ([a,b]) and for maslinic acid ([c,d]). $p < 0.05$ was considered significant. FOO, functional olive oil; OVOO, optimized virgin olive oil; VOO, virgin olive oil.

4. Discussion

The NUTRAOLEUM study is the first human nutritional clinical trial concerning the effects of VOO that is high in phenolic compounds and enriched with triterpenes, maslinic and oleanolic acids, from olive exocarp, on MS features and endothelial function risk biomarkers in comparison with standard VOO in healthy subjects.

The PREDIMED study reported that a MD supplemented with at least 50 g of dietary VOO caused a reversion of MS after a median follow-up of 4.8 years [25], reducing the rate of CVD events by 30% compared with a low-fat diet control group [26]. In addition, this MD enriched with VOO and without energy restrictions reduced the diabetes risk among individuals at high cardiovascular risk [27]. Consumption of VOO close to 2.7, 164 or 366 ppm/day of phenolic compounds in humans, a 0.03% of hydroxytyrosol in a rodent model, and 50 ppm/day of hydroxytyrosol in a murine model have been reported to improve the blood lipid profile, although results in mice were not conclusive [28], possibly due to differences in the phenolic content of the olive oil and the physio-pathology of the studied animals. Polyphenols from olive oils have been shown to provide additional benefits on HDLc, other than those provided by the MUFA content. However, contradictory data exists on these benefits. In 2015, a meta-analysis reported no effect on HDLc concentration after the intake of VOO with at least 150 ppm of phenolic compounds [29], while, in accordance with our results, a recent systematic review [30] concluded that plasma HDLc was increased in different studies consuming from 2.28 to 75 g/day of olive oil. In the Eurolive Study, a European multicenter study, three olive oils (refined, medium and high) differing in their phenolic compound content (2.7, 164 and 366 ppm/day of phenolic content, respectively) increased HDLc and decreased triacylglycerol concentrations [16]. The increase in HDLc was linear with the olive oil polyphenol content. This additional benefit has also been described in healthy and hypercholesterolemic subjects treated with polyphenol-enriched VOO [31] when excluding patients treated with hypolipidemic medication. Additionally, the increase of olive oil polyphenols in the lipoprotein fraction may increase HDL size, stability, and antioxidant status [32]. It has been reported that the daily intake of olive oils enriched with its own polyphenols (250 ppm or 500 ppm), as well as the intake of olive oil enriched in polyphenols from thyme (250 ppm/day) decrease LDLc and improve the lipoprotein subclass distribution and associated ratios [33]. Other authors have described that a one-year intervention with a MD enriched with VOO improved several LDL characteristics related to its atherogenicity (resistance against oxidation, size, composition, and cytotoxicity) but did not modify the plasma LDLc concentrations in a subsample of subjects at high cardiovascular risk in the PREDIMED study [34]. Our results are consistent with this null effect of VOO on LDLc. On the other hand, besides the weak increase in plasma triacylglycerols observed after interventions with both VOO and OVOO, this was without clinical significance given that levels were low at baseline and remain low at the end of the three interventions, and thus it did not increase cardiovascular risk in these healthy subjects (triacylglycerols < 150 mg/dL) [35]. Our results are in contrast with the triacylglycerol improvement reported in the EUROLIVE Study [16]. A recent meta-analysis and systematic review focused on high polyphenol VOO concluded no effect on plasma triacylglycerol concentrations [29]; in addition, Saibandith et al. [36] stated that the effect of olive oil polyphenols on plasma triacylglycerols remained unclear. However, longer studies are needed to clarify this issue.

To the best of our knowledge, this is the first clinical trial evaluating the effect of olive oil triterpenes on plasma lipids and endothelial function biomarkers. Previous animal studies have reported different effects of oleanolic acid on plasma lipids, depending on the experimental animal model [37]. Based on our results, FOO enriched with triterpenes did not modify plasma HDLc, LDLc, or triacylglycerols, but increased plasma total cholesterol concentrations, although no inter-group significance was found. However, although these modifications do not represent an increase in cardiovascular risk since the values are low enough to be considered safe (total cholesterol < 190 mg/dL) [35], further human clinical trials are needed to demonstrate the potential benefit of olive phenolic compounds and triterpenes on plasma lipid concentrations over longer intervention periods.

Endothelial dysfunction is a critical early event in the development of atherosclerosis [38]. An imbalance between vasodilating and vasoconstricting molecules, such as nitric oxide and endothelin-1, respectively, contributes to the pathogenesis of hypertension and its complications [39]. Our results indicate that plasma endothelin-1 levels decreased after the VOO, OVOO and FOO interventions, and these results were also confirmed throughout ex vivo blood culture experiments. Although endothelin-1 is mainly produced from vascular endothelial cell, several studies have suggested that blood cells, such as polymorphonuclear neutrophils [40] and T-Cells [41], and also macrophages [42] are responsible from circulating levels of endothelin-1. In addition, ex vivo experiment has demonstrated the release of the mature peptide after LPS and LPS + PMA stimulation [40]; Mencarelli et al. [43] have confirmed these results. As demonstrated here, endothelin-1 production was decreased after the three interventions. This effect may be beneficial for cardiovascular risk affected people, since the effect of endothelin-1 has been documented on endothelial and inflammatory cells, which contributes to pathophysiological processes such as vascular hypertrophy, cell proliferation, fibrosis and inflammation [44–46]. In humans, the consumption of VOO has shown benefits on blood pressure and endothelial function [47]. In agreement with our results, a meta-analysis stated that olive oils with at least 150 ppm of phenolic compounds exert a moderate effect on lowering SBP and no effects on DBP [29]. Regarding triterpenes, besides the weak SBP increase observed after this intervention, no clinical significance was observed as blood pressure remained under 130 mmHg and did not increase cardiovascular risk [35]. It is reported that SBP varies to a greater degree than DBP [48,49]. For this reason, we calculated pulse pressure and found no significant effect of FOO. A beneficial effect of triterpenes on endothelial function [50] and blood pressure [51] has been described in animal models of hypertension, but further studies are required to explore the mechanisms involved in the effect of specific components of VOO on endothelin-1 regulation.

In vitro studies showed that minor olive oil components, specifically hydroxytyrosol and its metabolites, down-regulate the secretion of E-selectin, *p*-selectin, sICAM-1, and sVCAM-1, affecting endothelial function [52]. However, and in agreement with our results, no differences in sICAM-1 or sVCAM-1 plasma concentrations were reported after 50 mL of VOO or refined olive oil consumption containing (161 or 14.67 ppm/day of phenolic compounds, respectively) in coronary heart disease patients [53]. Another study found a significant reduction in sICAM-1 but not in sVCAM-1 concentrations after the intake of 50 mL/day of olive oil [54]. Recently, it has been proposed that the intake of 25 mL/day of VOO containing 366 ppm of phenolic compounds modulates the expression of several genes related to the renin-angiotensin-aldosterone system [55]. Therefore, further longer studies are needed to reach final conclusions about the effect of VOO minor compounds on molecules modulating endothelial function.

One of the limitations of the present study is that young and healthy subjects are recruited as target population. The present intervention does not appear sufficient to draw definitive conclusions. Therefore, new studies in older subject affected by metabolic syndrome and endothelial dysfunction would be interesting in order to evaluate the beneficial effect of VOO components. Although no differences in dietary intakes were observed during the three interventions, measurements of dietary intake relied on self-reporting and were therefore subjective. Another limitation of this study is that dietary records for the washout periods were not recorded, thus we cannot analyzed dietary intakes during these periods. In addition, our subjects live in the south of Spain, where MD and VOO are highly consumed. Therefore, a 3-week intervention is not long enough to cause significant changes. Further studies are required to find conclusions related to the bioactive compounds presents in olive oils, and to explore the mechanisms involved in these effects of specific components of VOO on MS and endothelial function.

5. Conclusions

In conclusion, olive oil rich in polyphenols increased HDLc levels in females, although no differences were found at the end of the three interventions, and improved an endothelial function biomarker both in vivo and ex vivo. No additional benefits were obtained from triterpenes VOO enrichment after 3-wk supplementation. However, further longer studies are warranted on olive oil triterpenes and their health benefits in older subjects particularly in those affected by metabolic syndrome and endothelial dysfunction.

Supplementary Materials: The following are available online at http://www.mdpi.com/2072-6643/10/5/626/s1, Figure S1: Plasma endothelin-1 ex vivo secretion in whole blood cultures from healthy adults before and after 3 weeks of intervention with the three olive oils and PHA, LPS or PMA + IO stimulation. Table S1: CONSORT 2010 checklist of information to include when reporting a randomized trial.

Author Contributions: J.A.E.-C., B.G.-E., M.S.-F., R.d.l.T., M.F., M.-I.C., J.d.D.A., E.M.d.V., A.G., and M.D.M. designed the research. E.S.-R., S.B.-G., J.R.F.-N., M.A.C., and M.D.M. conducted the research. E.L.-C. and J.d.D.A. were responsible for the ex vivo analyses. M.R. carried out the olive oil analyses. R.d.l.T. carried out urine phenolic and triterpenic acid measurements. E.S.-R. carried out biochemical analyses. E.S.-R., E.L.-C., R.d.l.T., J.d.D.A., E.M.d.V. and M.D.M. analyzed the data and performed the statistical analysis. E.S.-R., E.L.-C., R.d.l.T., J.d.D.A., E.M.d.V., A.G. and M.D.M. had primary responsibility for the final content. All authors read and approved the final manuscript. This paper contains results included in the doctoral thesis of Estefanía Sánchez Rodríguez, which was written within the context of Nutrition and Food Sciences at the University of Granada.

Acknowledgments: The "NUTRAOLEUM Study" has been supported by the grant ITC-20131031 from the I+D FEDER-INTERCONNECTA (CDTI) and Junta de Andalucía, Spain". We thank ACER CAMPESTRES S.L., SAN FRANCISCO DE ASIS Coop and AGROINSUR S.L., for the funding provided. The authors thank Pilar Jiménez, Alberto Guarnido, María Molina and Elizabeth García for administering the questionnaires to the subjects; Isabel Mérida, Isabel Hinojosa, Agustín Martín García, and María Luz Abarca for collecting the biological samples; and Victoria Martín Laguna and Laura Campaña Martín for aliquoting the samples. The authors also thank María Cruz Rico Prados for sample analysis and Llenalia M. García Fernández for her contributions to the statistical analysis.

Conflicts of Interest: The authors declare no conflict of interest. The founding sponsors had no role in the design of the study; in the collection, analyses, or interpretation of data; in the writing of the manuscript, and in the decision to publish the results.

Appendix A

Analysis of Triterpenes in Urine

For the analysis of maslinic acid (MA) and oleanolic acid (OA), aliquots of 250 µL of urine were transferred into 15-mL screw-capped glass tubes and spiked with 1 ng/mL of d_3-OA, 20 µL of β-glucuronidase from *Escherichia coli* and 200 µL of 0.1 M phosphate buffer pH 6.0. After overnight incubation in a water bath at 37 °C, 50 mg of $NaHCO_3/Na_2CO_3$ (1:2, w/w) was added to each tube before extraction. The samples were then subjected to a liquid-liquid extraction with 2 mL of methyl *tert*-butyl ether. The mixture was homogenized in a shaker rotator for 20 min and centrifuged at 3500 rpm for 5 min at room temperature. The organic phase was transferred to clean tubes and evaporated (40 °C) under a stream of nitrogen. The extracts were then derivatized with 50 µL of 2-picolylamine (1 µg/µL in ACN). The reaction mixture was incubated for 10 min at 60 °C on a heating block and then dried under a nitrogen stream. Samples were reconstituted in 100 µL of ACN-H_2O MilliQ grade (1:1). Derivatized OA and MA in urine was quantified using an Acquity UPLC system, (Waters Associates, Milford, MA, USA) for the chromatographic separation, the column was coupled to a triple quadrupole (Quattro Premier) mass spectrometer provided with an orthogonal Z-spray-electrospray interface (ESI) (Waters Associates). Nitrogen was used as the drying and nebulizing gas. The desolvation gas flow was set to approximately 1200 L/h, and the cone gas flow was set to 50 L/h.

Capillary voltages of 3 kV and 2.5 kV were used in positive and negative ionization mode, respectively. The nitrogen desolvation temperature was set to 450 °C, and the source temperature was set to 120 °C. The collision gas was argon, and the flow rate was 0.21 mL/min.

The liquid chromatography separation was performed at 55 °C using an Acquity CSH phenyl-hexyl column (100 mm, 2.1 mm i.d., 1.7 µm) (Waters Associates) operating at a flow rate of 300 µL min^{-1}. Water and methanol, both containing formic acid (0.01% v/v) and ammonium formate (1 mM), were selected as mobile phase solvents. For the target detection of derivatized OA and MA, a gradient program was used to separate the analytes; the percentage of organic solvent was linearly changed as follows: 0 min, 70%; 0.5 min, 70%; 7 min, 98%; 9 min, 98%; 9.5 min, 70%; and 11 min, 70%.

References

1. Sarafidis, P.A.; Nilsson, P.M. The metabolic syndrome: A glance at its history. *J. Hypertens.* **2006**, *24*, 621–626. [CrossRef] [PubMed]
2. Alberti, K.G.; Zimmet, P.; Shaw, J. The metabolic syndrome—A new worldwide definition. *Lancet* **2005**, *366*, 1059–1062. [CrossRef]
3. Freitas Lima, L.C.; Braga, V.A.; do Socorro de França Silva, M.; Cruz, J.C.; Sousa Santos, S.H.; de Oliveira Monteiro, M.M.; Balarini, C.M. Adipokines, diabetes and atherosclerosis: An inflammatory association. *Front. Physiol.* **2015**, *6*, 1–15. [CrossRef] [PubMed]
4. Gardener, H.; Wright, C.B.; Gu, Y.; Demmer, R.T.; Boden-Albala, B.; Elkind, M.S.; Sacco, R.L.; Scarmeas, N. Mediterranean-style diet and risk of ischemic stroke, myocardial infarction, and vascular death: The Northern Manhattan Study. *Am. J. Clin. Nutr.* **2011**, *94*, 1458–1464. [CrossRef] [PubMed]
5. Mayneris-Perxachs, J.; Sala-Vila, A.; Chisaguano, M.; Castellote, A.I.; Estruch, R.; Covas, M.I.; Fitó, M.; Salas-Salvadó, J.; Martínez-González, M.A.; Lamuela-Raventós, R.; et al. Effects of 1-Year Intervention with a Mediterranean Diet on Plasma Fatty Acid Composition and Metabolic Syndrome in a Population at High Cardiovascular Risk. *PLoS ONE* **2014**, *9*, e85202. [CrossRef] [PubMed]

6. Estruch, R.; Ros, E.; Salas-Salvadó, J.; Covas, M.; Corella, D.; Arós, F.; Gómez-Gracia, E.; Ruiz-Gutiérrez, V.; Fiol, M.; Lapetra, J.; et al. Primary prevention of cardiovascular disease with a Mediterranean diet. *N. Engl. J. Med.* **2013**, *368*, 1279–1290. [CrossRef] [PubMed]

7. Schwingshackl, L.; Christoph, M.; Hoffmann, G. Effects of Olive Oil on Markers of Inflammation and Endothelial Function-A Systematic Review and Meta-Analysis. *Nutrients* **2015**, *7*, 7651–7675. [CrossRef] [PubMed]

8. Covas, M.I.; de la Torre, K.; Farré-Albaladejo, M.; Kaikkonen, J.; Fitó, M.; López-Sabater, C.; Pujadas-Bastardes, M.A.; Joglar, J.; Weinbrenner, T.; Lamuela-Raventós, R.M.; et al. Postprandial LDL phenolic content and LDL oxidation are modulated by olive oil phenolic compounds in humans. *Free Radic. Biol. Med.* **2006**, *40*, 608–616. [CrossRef] [PubMed]

9. Tresserra-Rimbau, A.; Medina-Remón, A.; Pérez-Jiménez, J.; Martínez-González, M.A.; Covas, M.I.; Corella, D.; Salas-Salvadó, J.; Gómez-Gracia, E.; Lapetra, J.; Arós, F.; et al. Dietary intake and major food sources of polyphenols in a Spanish population at high cardiovascular risk: The PREDIMED study. *Nutr. Metab. Cardiovasc. Dis.* **2013**, *23*, 953–959. [CrossRef] [PubMed]

10. Storniolo, C.E.; Roselló-Catafau, J.; Pintó, X.; Mitjavila, M.T.; Moreno, J.J. Polyphenol fraction of extra virgin olive oil protects against endothelial dysfunction induced by high glucose and free fatty acids through modulation of nitric oxide and endothelin-1. *Redox Biol.* **2014**, *2*, 971–977. [CrossRef] [PubMed]

11. Sánchez-Quesada, C.; López-Biedma, A.; Warleta, F.; Campos, M.; Beltrán, G.; Gaforio, J.J. Bioactive Properties of the Main Triterpenes Found in Olives, Virgin Olive Oil, and Leaves of Olea europaea. *J. Agric. Food Chem.* **2013**, *61*, 12173–12182. [CrossRef] [PubMed]

12. Rodríguez-Rodríguez, R. Oleanolic acid and related triterpenoids from olives on vascular function: Molecular mechanisms and therapeutic perspectives. *Curr. Med. Chem.* **2015**, *22*, 1414–1425. [CrossRef] [PubMed]

13. EFSA Panel on Dietetic Products, Nutrition, and Allergies (NDA). General guidance for stakeholders on the evaluation of Article 13.1, 13.5 and 14 health claims. *EFSA J.* **2011**, *9*, 1–24.

14. Biel, S.; Mesa, M.-D.; de la Torre, R.; Espejo, J.-A.; Fernández-Navarro, J.-R.; Fitó, M.; Sánchez-Rodriguez, E.; Rosa, C.; Marchal, R.; Alche, J.D.; et al. The NUTRAOLEOUM Study, a randomized controlled trial, for achieving nutritional added value for olive oils. *BMC Complement. Altern. Med.* **2016**, *16*, 404. [CrossRef] [PubMed]

15. FDA. U.S. Food and Drug Administration. Available online: https://www.fda.gov/food/labelingnutrition/ucm073992.htm#cardio (accessed on 28 March 2018).

16. Covas, M.-I.; Nyyssönen, K.; Poulsen, H.E.; Kaikkonen, J.; Zunft, H.-J.F.; Kiesewetter, H.; Gaddi, A.; de la Torre, R.; Mursu, J.; Bäumler, H.; et al. The Effect of Polyphenols in Olive Oil on Heart Disease Risk Factors. *Ann. Intern. Med.* **2006**, *145*, 333–341. [CrossRef] [PubMed]

17. Fielding, C.J.; Havel, R.J.; Todd, K.M.; Yeo, K.E.; Schloetter, M.C.; Weinberg, V.; Frost, P.H. Effects of dietary cholesterol and fat saturation on plasma lipoproteins in an ethnically diverse population of healthy young men. *J. Clin. Investig.* **1995**, *95*, 611–618. [CrossRef] [PubMed]

18. Yang, Y.J.; Kim, M.K.; Hwang, S.H.; Ahn, Y.; Shim, J.E.; Kim, D.H. Relative validities of 3-day food records and the food frequency questionnaire. *Nutr. Res. Pract.* **2010**, *4*, 142–148. [CrossRef] [PubMed]

19. Base de Datos de Composición de Alimentos (BEDCA). Available online: http://www.bedca.net/ (accessed on 28 March 2018).

20. Huisman, H.W.; Schutte, A.E.; van Rooyen, J.M.; Schutte, R.; Malan, L.; Fourie, C.M.T.; Malan, N.T. The Association of Red Blood Cell Counts with Endothelin-1 in African and Caucasian Women. *Clin. Exp. Hypertens.* **2009**, *31*, 1–10. [CrossRef] [PubMed]

21. Walter, R.; Mark, M.; Gaudenz, R.; Harris, L.G.; Reinhart, W.H. Influence of nitrovasodilators and endothelin-1 on rheology of human blood in vitro. *Br. J. Pharmacol.* **1999**, *128*, 744–750. [CrossRef] [PubMed]

22. Pozo, O.J.; Pujadas, M.; Gleeson, S.B.; Mesa-García, M.D.; Pastor, A.; Kotronoulas, A.; Fitó, M.; Covas, M.I.; Navarro, J.R.F.; Espejo, J.A.; et al. Liquid chromatography tandem mass spectrometric determination of triterpenes in human fluids: Evaluation of markers of dietary intake of olive oil and metabolic disposition of oleanolic acid and maslinic acid in humans. *Anal. Chim. Acta* **2017**, *990*, 84–95. [CrossRef] [PubMed]

23. Senn, S. *Cross-over Trials in Clinical Research*, 2nd ed.; John Wiley & Sons, Ltd.: Chichester, UK, 2002; pp. 35–53.

24. Liu, G.F.; Lu, K.; Mogg, R.; Mallich, M.; Mehrotra, D.V. Should baseline be a covariate or dependent variable in analyses of change from baseline in clinical trials? *Stat. Med.* **2009**, *28*, 2509–2530. [CrossRef] [PubMed]

25. Estruch, R.; Salas-Salvadó, J. Towards an even healthier mediterranean diet. *Nutr. Metab. Cardiovasc. Dis.* **2013**, *23*, 1163–1166. [CrossRef] [PubMed]

26. Babio, N.; Toledo, E.; Estruch, R.; Ros, E.; Martínez-González, M.A.; Castañer, O.; Bulló, M.; Corella, D.; Arós, F.; Gómez-Gracia, E.; et al. Mediterranean diets and metabolic syndrome status in the PREDIMED randomized trial. *CMAJ* **2014**, *186*, E649–E657. [CrossRef] [PubMed]

27. Salas-Salvadó, J.; Bulló, M.; Estruch, R.; Ros, E.; Covas, M.-I.; Ibarrola-Jurado, N.; Corella, D.; Arós, F.; Gómez-Gracia, E.; Ruiz-Gutiérrez, V.; et al. Prevention of Diabetes with Mediterranean Diets. *Ann. Intern. Med.* **2014**, *160*, 1–10. [CrossRef] [PubMed]

28. Peyrol, J.; Riva, C.; Amiot, M. Hydroxytyrosol in the Prevention of the Metabolic Syndrome and Related Disorders. *Nutrients* **2017**, *9*, 306. [CrossRef] [PubMed]

29. Hohmann, C.D.; Cramer, H.; Michalsen, A.; Kessler, C.; Steckhan, N.; Choi, K.; Dobos, G. Effects of high phenolic olive oil on cardiovascular risk factors: A systematic review and meta-analysis. *Phytomedicine* **2015**, *22*, 631–640. [CrossRef] [PubMed]

30. Rondanelli, M.; Giacosa, A.; Morazzoni, P.; Guido, D.; Grassi, M.; Morandi, G.; Bologna, C.; Riva, A.; Allegrini, P.; Perna, S. MediterrAsian Diet Products that Could Raise HDL-Cholesterol: A Systematic Review. *BioMed. Res. Int.* **2016**, *2016*, 1–15. [CrossRef] [PubMed]

31. Farràs, M.; Castañer, O.; Martín-Peláez, S.; Hernáez, Á.; Schröder, H.; Subirana, I.; Muñoz-Aguayo, D.; Gaixas, S.; de la Torre, R.; Farré, M.; et al. Complementary phenol-enriched olive oil improves HDL characteristics in hypercholesterolemic subjects. A randomized, double-blind, crossover, controlled trial. The VOHF study. *Mol. Nutr. Food Res.* **2015**, *59*, 1758–1770. [CrossRef] [PubMed]

32. Hernaez, A.; Fernandez-Castillejo, S.; Farras, M.; Catalan, U.; Subirana, I.; Montes, R.; Sola, R.; Munoz-Aguayo, D.; Gelabert-Gorgues, A.; Diaz-Gil, O.; et al. Olive Oil Polyphenols Enhance High-Density Lipoprotein Function in Humans: A Randomized Controlled Trial. *Arterioscler. Thromb. Vasc. Biol.* **2014**, *34*, 2115–2119. [CrossRef] [PubMed]

33. Fernández-Castillejo, S.; Valls, R.-M.; Castañer, O.; Rubió, L.; Catalán, Ú.; Pedret, A.; Macià, A.; Sampson, M.L.; Covas, M.-I.; Fitó, M.; et al. Polyphenol rich olive oils improve lipoprotein particle atherogenic ratios and subclasses profile: A randomized, crossover, controlled trial. *Mol. Nutr. Food Res.* **2016**, *60*, 1544–1554. [CrossRef] [PubMed]

34. Hernáez, Á.; Castañer, O.; Goday, A.; Ros, E.; Pintó, X.; Estruch, R.; Salas-Salvadó, J.; Corella, D.; Arós, F.; Serra-Majem, L.; et al. The Mediterranean Diet decreases LDL atherogenicity in high cardiovascular risk individuals: A randomized controlled trial. *Mol. Nutr. Food Res.* **2017**, *61*, 1601015. [CrossRef] [PubMed]

35. Nordestgaard, B.G.; Langsted, A.; Mora, S.; Kolovou, G.; Baum, H.; Bruckert, E.; Watts, G.F.; Sypniewska, G.; Wiklund, O.; Borén, J.; et al. Fasting is not routinely required for determination of a lipid profile: Clinical and laboratory implications including flagging at desirable concentration cut-points—A joint consensus statement from the European Atherosclerosis Society and European Federation of Clinical Chemistry and Laboratory Medicine. *Eur. Heart J.* **2016**, *37*, 1944–1958. [PubMed]

36. Saibandith, B.; Spencer, J.; Rowland, I.; Commane, D. Olive Polyphenols and the Metabolic Syndrome. *Molecules* **2017**, *22*, 1082. [CrossRef] [PubMed]

37. Luo, H.; Liu, J.; Ouyang, Q.; Xuan, C.; Wang, L.; Li, T.; Liu, J. The effects of oleanolic acid on atherosclerosis in different animal models. *Acta Biochim. Biophys. Sin.* **2017**, *49*, 349–354. [CrossRef] [PubMed]

38. Ross, R. The pathogenesis of atherosclerosis: A perspective for the 1990s. *Nature* **1993**, *362*, 801–809. [CrossRef] [PubMed]

39. Gkaliagkousi, E.; Gavriilaki, E.; Triantafyllou, A.; Douma, S. Clinical Significance of Endothelial Dysfunction in Essential Hypertension. *Curr. Hypertens. Rep.* **2015**, *17*, 85. [CrossRef] [PubMed]

40. Cambiaggi, C.; Mencarelli, M.; Muscettola, M.; Grasso, G. Gene expression of endothelin-1 (ET-1) and release of mature peptide by activated human neutrophils. *Cytokine* **2001**, *14*, 230–233. [CrossRef] [PubMed]

41. Shinagawa, S.; Okazaki, T.; Ikeda, M.; Yudoh, K.; Kisanuki, Y.Y.; Yanagisawa, M.; Kawahata, K.; Ozaki, S. T cells upon activation promote endothelin 1 production in monocytes via IFN-γ and TNF-α. *Sci. Rep.* **2017**, *7*, 14500. [CrossRef] [PubMed]

42. Massai, L.; Carbotti, P.; Cambiaggi, C.; Mencarelli, M.; Migliaccio, P.; Muscettola, M.; Grasso, G. Prepro-endothelin-1 mRNA and its mature peptide in human appendix. *Gastrointest. Liver Physiol.* **2003**, *284*, G340–G348. [CrossRef] [PubMed]

43. Mencarelli, M.; Pecorelli, A.; Carbotti, P.; Valacchi, G.; Grasso, G.; Muscettola, M. Endothelin receptor A expression in human inflammatory cells. *Regul. Pept.* **2009**, *158*, 1–5. [CrossRef] [PubMed]

44. Achmad, T.H.; Rao, G.S. Chemotaxis of human boold monocytes toward endothelin-1 and the influence of calcium channel blockers. *Biochem. Biophys. Res. Commun.* **1992**, *189*, 994–1000. [CrossRef]

45. Ruetten, H.; Thiemermann, C. Endothelin-1 stimulates the biosynthesis of tumour necrosis factor in macrophages: ET-receptors, signal transduction and inhibitionby dexamethasone. *J. Physiol. Pharmacol.* **1997**, *48*, 675–688. [PubMed]

46. Zouki, C.; Baron, C.; Fournie, A.; Filep, J.G. Endothelin-1 enhances neutrophil adhesion to human coronary artery endothelial cells: Role of ETA receptors and platelet activating factor. *Br. J. Pharmacol.* **1999**, *127*, 969–979. [CrossRef] [PubMed]

47. Zern, T.L.; Fernandez, M.L. Cardioprotective effects of dietary polyphenols. *J. Nutr.* **2005**, *135*, 2291–2294. [CrossRef] [PubMed]

48. Musini, V.M.; Wright, J.M. Factors affecting blood pressure variability: Lessons learned from two systematic reviews of randomized controlled trials. *PLoS ONE* **2009**, *4*, e5673. [CrossRef] [PubMed]

49. Handler, J. The Importance of Accurate Blood Pressure Measurement. *Perm. J.* **2009**, *13*, 51–54. [CrossRef] [PubMed]

50. Rodriguez-Rodriguez, R.; Herrera, M.D.; de Sotomayor, M.A.; Ruiz-Gutierrez, V. Pomace Olive Oil Improves Endothelial Function in Spontaneously Hypertensive Rats by Increasing Endothelial Nitric Oxide Synthase Expression. *Am. J. Hypertens.* **2007**, *20*, 728–734. [CrossRef] [PubMed]

51. Valero-Muñoz, M.; Martín-Fernández, B.; Ballesteros, S.; de la Fuente, E.; Quintela, J.C.; Lahera, V.; de las Heras, N. Protective effect of a pomace olive oil concentrated in triterpenic acids in alterations related to hypertension in rats: Mechanisms involved. *Mol. Nutr. Food Res.* **2014**, *58*, 376–383. [CrossRef] [PubMed]

52. Dell'Agli, M.; Fagnani, R.; Mitro, N.; Scurati, S.; Masciadri, M.; Mussoni, L.; Galli, G.V.; Bosisio, E.; Crestani, M.; De Fabiani, E.; et al. Minor Components of Olive Oil Modulate Proatherogenic Adhesion Molecules Involved in Endothelial Activation. *J. Agric. Food Chem.* **2006**, *54*, 3259–3264. [CrossRef] [PubMed]

53. Fitó, M.; Cladellas, M.; de la Torre, R.; Martí, J.; Muñoz, D.; Schröder, H.; Alcántara, M.; Pujadas-Bastardes, M.; Marrugat, J.; López-Sabater, M.C.; et al. Anti-inflammatory effect of virgin olive oil in stable coronary disease patients: A randomized, crossover, controlled trial. *Eur. J. Clin. Nutr.* **2007**, *62*, 570–574. [CrossRef] [PubMed]

54. Papageorgiou, N.; Tousoulis, D.; Psaltopoulou, T.; Giolis, A.; Antoniades, C.; Tsiamis, E.; Miliou, A.; Toutouzas, K.; Siasos, G.; Stefanadis, C. Divergent anti-inflammatory effects of different oil acute consumption on healthy individuals. *Eur. J. Clin. Nutr.* **2011**, *65*, 514–519. [CrossRef] [PubMed]

55. Martín-Peláez, S.; Castañer, O.; Konstantinidou, V.; Subirana, I.; Muñoz-Aguayo, D.; Blanchart, G.; Gaixas, S.; de la Torre, R.; Farré, M.; Sáez, G.T.; et al. Effect of olive oil phenolic compounds on the expression of blood pressure-related genes in healthy individuals. *Eur. J. Nutr.* **2017**, *56*, 663–670. [CrossRef] [PubMed]

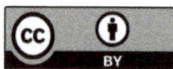

nutrients

MDPI

Article

The Effect of Low-Carbohydrate Diet on Glycemic Control in Patients with Type 2 Diabetes Mellitus

Li-Li Wang [1], Qi Wang [1], Yong Hong [1], Omorogieva Ojo [2], Qing Jiang [1], Yun-Ying Hou [1], Yu-Hua Huang [3] and Xiao-Hua Wang [1,*]

[1] School of Nursing, Medical College, Soochow University, Suzhou 215006, China; wanglili83476@suda.edu.cn (L.-L.W.); xuweipan@whu.edu.cn (Q.W.); 20175231003@stu.suda.edu.cn (Y.H.); jiangqing2015@suda.edu.cn (Q.J.); houyunying@suda.edu.cn (Y.-Y.H.)
[2] Department of Adult Nursing and Paramedic Science, University of Greenwich, London SE9 2UG, UK; o.ojo@greenwich.ac.uk
[3] Medical College, Soochow University, Suzhou 215006, China; Huangyuhua@suda.edu.cn
* Correspondence: wangxiaohua@suda.edu.cn; Tel.: +86-138-1488-0208

Received: 8 April 2018; Accepted: 17 May 2018; Published: 23 May 2018

Abstract: Objective: In China, a low-fat diet (LFD) is mainly recommended to help improve blood glucose levels in patients with type 2 diabetes mellitus (T2DM). However, a low-carbohydrate diet (LCD) has been shown to be effective in improving blood glucose levels in America and England. A few studies, primarily randomized controlled trials, have been reported in China as well. Method: Firstly, we designed two 'six-point formula' methods, which met the requirements of LCD and LFD, respectively. Fifty-six T2DM patients were recruited and randomly allocated to the LCD group ($n = 28$) and the LFD group ($n = 28$). The LCD group received education about LCD's six-point formula, while the LFD group received education about LFD's six-point formula. The follow-up time was three months. The indicators for glycemic control and other metabolic parameters were collected and compared between the two groups. Results: Forty-nine patients completed the study. The proportions of calories from three macronutrients the patients consumed met the requirements of LCD and LFD. Compared to the LFD group, there was a greater decrease in HbA1c level in the LCD group (-0.63% vs. -0.31%, $p < 0.05$). The dosages of insulin and fasting blood glucoses (FBG) in the third month were lower than those at baseline in both groups. Compared with baseline values, body mass index (BMI) and total cholesterol (TC) in the LCD group were significantly reduced in the third month ($p < 0.05$); however, there were no statistically significant differences in the LFD group. Conclusions: LCD can improve blood glucose more than LFD in Chinese patients with T2DM. It can also regulate blood lipid, reduce BMI, and decrease insulin dose in patients with T2DM. In addition, the six-point formula is feasible, easily operable, and a practical educational diet for Chinese patients with T2DM.

Keywords: diabetes mellitus; diet; carbohydrate; blood glucose; HbA1c; fasting blood glucose; postprandial blood glucose

1. Introduction

Dietary intervention is a strategy to manage diabetes mellitus (DM) [1], as it can reduce the burden on islet cells and thus improve blood glucose levels, lipid profiles, and cognitive status [2–4]. However, good adherence to diabetic diets is the premise of diet therapy. In China, a low-fat diet (LFD) is mainly recommended to help improve blood glucose levels in patients with type 2 diabetes mellitus (T2DM) [5]. Studies have shown that LFD could reduce glycated hemoglobin (HbA1c) by as much as 0.8–2.8% [6–8].

On the other hand, a low-carbohydrate diet (LCD) is a dietary strategy that refers to carbohydrate intake of between 30–200 g/day or calories from carbohydrates/total calories of <45%, supplementing instead with fat or protein [9]. This has been found to be effective in the treatment of obesity, and apart from significantly reducing weight, it can also effectively improve blood lipid and insulin resistance [10]. In recent years, the American Diabetes Association and Diabetes UK have both confirmed the effectiveness of LCD in reducing weight, improving blood glucose, and regulating blood lipid in patients with DM [11,12]. In Japan, Yamada [13] reported that HbA1c and triglyceride (TG) levels in patients with T2DM decreased significantly in the LCD group without calorie-restriction, compared to the LFD group with calorie-restriction. This indicates that LCD made patients with DM have less desire to eat due to a feeling of satiety. However, only limited studies relating to the use of LCD in patients with DM, especially randomized controlled trials, have been reported in China.

Based on research evidence, only 29.8% of Chinese patients with T2DM comply with a diabetic diet advised by their doctors and dietitians [14]. In addition, we found that certain types of foods were strictly limited and patients with DM were finding it hard to understand the caloric values of foods consumed, thus making it difficult to adhere to the diet. Thus, it is necessary to develop an easy and more effective method to support these patients. Firstly, we designed the 'six-point formula' to help patients master LCD and LFD. We then let them record details of their diets and hand over to us the task of calculating the caloric values of foods. Based on this, we explored the effect of two DM diets (LCD and LFD) on hyperglycemia.

2. Materials and Methods

2.1. Subjects

Participants with T2DM were recruited from the community and the First Affiliated Hospital of Soochow University. The inclusion criteria were the following: Patients older than 18 years, had been diagnosed with T2DM, had no change in oral antidiabetic drugs or insulin in half a month before the intervention, were able to communicate, had volunteered to participate in this study, and are able to provide informed consent. Those excluded were patients who ate nuts regularly ($\geq$4 day/week) [15]; were allergic to food, especially nuts; had difficulty in chewing nuts (such as those with few teeth); received other dietary interventions or had severe conditions including indigestion, heart failure, renal failure, malignant tumours, severe cerebrovascular disease, ketosis, digestive dysfunction, liver dysfunction or severe gallbladder and pancreatic diseases; and those whose fasting blood glucose (FBG) were more than 16.7 mmol/L [16] during the interventions.

2.2. Study Design

This study is a prospective, single-blind randomized controlled trial (RCT) performed between December 2015 to December 2016. The recruited patients were randomly allocated to receive either LCD or LFD using a table of random numbers. Before the intervention, all subjects underwent a one-week [17] washout period to diminish the effect of background diets on the study. The patients were blinded when assigned to groups. This study followed the Declaration of Helsinki and the Guidelines for Good Clinical Practice and was approved by the ethics committee of the First Affiliated Hospital of Soochow University (No. 2015106). All enrolled patients signed a consent form.

2.3. Sample Size Calculation

Evidence from the literature showed that changes in the HbA1c level for six months were 0.6 ± 0.5% in the LCD group and 0.2 ± 0.5% in the calorie-restricted group [13]. Therefore, we calculated 25 patients for each group, with α = 0.05 and power = 0.80. In view of the sample loss of 10%, the number for each group was 28. Finally, we recruited 28 patients for each group in the study.

2.4. Biochemical Parameters and Analyses

Glycated hemoglobin provides an estimate of glycemic control for the past three months and is predictive of clinical outcomes [18]. HbA1c was measured at baseline and at the end of the third month. Blood samples were obtained to measure HbA1c at the nursing School of Soochow University and measured by high-performance liquid chromatography using Afinion AS100 Analyzer (Alere, Inc., Shanghai, China) in the molecular laboratory of the nursing school of Soochow University. Fasting blood glucose (FBG) and postprandial 2-h blood glucose levels were measured by collecting the peripheral blood from fingers using rapid glycaemic apparatus by patients once a week at home.

Fasting blood samples were also collected for various biochemical assays, including total cholesterol (TC), performed as per the experimental protocol in hospitals.

Hypoglycemic episodes in this study were determined by the self-reported hypoglycemic symptoms of patients with or without a measured plasma glucose concentration <70 mg/dL (3.9 mmol/L) or only a measured plasma glucose concentration <70 mg/dL (3.9 mmol/L). Therefore, all episodes of abnormal low plasma glucose concentration that exposed the individual to potential harm and other clinical incidents, including severe hypoglycemia, documented symptomatic hypoglycemia, asymptomatic hypoglycemia, probable symptomatic hypoglycemia and relative hypoglycemia referred to the self-reported hypoglycemic symptoms of patients without a measured plasma glucose concentration <70 mg/dL (3.9 mmol/L), were considered [19]. In this study, the modification of hypoglycemic agents referred to change in the quantities of insulin dosages the participants used at baseline and in the third month. Researchers collected data of modification of hypoglycemic agents at every follow up.

2.5. Anthropometric Measurements

Body mass index (BMI) was calculated as weight (in kilograms) divided by height (in meters squared). At baseline and in the third month, the weight and height of patients were measured by a unified measuring device at the nursing school of Soochow University.

2.6. Diet Record

Patients maintained a diet record, including a detailed diet of any day over the weekend and two working days. The composition of the diets was calculated using the Chinese CDC nutrition calculator V2.63 software (Development team of Fei Hua nutrition software, Beijing, China) and the quantities and distributions of energy from three macronutrients intake was determined. This also enabled an understanding of the patients' dietary adherence.

2.7. Intervention

Firstly, our team developed a preliminary dietary education handbook for patients with T2DM based on evidence from literature and guidelines regarding T2DM dietary management [5,20]. Secondly, two endocrinologists, four diabetic nurse specialists, and one dietician reviewed and modified the handbook. Finally, five T2DM inpatients of different ages and educational levels reviewed the handbook to ensure that patients with T2DM understood it and that it could help improve their dietary adherence. The major content of the handbook was a concise formula that included six points. Detailed contents of the six-point formula are shown in Figure 1. Other educational contents about foods included how to distinguish vegetables and staple food (such as potato and broad bean); ways to cook food; and symptoms, prevention and treatment of hypoglycemia.

In the one-on-one education session, the researcher and the patients reviewed the handbook. Using the LCD handbook, the researcher focused on instructing patients to restrict intake of staple food/meal (1 Liang) per day in the LCD group. The reduced staple food/meal was replaced by consuming 60 g/day nuts for males and 50 g/day for females, respectively. Nuts were uniformly purchased, weighed, vacuum-packed, and distributed every two weeks.

For patients in the LFD group, we provided participants with a handbook about LFD, and instructed them on a pithy formula of six points.

Follow up was conducted once a week in the first month of the intervention and once every two weeks in the second and third months. The duration of follow up was about 10 min. The main focus of the follow-up was to review the patients' compliance to the diet program and to support them to adhere to it (in patients with poor compliance). It also involved collecting data of the modification of hypoglycemic agents and the occurrence of hypoglycemia. If a patient's diet did not meet the requirements of the dietary program in the intervention period, they were excluded from the study.

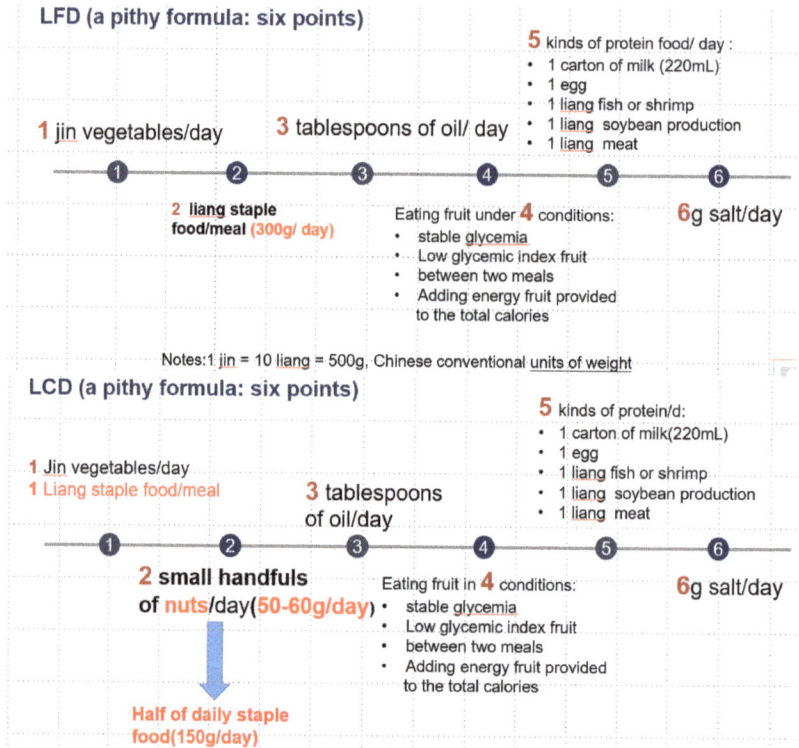

Figure 1. The detailed contents of the six-point formula of two groups. Notes: 1 jin = 10 liang = 500 g, Chinese conventional units of weight. Staple food/meal refers to foods rich in carbohydrates, mainly three kinds of steamed bread, noodles and rice in China. LFD: Low-fat diet; LCD: Low-carbohydrate diet.

2.8. Statistical Analysis

Statistical analyses were performed using SPSS 18.0 software (SPSS, Inc., Chicago, IL, USA). For continuous variables, the results were described as the mean ± standard deviation (SD) and comparisons were performed using Independent Samples *t*-test, paired samples *t*-test or the Wilcoxon rank-sum test. For categorical variables, the results were presented as frequency (percentages); comparisons between groups were made using the Chi-squared test or Fisher's exact test. The trends in the FBG and postprandial 2 h blood glucose in two groups during the intervention were described by the fold line diagram. Intention-To-Treat (ITT) of HbA1c was performed to ensure the reliability of research results. A *p* value of < 0.05 was considered statistically significant.

3. Results

3.1. Study Participants

On the basis of inclusion and exclusion criteria, 56 T2DM participants were recruited and randomly allocated to the LCD group (n = 28) and the LFD group (n = 28). Four participants in the LCD group and three participants in the LFD group withdrew from the study. In the LCD group, two participants didn't like nuts, one showed poor adherence (<4 day/week, and one was lost during follow-up. In the LFD group, two showed poor adherence to the diet program (<4 day/week) and one was lost during follow-up. Finally, the data of 24 in the LCD group and 25 in the LFD group were analyzed (Figure 2). The mean age of patients were (63.94 ± 10.79) years and 26 (53.1%) were men. The general characteristics of the enrolled participants in each group are shown in Table 1 There were no statistically significant differences in any of the parameters between the two groups (p > 0.05).

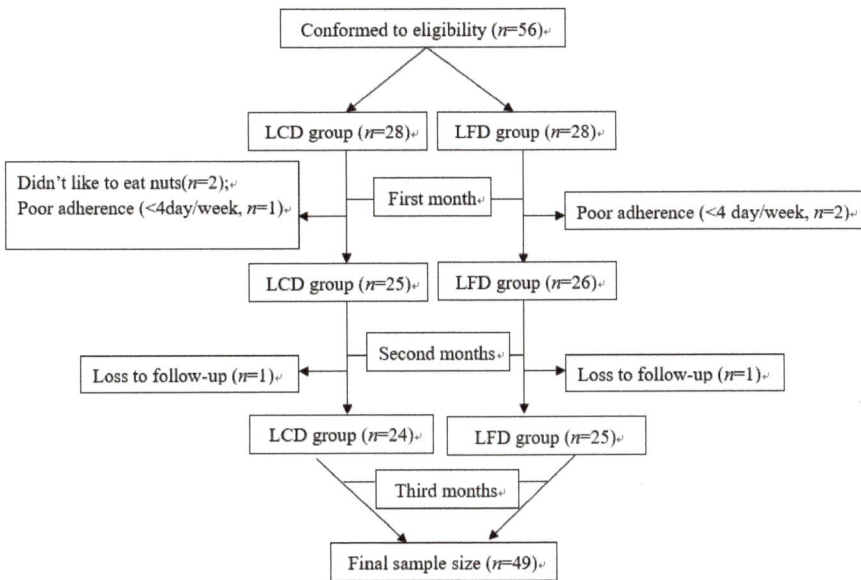

Figure 2. Flow diagram of the patients.

Table 1. Baseline characteristics.

Variables		LCD (n = 24) $\bar{x} \pm$ SD/n (%)	LFD (n = 25) $\bar{x} \pm$ SD/n (%)	t/χ^2	p
Demographic data					
Age, years		66.79 ± 9.12	61.20 ± 11.71	1.860 [a]	NS
Gender, Male		13 (54.2)	13 (52.0)	0.023 [b]	NS
Marital Status	Married	23 (95.8)	22 (88)		
	Unmarried	0 (0)	1 (4.0)	1.728 [c]	NS
	Widowhood	1 (4.2)	2 (8.0)		
Education level, years		9.63 ± 4.10	8.36 ± 3.12	1.219 [a]	NS

Table 1. *Cont.*

Variables		LCD (*n* = 24)	LFD (*n* = 25)	*t*/χ^2	*p*
		$\bar{x} \pm$ SD/*n* (%)	$\bar{x} \pm$ SD/*n* (%)		
Occupation status	On the job	4 (16.7)	10 (40.0)	3.267 [b]	NS
	Retirement	20 (83.3)	15 (60.0)		
Residential status	Living by oneself	1 (4.2)	4 (16.0)	3.733 [c]	NS
	Living with spouse	21 (87.4)	19 (76.0)		
	Living with children	1 (4.2)	2 (8.0)		
	Living with mother	1 (4.2)	0 (0)		
Medical insurance, No		1 (4.2)	1 (4.0)	0.001 [b]	NS
Family Support	Value	19 (79.2)	14 (56.0)	2.988 [b]	NS
	Ordinary	5 (20.8)	11 (44.0)		
Exercise	Never exercise	1 (4.2)	2 (8.0)	0.400 [c]	NS
	Never regular exercise	11 (45.8)	12 (48.0)		
	Regular exercise	12 (50.0)	11 (44.0)		
Clinical data					
Smoking, yes		2 (8.3)	5 (20.0)	1.361 [d]	NS
SBP, mmHg		131.42 $\pm$ 10.89	130.84 $\pm$ 14.83	0.155 [a]	NS
DBP, mmHg		77.54 $\pm$ 10.48	76.40 $\pm$ 10.43	0.382 [a]	NS
Family history of diabetes, yes		12 (50.0)	9 (36.0)	0.980 [b]	NS
Diabetes duration, years		12.79 $\pm$ 6.49	9.10 $\pm$ 6.52	1.985 [a]	NS
Oral antilipemic agents, yes		8 (33.3)	11 (44.0)	0.587 [a]	NS
Oral antidiabetic drugs or/and insulin		22 (91.7)	22 (88.0)	- [d]	NS
Complications, yes		9 (37.5)	5 (20.0)	1.838 [b]	NS
Accompanying diseases, yes		17 (70.8)	19 (76.0)	0.168 [b]	NS

p value for comparison between treatments diets by Independent Samples *t*-test or Chi-square test. [a] *t*-test; [b] Chi-square test; [c] Likelihood Ratio; [d] Fisher's Exact Test. NS: Differences are not significant; SBP: Systolic blood pressure; DBP: Diastolic blood pressure.

3.2. Dietary Adherence

3.2.1. Comparison of Dietary Adherence

Dietary adherence was assessed mainly from two aspects: the days of adherence to the dietary program per week and macro-nutrient allocation and their quantities. The Wilcoxon rank-sum test was performed to compare dietary compliance in the two groups (LCD versus LFD). The result showed that there was no difference in self-reported dietary compliance per week (*p* > 0.05, Table 2).

Table 2. Comparison of dietary adherence between the two groups.

	LCD (*n* = 24)	LFD (*n* = 25)	Z	*p*
4 d/W	3 (12.5)	7 (28.0)	4.449	NS
5~6 d/W	7 (29.2)	10 (40.0)		
7 d/W	14 (58.3)	8 (32.0)		

p value for comparison by Wilcoxon rank-sum test. Z: Wilcoxon rank-sum test; NS: Differences are not significant.

3.2.2. Proportions of Calories from Three Macronutrients the Patients Consumed

Prior to the intervention, the total energy and the proportions of calories from the three major nutrients were not significantly different between the two groups (LCD versus LFD). After the intervention, compared to the LFD group, the calories from carbohydrates decreased, while those from fat significantly increased in the LCD group (*p* < 0.05). In addition, the percentage of calories from carbohydrates (39%) met the standard of LCD (<45%). The 26% of calories from fat met the standard of LFD, while the calories from protein were almost similar in the two groups (*p* > 0.05, Table 3) (Figure 3).

Table 3. Comparison of the calories from three macronutrients consumed by the patients.

	Variables	LCD (*n* = 24)	LFD (*n* = 25)	*T*	*p*
Baseline	Total calorie intake/day	1796.0 ± 186.6	1768.8 ± 138.7	0.421	NS
	Carbohydrate-calorie (Kcal)	948.8 ± 130.9	922.5 ± 145.1	0.485	NS
	Fat-calorie (Kcal)	538.9 ± 92.4	542.0 ± 94.8	−0.084	NS
	Protein-calorie (Kcal)	306.6 ± 56.7	303.3 ± 41.8	0.166	NS
3rd month	Total calorie intake/day	1808.0 ± 190.7	1731.5 ± 109.6	1.257	NS
	Carbohydrate-calorie (Kcal)	695.2 ± 106.6	970.2 ± 101.1	−6.747	<0.001 **
	Fat-calorie (Kcal)	763.1 ± 99.1	442.8 ± 52.0	10.320	<0.001 **
	Protein-calorie (Kcal)	350.3 ± 64.4	317.4 ± 52.0	1.433	NS

p value for comparison by Independent Samples *t*-test. ** *p* < 0.01 NS: Differences are not significant.

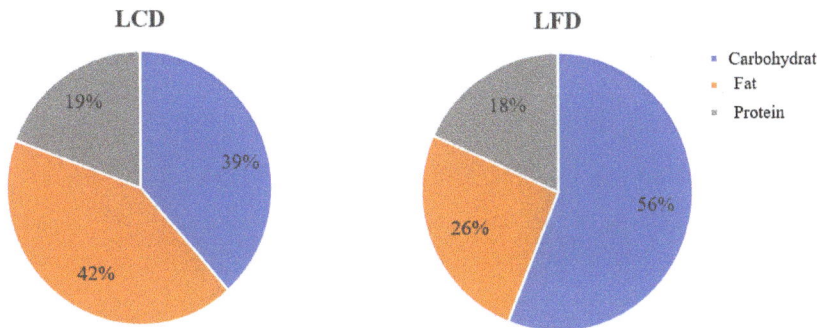

Figure 3. The percentage of the calories from carbohydrates (39%) met the standard of LCD (<45%) in the LCD group, while the 26% calories from fat met the standard of LFD. LCD: Low-carbohydrate diet; LFD: Low-fat diet

3.3. Effect of LCD on Glycemic Control

Glycated Hemoglobin

Compared to the baseline, HbA1c levels in both the LCD group and LFD group decreased significantly (0.63 ± 1.18% and 0.31 ± 0.70%), respectively. At the baseline, HbA1c levels were not significantly different between the two groups. However, after the intervention, HbA1c levels in the LCD group decreased significantly (*p* < 0.05, Table 4), when compared to the LFD group. The Intention-To-Treat (ITT) in relation to HbA1c levels was performed to ensure the stability of the above results. The ITT results were found to be in agreement with the earlier findings (Table 5).

Table 4. Comparison of glycated hemoglobin (%) between the two groups.

Study Period	LCD (*n* = 24)	LFD (*n* = 25)	*t*	*p*
Baseline	7.43 ± 1.39	7.79 ± 1.20	−0.971	NS
3rd month	6.80 ± 0.83	7.48 ± 1.15	−2.350	0.023 *
MD	0.63 ± 1.18	0.31 ± 0.70	-	-
t	2.601	2.213	-	-
p	0.016 *	0.037 *	-	-

p value for comparison by Independent Samples *t*-test or paired samples *t*-test. * *p* < 0.05. NS: Differences are not significant.

Table 5. Comparison of glycated hemoglobin (%) between the two groups in ITT.

Study Period	LCD (*n* = 28)	LFD (*n* = 28)	*T*	*p*
Baseline	7.39 ± 1.29	8.16 ± 1.59	−1.994	NS
3rd month	6.85 ± 0.79	7.89 ± 1.63	−3.017	0.004 **
MD	0.54 ± 1.12	0.28 ± 0.67	-	-
t	2.556	2.194	-	-
p	0.017 *	0.037 *	-	-

p value for comparison by Independent Samples *t*-test or paired samples *t*-test. * $p < 0.05$; ** $p < 0.01$; ITT: Intention-To-Treat; NS: Differences are not significant.

3.4. Fasting Blood Glucose

3.4.1. Changing Trends of Fasting Blood Glucose

The changing trends of the FBG in the two groups during the intervention are described by the fold line diagram (Figure 4). The results showed that the change of FBG in the LCD group decreased significantly for the first four weeks and then decreased steadily after the fourth week. In contrast, the FBG in the LFD group demonstrated dynamic fluctuation, although it was lower than the baseline value.

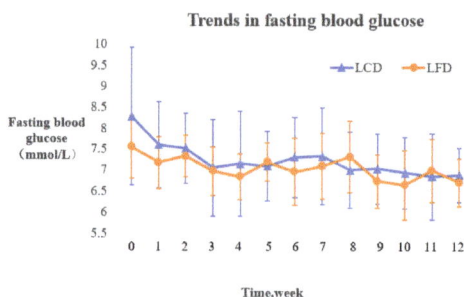

Figure 4. The changing trends of the FBG in the LCD and LFD Groups. FBG: fasting blood glucoses

3.4.2. Comparison of Fasting Blood Glucose levels

Compared to the baseline, FBG levels of the two groups significantly improved ($p < 0.01$). But the differences between the two groups with respect to FBG was not statistically significant ($p > 0.05$) (Table 6).

Table 6. Comparison of fasting blood glucose (mmol/L) between the two groups.

Study Period	LCD (*n* = 24)	LFD (*n* = 25)	*t*	*p*
Baseline	8.28 ± 1.64	7.55 ± 0.75	1.469	NS
3rd month	6.87 ± 0.65	6.70 ± 0.57	0.793	NS
t	4.873	3.889	-	-
p	<0.001 **	0.003 **	-	-

p value for comparison by Independent Samples *t*-test or paired samples *t*-test. ** $p < 0.01$. NS: Differences are not significant.

3.5. Postprandial Two-Hour Blood Glucose

3.5.1. Trends in Postprandial Two-Hour Blood Glucose

The changing trends of the postprandial 2-h blood glucose of the two groups during the intervention are described by the fold line diagram (Figure 5.). Both groups showed fluctuation in this indicator.

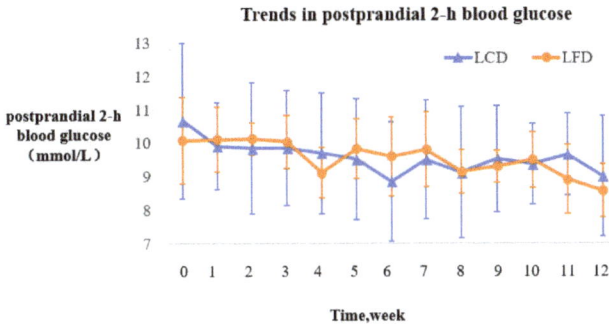

Figure 5. The changing trends of the postprandial 2-h blood glucose in the LCD and LFD Groups.

3.5.2. Comparison of Postprandial Two-Hour Blood Glucose

Compared to the baseline, the postprandial 2-h blood glucose in the two groups improved significantly ($p < 0.01$). However, there was no significant difference between the two groups ($p > 0.05$) (Table 7).

Table 7. Comparison of postprandial 2-h blood glucose (mmol/L) in the groups.

Study Period	LCD (*n* = 24)	LFD (*n* = 25)	*t*	*p*
Baseline	10.67 ± 2.33	10.08 ± 1.29	0.818	NS
3rd month	9.00 ± 1.80	8.58 ± 0.80	0.761	NS
t	4.690	3.786	-	-
p	<0.001 **	0.003 **	-	

p value for comparison between treatments diets by Independent Samples *t*-test or paired samples *t*-test. ** $p < 0.01$. NS: Differences are not significant.

3.6. Effect of LCD on Other Metabolic and Anthropometric Indicators

Compared to the baseline, body mass index (BMI) and total cholesterol (TC) in the LCD group improved significantly in the third month ($p < 0.05$). However, there were no similar results in the LFD group. After the intervention, the metabolic indicators were not significantly different between the two groups (Table 8).

Table 8. Comparison of other metabolic indicators between the two groups.

Variables	Study Period	LCD (*n* = 24)	LFD (*n* = 25)	*t*	*p*
BMI (Kg/m^2)	Baseline	24.29 ± 3.36	24.62 ± 5.17	−0.261	NS
	3rd month	23.52 ± 2.70	23.47 ± 3.11	0.060	NS
	t	2.756	1.235	-	-
	p	0.011 *	NS	-	-
TC (mmol/L)	Baseline	4.85 ± 0.87	4.55 ± 1.04	1.101	NS
	3rd month	4.49 ± 0.86	4.63 ± 0.99	−0.521	NS
	t	2.540	−0.363	-	-
	p	0.018 *	NS	-	-

p value for comparison by Independent Samples *t*-test or paired samples *t*-test. * $p < 0.05$; BMI: Body mass index; TC: total cholesterol. NS: Differences are not significant.

3.7. Hypoglycemia and Medication Changes

3.7.1. Frequency of Hypoglycemia

The frequencies of hypoglycemia during the three-month period in the two groups showed no significant differences ($p > 0.05$), before and after the intervention. In addition, there were no significant differences ($p > 0.05$) between the two groups before and after the interventions (Table 9)

Table 9. Comparison of the frequencies of hypoglycemia between the two groups.

Time	LCD (*n* = 24)	LFD (*n* = 25)	*t*	*P*
Baseline	0.21 ± 0.59	0.52 ± 0.77	−1.596	NS
3rd month	0.04 ± 0.20	0.36 ± 0.86	−1.798	NS
t	1.282	0.778	-	-
p	NS	NS	-	-

p value for comparison by Independent Samples *t*-test or paired samples *t*-test. NS: Differences are not significant.

3.7.2. The Dosages of Insulin Used

When compared to the baseline, the dosage of insulin used in the two groups decreased significantly after the intervention ($p < 0.05$, Table 10), although there was no significant difference between the two groups ($p > 0.05$).

Table 10. Comparison of insulin dose (insulin unit, IU) between the two groups.

Times	LCD (*n* = 7)	LFD (*n* = 13)	*t*	*P*
Baseline	31.14 ± 16.38	29.00 ± 12.27	0.332	NS
3rd month	28.29 ± 13.74	26.62 ± 11.20	0.294	NS
t	2.765	3.023	-	-
p	0.033 *	0.011 *	-	-

p value for comparison by paired samples *t*-test. * $p < 0.05$. NS: Differences are not significant.

3.7.3. The Changes of Other Antidiabetic Drugs

There was no significant difference between the two groups in the third month ($p > 0.05$, Table 11).

Table 11. Comparison of other antidiabetic drugs between the two groups.

	LCD (*n* = 23)	LFD (*n* = 11)	χ^2	*p*
No change	20 (87.0%)	11 (100%)		
Reduction	2 (8.7%)	0 (0)	2.482	NS
Addition	1 (4.3%)	0 (0)		

p value for comparison between treatments diets by Chi-square test. NS: Differences are not significant.

4. Discussion

The use of LCD in human nutrition and health is a dietary strategy that ensures that carbohydrate intake is restricted. However, in a Chinese dietary plan, most staple foods have high glycemic index [20,21]. Therefore, it would seem that LCD may not be accepted easily among Chinese patients with diabetes mellitus (DM). In consideration, we initially designed the 'six-point formula' to help patients improve dietary adherence. We found that the participants showed good adherence to the intervention, and no significant difference with respect to dietary adherence between two groups (LCD versus LFD) was observed. The proportions of energy provided by the three macronutrients met the requirements of LCD and LFD. It was indicated that the 'six-point formula' of the DM diet was feasible for Chinese T2DM patients.

4.1. Effect of LCD on Glycemic Control

High levels of HbA1c, FBG, and postprandial 2h blood glucose levels are some of the most difficult challenges faced by patients with T2DM and these parameters could be used as the main indicators to establish glycemic control [5].

HbA1c levels can reflect blood glucose levels in 2~3 months before blood extraction and long-term glycemic control of patients [5]. The result of this study showed that HbA1c levels in LCD (8.5%) decreased significantly ($p < 0.05$) compared to that in LFD (4%). The reason might be due to the decreased level of high glycemic index foods, the total amount of foods rich in carbohydrates, and the increased intake of nuts, which could help improve hyperglycemia and insulin sensitivity [22–24]. Yamada et al. [13] showed that HbA1c levels were significantly decreased by as much as 7.9% in the LCD group and by only 2.6% in the calorie-restricted group. Mayer et al. [25] also found LCD led to a relative improvement in HbA1c than LFD. However, some studies have shown that LFD could decrease HbA1c by 0.8–2.08% [7,8]. These values were less than the result of our study, which might be due to the effect of the 'six-point formula' that was simple and easy to remember, helped patients master the methods of the DM diet better, and improved dietary compliance and hyperglycemia.

Fasting blood glucose and postprandial 2-h blood glucose are important indicators for the diagnosis and monitoring of DM [5]. The fold line diagram in this study showed that FBG significantly decreased during the first four weeks in the two groups. While FBG steadily decreased in the LCD group, there was dynamic fluctuation after the initial first month in the LFD group. A reason for the same might be that the patients in the two groups showed keen interest in the 'six-point formula' at the beginning of the intervention, which helped improve their dietary adherence and promote FBG control. In addition, nuts could stabilize blood glucose levels [23,26,27], which may have contributed to the steady decrease of FBG in the LCD group. Postprandial 2h blood glucose obviously decreased in the LCD group, which might have resulted from its relationship to limited carbohydrates [20,22].

4.2. Other Metabolic Indicators

Nuts are high-fat diets with high-energy levels, but they do not increase the weight of patients [27] because they increase a feeling of satiety and lead to a strong dietary compensation effect [28]. In addition, energy absorption efficiency of the nuts is low and the total energy does not increase [28]. This study further confirmed that BMI in the LCD group decreased. The result is in agreement with the results of Li et al. [23] and Barbour et al. [29].

Diabetes is significantly related to dyslipidemia [5]. While we pay attention to blood glucose levels, it is also necessary to regulate blood lipids. Lovejoy et al. [30] found that TC level in diets enriched in almonds was lower by 21%. Our study found that the TC level decreased significant by 7.4% in the LCD group, which might be related to the effect of some ingredients of the nuts consumed [27].

4.3. Hypoglycemia and Medication Changes

We found that the insulin dose used by patients in the LCD group during the intervention period decreased, consistent with a study by Westman et al. [31], which found that patients could reduce or terminate the use of hypoglycemic agents by controlling the intake of carbohydrates. But there were no significant differences between group comparisons.

In this study, hypoglycemia is used as a safety indicator. Although there was no statistical change in the frequency of hypoglycemia in within-group comparison and no difference in between-group comparison, the frequencies of hypoglycemia were reduced in the two groups.

5. Limitation

There are some limitations to the study. Firstly, the method used to evaluate the energy intake of food may not have been robust enough. At the baseline, we obtained data of caloric intake from patients' memories, which meant that it was probably underestimated. Secondly, measurement differences might exist in FBG and postprandial 2-h blood glucose levels, which were measured at home by the patients themselves using different blood glucose meters. Thirdly, the prolonged effect of LCD on the prognosis of DM was not observed due to short follow-up time. Finally, a control group without a treatment was not considered in the study design.

6. Conclusions

LCD can improve blood glucose more than LFD in Chinese patients with T2DM. It can also regulate blood lipids, reduce BMI, and decrease insulin doses in patients with T2DM. In addition, the six-point formula is feasible, easily operable, and is a practical educational diet for Chinese patients with T2DM.

Author Contributions: L.-L.W. and Q.W. collected and analyzed data and wrote the initial draft, which was revised by X.-H.W., Y.-H.H., Y.H., O.O., Q.J., Y.-Y.H. All authors participated in research design and quality control. L.-L.W. and Q.W. contributed equally to this study. X.-H.W. was the corresponding author.

Acknowledgments: We thank the patients with T2DM who participated in the study. Thanks also to Huijuan Zhou, Xiaoyan Zhang and Li Wang, who provided us with study sites to ensure that the study was conducted. This study was supported by Suzhou Science and Technology Project, China (Grant number SYS201513).

Conflicts of Interest: The authors declare no conflict of interest.

References

1. Breen, C.; Ryan, M.; Gibney, M.J.; O'Shea, D. Diabetes-related nutrition knowledge and dietary intake among adults with type 2 diabetes. *Br. J. Nutr.* **2015**, *114*, 439–447. [CrossRef] [PubMed]
2. Ley, S.H.; Hamdy, O.; Mohan, V.; Hu, F.B. Prevention and management of type 2 diabetes: Dietary components and nutritional strategies. *Lancet* **2014**, *383*, 1999–2007. [CrossRef]
3. Seetharaman, S.; Andel, R.; McEvoy, C.; Aslan, A.K.D.; Finkel, D.; Pedersen, N.L. Blood Glucose, Diet-Based Glycemic Load and Cognitive Aging Among Dementia-Free Older Adults. *J. Gerontol. A Biol. Sci. Med. Sci.* **2015**, *70*, 471. [CrossRef] [PubMed]
4. Seetharaman, S. The Influences of Dietary Sugar and Related Metabolic Disorders on Cognitive Aging and Dementia. *Mol. Basis Nutr. Aging* **2016**, 331–344. [CrossRef]
5. Chinese Diabetes Society. Guidelines for the prevention and treatment of type 2 diabetes in China. *Chin. Med. J.* **2017**, *10*, 4–67.
6. Cao, A.H.; Sun, L.Z.; Cui, J.W. Effects of A Low-Carbohydrate Diet and A Low-Fat Diet on Weight and Glycemic Control in Type 2 Diabetics Mellitus. *Chin. Gener. Pract.* **2011**, *14*, 52–56.
7. Cao, A.L.; Xin, B. Effects of low-fat diet on body mass, blood lipids and sugar control in obese patients with type 2 diabetes mellitus. *Clin. Focus* **2012**, *27*, 1025–1031.
8. Wang, Y.L.; Yao, Y.N.; Yang, X.L. Clinical study of the changing of bodyweight (BW) and fasting blood glucose (FBG) in obese patients with type 2 diabetes on a low-carbohydrate diet (LCD). *J. Xinjiang Med. Univ.* **2009**, *32*, 914–916.
9. Hite, A.H.; Berkowitz, V.G.; Berkowitz, K. Low-carbohydrate diet review: Shifting the paradigm. *Nutr. Clin. Pract.* **2011**, *26*, 300. [CrossRef] [PubMed]
10. Forsythe, C.E.; Phinney, S.D.; Fernandez, M.L.; Quann, E.E.; Wood, R.J.; Bibus, D.M.; Kraemer, W.J.; Feinman, R.D.; Volek, J.S. Comparison of Low Fat and Low Carbohydrate Diets on Circulating Fatty Acid Composition and Markers of Inflammation. *Lipids* **2008**, *43*, 65–77. [CrossRef] [PubMed]
11. Dyson, P.A.; Kelly, T.; Deakin, T.; Duncan, A.; Frost, G.; Harrison, Z.; Khatri, D.; Kunka, D.; McArdle, P.; Mellor, D. Diabetes UK evidence-based nutrition guidelines for the prevention and management of diabetes. *Diabet. Med.* **2011**, *28*, 1282–1288. [CrossRef] [PubMed]
12. Wheeler, M.L.; Dunbar, S.A.; Jaacks, L.M.; Wahida, K.; Mayer-Davis, E.J.; Judith, W.R., Jr.; William, S. Macronutrients, Food Groups, and Eating Patterns in the Management of Diabetes. *Diabet. Care* **2010**, *35*, 434–445. [CrossRef] [PubMed]

13. Yamada, Y.; Uchida, J.; Izumi, H.; Tsukamoto, Y.; Inoue, G.; Watanabe, Y.; Irie, J.; Yamada, S. A non-calorie-restricted low-carbohydrate diet is effective as an alternative therapy for patients with type 2 diabetes. *Int. Med.* **2012**, *53*, 13. [CrossRef]

14. Zhu, H.M.; Ji, C. The status and compliance of medical nutrition education in patients with type 2 diabetes. *J. Nurs.* **2015**, 50–52.

15. Asghari, G.; Ghorbani, Z.; Mirmiran, P.; Azizi, F. Nut consumption is associated with lower incidence of type 2 diabetes: The Tehran Lipid and Glucose Study. *Diabet. Metab.* **2017**, *43*, 18. [CrossRef] [PubMed]

16. Chen, L. A brief discussion on the increase of fasting blood glucose. *Health Guide* **2014**, *20*, 34–35.

17. Daving, Y.; Andrén, E.; Nordholm, L.; Grimby, G. Reliability of an interview approach to the Functional Independence Measure. *Clin. Rehabil.* **2001**, *15*, 301. [CrossRef] [PubMed]

18. Turner, R.; Holman, R.; Cull, C.; Stratton, I.; Matthews, D.; Frighi, V.; Manley, S.; Neil, A.; McElroy, K.; Wright, D. Intensive blood-glucose control with sulphonylureas or insulin compared with conventional treatment and risk of complications in patients with type 2 diabetes (UKPDS 33). UK Prospective Diabetes Study (UKPDS) Group. *Lancet* **1998**, *352*, 837.

19. Association WOHAD. Defining and reporting hypoglycemia in diabetes: A report from the American Diabetes Association Workgroup on Hypoglycemia. *Diabet. Care* **2005**, *28*, 1245.

20. Cai, W. *Modern Nutrition*; Fudan University Press: Shanghai, China, 2011.

21. Akhoundan, M.; Shadman, Z.; Jandaghi, P.; Aboeerad, M.; Larijani, B.; Jamshidi, Z.; Ardalani, H.; Nikoo, M.K. The Association of Bread and Rice with Metabolic Factors in Type 2 Diabetic Patients. *PLoS ONE* **2016**, *11*, e0167921. [CrossRef] [PubMed]

22. Cohen, A.E.; Johnston, C.S. Almond ingestion at mealtime reduces postprandial glycemia and chronic ingestion reduces hemoglobin A in individuals with well-controlled type 2 diabetes mellitus. *Metab. Clin. Exp.* **2011**, *60*, 1312. [CrossRef] [PubMed]

23. Li, S.C.; Liu, Y.H.; Liu, J.F.; Chang, W.H.; Chen, C.M.; Chen, C.Y. Almond consumption improved glycemic control and lipid profiles in patients with type 2 diabetes mellitus. *Metab. Clin. Exp.* **2011**, *60*, 474–479. [CrossRef] [PubMed]

24. Sacks, F.M.; Carey, V.J.; Anderson, C.A.; Miller, E.R.; Copeland, T.; Charleston, J.; Harshfield, B.J.; Laranjo, N.; McCarron, P.; Swain, J. Effects of high vs low glycemic index of dietary carbohydrate on cardiovascular disease risk factors and insulin sensitivity: The OmniCarb randomized clinical trial. *JAMA* **2014**, *312*, 2531–2541. [CrossRef] [PubMed]

25. Mayer, S.B.; Jeffreys, A.S.; Olsen, M.K.; McDuffie, J.R.; Feinglos, M.N., Jr.; Yancy, W.S. Two Diets with Different Hemoglobin A1c and Antiglycemic Medication Effects Despite Similar Weight Loss in Type 2 Diabetes. *Diabet. Obes. Metab.* **2014**, *16*, 90–93. [CrossRef] [PubMed]

26. Liu, J.F.; Liu, Y.H.; Chen, C.M.; Chang, W.H.; Chen, C.O. The effect of almonds on inflammation and oxidative stress in Chinese patients with type 2 diabetes mellitus: A randomized crossover controlled feeding trial. *Eur. J. Nutr.* **2013**, *52*, 927–935. [CrossRef] [PubMed]

27. Vadivel, V.; Kunyanga, C.N.; Biesalski, H.K. Health benefits of nut consumption with special reference to body weight control. *Nutrition* **2015**, *28*, 1089–1097. [CrossRef] [PubMed]

28. Tan, S.Y.; Dhillon, J.; Mattes, R.D. A review of the effects of nuts on appetite, food intake, metabolism, and body weight. *Am. J. Clin. Nutr.* **2014**, *100* (Suppl. 1), 412S–422S. [CrossRef] [PubMed]

29. Barbour, J.A.; Howe, P.R.; Buckley, J.D.; Bryan, J.; Coates, A.M. Effect of 12 Weeks High Oleic Peanut Consumption on Cardio-Metabolic Risk Factors and Body Composition. *Nutrients* **2015**, *7*, 7381–7398. [CrossRef] [PubMed]

30. Lovejoy, J.C.; Most, M.M.; Lefevre, M.; Greenway, F.L.; Rood, J.C. Effect of diets enriched in almonds on insulin action and serum lipids in adults with normal glucose tolerance or type 2 diabetes. *Am. J. Clin. Nutr.* **2002**, *76*, 1000–1006. [CrossRef] [PubMed]

31. Westman, E.C.; Feinman, R.D.; Mavropoulos, J.C.; Vernon, M.C.; Volek, J.S.; Wortman, J.A.; Yancy, W.S.; Phinney, S.D. Low-carbohydrate nutrition and metabolism. *Am. J. Clin. Nutr.* **2007**, *86*, 276–284. [CrossRef] [PubMed]

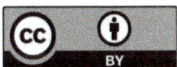

nutrients   [MDPI]

Article

SunGold Kiwifruit Supplementation of Individuals with Prediabetes Alters Gut Microbiota and Improves Vitamin C Status, Anthropometric and Clinical Markers

Renée Wilson [1], Jinny Willis [2], Richard B. Gearry [1,3], Alan Hughes [4], Blair Lawley [4], Paula Skidmore [5], Chris Frampton [1], Elizabeth Fleming [5], Angie Anderson [5], Lizzie Jones [5], Gerald W. Tannock [3,4,6] and Anitra C. Carr [7,*]

[1] Department of Medicine, University of Otago, Christchurch 8140, New Zealand; renee.wilson@postgrad.otago.ac.nz (R.W.); richard.gearry@cdhb.health.nz (R.B.G.); chris.frampton@otago.ac.nz (C.F.)

[2] New Zealand Nursing Organisation, Christchurch 8140, New Zealand; jinny.willis@nzno.org.nz

[3] Microbiome Otago, University of Otago, Dunedin 9054, New Zealand; gerald.tannock@otago.ac.nz

[4] Department of Microbiology and Immunology, University of Otago, Dunedin 9054, New Zealand; alan.hughes@otago.ac.nz (A.H.); blair.lawley@otago.ac.nz (B.L.)

[5] Department of Human Nutrition, University of Otago, Dunedin 9054, New Zealand; paula.skidmore@otago.ac.nz (P.S.); liz.fleming@otago.ac.nz (E.F.); angie.anderson@otago.ac.nz (A.A.); lizzieig71@gmail.com (L.J.)

[6] Riddet Centre of Research Excellence, Massey University, Palmerston North 4442, New Zealand

[7] Department of Pathology & Biomedical Science, University of Otago, Christchurch 8140, New Zealand

* Correspondence: anitra.carr@otago.ac.nz; Tel.: +64-3-364-0649

Received: 11 June 2018; Accepted: 2 July 2018; Published: 12 July 2018

Abstract: Kiwifruit are a nutrient dense food and an excellent source of vitamin C. Supplementation of the diet with kiwifruit enhances plasma vitamin C status and epidemiological studies have shown an association between vitamin C status and reduced insulin resistance and improved blood glucose control. In vitro experiments suggest that eating kiwifruit might induce changes to microbiota composition and function; however, human studies to confirm these findings are lacking. The aim of this study was to investigate the effect of consuming two SunGold kiwifruit per day over 12 weeks on vitamin C status, clinical and anthropometric measures and faecal microbiota composition in people with prediabetes. This pilot intervention trial compared baseline measurements with those following the intervention. Participants completed a physical activity questionnaire and a three-day estimated food diary at baseline and on completion of the trial. Venous blood samples were collected at each study visit (baseline, 6, 12 weeks) for determination of glycaemic indices, plasma vitamin C concentrations, hormones, lipid profiles and high-sensitivity C-reactive protein. Participants provided a faecal sample at each study visit. DNA was extracted from the faecal samples and a region of the 16S ribosomal RNA gene was amplified and sequenced to determine faecal microbiota composition. When week 12 measures were compared to baseline, results showed a significant increase in plasma vitamin C (14 μmol/L, $p < 0.001$). There was a significant reduction in both diastolic (4 mmHg, $p = 0.029$) and systolic (6 mmHg, $p = 0.003$) blood pressure and a significant reduction in waist circumference (3.1 cm, $p = 0.001$) and waist-to-hip ratio (0.01, $p = 0.032$). Results also showed a decrease in HbA1c (1 mmol/mol, $p = 0.005$) and an increase in fasting glucose (0.1 mmol/L, $p = 0.046$), however, these changes were small and were not clinically significant. Analysis of faecal microbiota composition showed an increase in the relative abundance of as yet uncultivated and therefore uncharacterised members of the bacterial family *Coriobacteriaceae*. Novel bacteriological investigations of *Coriobacteriaceae* are required to explain their functional relationship to kiwifruit polysaccharides and polyphenols.

Keywords: vitamin C; blood pressure; waist circumference; glucose; glycaemic control; HbA1c; kiwifruit; gut microbiota; *Coriobacteriaceae*

1. Introduction

Diabetes is one of the largest global health crises, affecting 415 million adults worldwide, with type 2 diabetes mellitus (T2DM) accounting for at least 90% of all cases of diabetes [1]. People with diabetes are at a higher risk of developing a number of disabling and life-threatening health conditions [1]. Prediabetes reflects a stage between normal glucose tolerance (NGT) and T2DM. Those with prediabetes are at high risk of progressing to T2DM, although this is not inevitable [2]. In routine practice, prediabetes is characterized by an increase in HbA1c. Results from the 2008/2009 New Zealand Adult Nutrition Survey (NZANS) provided data on the prevalence of diabetes and prediabetes using the American Diabetes Association (ADA) criteria and found that the prevalence of diabetes and prediabetes in New Zealand was 7.0% and 25.5% respectively [3]. The alarmingly high prevalence of people with prediabetes necessitates further research to explore modifiable causative factors for prediabetes.

Hyperglycaemia (elevated blood glucose concentrations) and insulin resistance are implicated in the pathogenesis of micro- and macrovascular complications [4]. Maintaining normal blood glucose levels through diet is one of the main goals in the management of a glucose metabolism disorder (diabetes or prediabetes) [5]. Higher plasma vitamin C is associated with reduced insulin resistance and improved blood glucose control [6–10]. Since hyperglycaemia is associated with increased oxidative stress, a role for antioxidants such as vitamin C in the prevention of T2DM and/or the reduction of complications is a reasonable proposition. However, there have been mixed findings reported in randomised controlled trials (RCTs) of supplementation with vitamin C on glycaemic control and insulin sensitivity [11–13]. A recent meta-analysis of 15 RCTs investigating vitamin C supplementation and insulin resistance and biomarkers of glycaemic control (fasting glucose, HbA1c) found that doses of $\geq$200 mg/day vitamin C significantly reduced glucose concentrations in patients with T2DM, particularly if the intervention was for more than 30 days and in older individuals [14]. Furthermore, a recent 12 month RCT found that treating those with T2DM with both metformin and vitamin C was more effective at reducing HbA1c and risk factors for diabetes-related long-term complications than treating with metformin alone [15].

SunGold kiwifruit are one of the best dietary sources of vitamin C (160 mg/100 g) among fruit and vegetables [16]. Regular consumption of two SunGold kiwifruit has been shown to significantly increase the plasma vitamin C levels in men with inadequate levels of plasma vitamin C [17]. Virtually all fruits represent a source of sugars and therefore moderate consumption is recommended in people with T2DM. However, there are differing amounts of sugar and other nutrients in various fruit and portion sizes vary markedly. Kiwifruit, eaten as a whole fruit, have a low glycaemic impact and are, therefore, thought to be a suitable choice for those with prediabetes and T2DM [18].

In addition to having a positive effect on glycaemic control, gold kiwifruit contain dietary fibre (1.4 g/100 g in raw Zespri SunGold kiwifruit) [16] and polyphenols which resist digestion by human enzymes and are degraded by bacteria in the digestive tract, stimulating the growth or activity of certain bacteria in the colon. The fibre in kiwifruit comprises both soluble (e.g., pectin) and insoluble (e.g., hemicelluloses and celluloses) components which make up cell walls [19].

T2DM has been reported to be associated with an alteration in the usual balance of bowel bacterial species, described as a bacterial dysbiosis [20]. Differences in the gut microbiota have been demonstrated between individuals with T2DM and healthy individuals in previous research [21,22]. Further, the finding of differences in gut microbiota between healthy individuals, individuals with prediabetes and those with T2DM suggests a potential association between gut ecology and the progression from normal glucose tolerance to T2DM [23]. A logical extension is the hypothesis that manipulation, by dietary change, of the relative abundances of particular bacterial taxa within the gut microbiota could play a role in managing T2DM [24].

On the basis of in vitro experiments, SunGold Kiwifruit consumption has been speculated to affect the composition and functioning of the bowel microbiota [25]. However, the outcomes of this study need to be confirmed in human intervention studies. Therefore, the aim of the present study was to determine whether gold kiwifruit consumption by a prediabetic cohort altered gut microbiota composition, increased plasma vitamin C concentrations and improved glycaemic control or prevented further deterioration of glucose intolerance.

2. Materials and Methods

2.1. Study Participants

The study was approved by the Southern Health and Disability Ethics Committee (consent no. 16/STH/87) and was included in the Australian New Zealand Clinical Trials Registry (ACTRN12616000858493). Written informed consent was obtained from all participants. Individuals ≥18 years meeting the inclusion criteria detailed below were recruited by a range of methods including: advertisements in local newspapers, flyers in general practice and other primary care health settings, e-mailing staff at local large businesses including the Canterbury District Health Board (CDHB), participants from previous studies were contacted, study information was posted to those who had attended prediabetes education classes and flyers placed at local businesses in Christchurch, New Zealand.

A total of 41 individuals underwent a screening questionnaire and venous blood test to measure HbA1c to ascertain eligibility for the study. Twenty-six participants were enrolled and 24 participants completed the study. Four participants (one of whom did not complete the trial) were excluded from the gut microbiota analyses due to starting a course of antibiotics during the trial. One patient left the study due to a family bereavement. Another participant was admitted to hospital for a pre-existing condition and had to conclude involvement in the study.

2.1.1. Inclusion Criteria

Participants (≥18 years) who met the ADA diagnostic criteria for prediabetes (HbA1c result of 39–46 mmol/mol) at baseline were recruited. HbA1c is routinely used as the diagnostic test for diabetes in New Zealand [26]. The red blood cell has a 90–120 day lifespan and during this time haemoglobin is glycated in proportion to the mean exposure to glucose [26]. Accordingly, a three-month intervention period was chosen for this trial.

2.1.2. Exclusion Criteria

Individuals unable to give informed consent, those with an HbA1c outside the diagnostic range for prediabetes (HbA1c result of 39–46 mmol/mol), those with a previous diagnosis of diabetes, or those on diabetes medications such as Metformin. In addition, individuals who had taken antibiotics in the last month, those with a medical history of significant gastrointestinal disease (for example, inflammatory bowel disease), previous bowel resection, those with a known kiwifruit allergy, women who were pregnant, breastfeeding or planning a pregnancy and those planning to travel overseas in the three months post selection (trial period) were also excluded.

2.2. Study Design

This was a pilot intervention trial where baseline measurements were used as the control measures for comparison. Participants were screened with a questionnaire and venous blood test to measure HbA1c. If eligible they started a lead in phase where they were asked to not eat any kiwifruit (green or gold) for seven days. During this time, they also completed an estimated food diary by writing down everything they ate or drank over three non-consecutive days (two weekdays and one weekend day) to analyse their usual dietary intake.

After the lead-in phase, Zespri SunGold kiwifruit (Gold3, *Actinidia chinensis*) were delivered to participants weekly. Participants were provided with twice as many fruit as were required and were advised that extra fruit could be shared with family and friends but to ensure that they had enough to last them until the next delivery. The participants were asked to store the fruit in a refrigerator or cool place. The kiwifruit were selected to be of the same size and quality. The average weight of one SunGold kiwifruit was 132 g (whole fruit) and 95 g for the flesh (28% accounts for the skin, [16]). Participants were asked to consume the flesh of two SunGold kiwifruit every day for twelve weeks. Strategies to avoid forgetting the fruit were discussed such as eating them at the same time every day and having two kiwifruit out on the bench every day so the participants knew whether or not they had eaten them. Participants were asked not to eat any kiwifruit other that the two study fruit during the 12 weeks. As the study was a free-living situation, participants were asked to consume the fruit as part of their usual diet. Participants were asked not to eat the skin and to eat the flesh raw and not crushed or blended in a smoothie. Participants were asked to maintain their normal dietary and lifestyle habits for the duration of the trial.

Following screening and the lead-in week there were three study visits; baseline, week six and week twelve (Figure 1). Table 1 shows the information that was collected at each study visit.

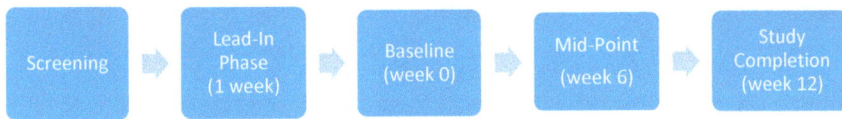

Figure 1. Study timeline.

Table 1. Information and samples collected at each study visit.

	Lead-In Phase	Week 0 (Baseline)	Week 6 (Study Mid-Point)	Week 12 (Study Completion)
Questionnaires	Food diary	Demography Medical history Medications Supplements Anthropometry Physical activity	Changes to medications and supplements Anthropometry	Changes to medications and supplements Anthropometry Physical activity Food diary
Blood Tests		Fasting glucose vitamin C HbA1c Lipids Hormones hs-CRP	Fasting glucose	Fasting glucose vitamin C HbA1c Lipids Hormones hs-CRP

2.3. Anthropometric Measures

2.3.1. Weight (kg)

Participants were asked to remove their footwear and heavy outer clothing such as jackets and were weighed to the nearest 0.1 kg on calibrated Tanita scales (Model BWB-800A, Tanita Corporation, Tokyo, Japan).

2.3.2. Height (m)

Measured once at baseline to the nearest mm using calibrated height measures.

2.3.3. BMI (kg/m^2)

Calculated by weight in kilograms divided by height in metres squared.

2.3.4. Waist Circumference (cm)

The WHO STEPwise Approach to Surveillance protocol for measuring waist circumference was used. The measurement was made at the approximate midpoint between the lower margin of the last palpable rib and the top of the iliac crest [27]. The tightness of the tape was controlled by using a Gulick II Measuring tape (Model 67020, Country Technology Inc., Gays Mills, WI, USA). Three measurements were taken at each study visit. The measurements for each participant were averaged. The coefficient of variation associated with the measurement error for waist circumference was 0.65%.

2.3.5. Hip Circumference (cm)

Measured to the nearest mm around the widest portion of the buttocks with the tape parallel to the floor using a Gulick II Measuring tape, as described above. Three measurements were taken at each study visit. The measurements for each participant were averaged. The coefficient of variation associated with the measurement error for hip circumference was 1.86%.

2.3.6. Waist-To-Hip Ratio

Calculated by dividing the waist circumference by the hip measurement.

2.3.7. Fat Mass (%)

Measured using the BIA 450 Bioimpedance Analyser (Biodynamics Corporation, Seattle, WI, USA). Patient assessments were conducted using a connection between the individual's wrist and ankle and the analyser, using standard ECG sensor pad electrodes (CONMED Corporation, Utica, NY, USA). One participant had a pacemaker so was excluded from this measure.

2.3.8. Blood Pressure (mmHg)

Measured using an automated blood pressure monitor (Bp TRU, BTM-300, Omron Healthcare Co., Ltd., Muko, Kyoto, Japan). Three measurements were taken at each study visit. The measurements for each participant were averaged. The coefficient of variation associated with the measurement error for systolic and diastolic blood pressure were 2.99% and 5.16% respectively.

2.4. Blood Parameters

Venous blood samples were collected after a 12-hour fast and were analysed for fasting glucose as an additional measure of glycaemic control. EDTA plasma was collected and immediately stored on ice and centrifuged for 10 minutes at 1000× *g* (2500 rpm) at 4 °C. The plasma was removed and immediately frozen at −80 °C for batch analysis of vitamin C.

2.4.1. Glucose

Fasting glucose was measured in blood collected in fluoride oxalate venoject tubes by standard methods (Glucose Hexokinase Enzymatic Assay, Abbott c series analyser, Abbott Park, IL, USA) at an IANZ laboratory. The coefficient of variation associated with the measurement of glucose in plasma is 1.5% at 6.78 mmol/L [28].

2.4.2. Vitamin C

Frozen plasma samples were rapidly defrosted, acidified and stabilised with perchloric acid and a metal chelator. The supernatants were then treated with a reducing agent prior to analysis to recover any vitamin C that had become oxidised during handling or storage [29]. The samples were analysed by the gold standard method of high performance liquid chromatography with electrochemical detection as described previously [17,29].

2.4.3. HbA1c

Determined in EDTA blood by standard methods (Bio-rad Variant HPLC, Bio-Rad, Hercules, CA, USA) at an IANZ laboratory. The coefficient of variation associated with the measurement of HbA1c at the IANZ is 0.66% at HbA1c of 38 mmol/mol [30].

2.4.4. Lipid Parameters

Total cholesterol, HDL-cholesterol, LDL-cholesterol and triglycerides were determined in lithium heparin blood by standard methods (Abbott c series analyser, Abbott Park, IL, USA) at an IANZ laboratory.

2.4.5. hs-CRP

The inflammatory marker hs-CRP was measured using end-point nephelometry at an IANZ laboratory.

2.4.6. Hormones

EDTA plasma was collected and centrifuged for 10 minutes at $1000 \times g$ (2500 rpm) at 4 °C. The plasma was frozen at −80 °C and stored for batched analyses. Ghrelin, leptin and adiponectin were determined by the Christchurch Heart Institute, Department of Medicine, University of Otago, Christchurch.

Ghrelin was measured by an in-house RIA following extraction from plasma using Sep Pak C18 cartridges, as described previously [31]. The assay recognises the total circulating ghrelin (i.e., both octanoyl and non-octanoyl forms). The cross reactivities of other peptides in the assay, including vasointestinal peptide, prolactin, galanin, growth hormone releasing hormone, neuropeptide Y, brain natriuretic peptide, atrial natriuretic peptide, endothelin-1 and angiotensin II were all less than 0.03%. The RIA had a mean detection limit of 10.8 ± 0.8 pmol/L and mean ED50 of 136.2 ± 10.0 pmol/L over 23 consecutive assays.

Leptin and adiponectin were measured using commercial ELISA from BioVendor (Brno, Czech Republic), Research and Diagnostic products (RD191001100 Human Leptin ELISA and RD191023100 Human Adiponectin ELISA) according to the manufacturer's instructions.

Insulin was measured using the Roche Cobas e411 method in an IANZ laboratory. After storage at −80 °C, thawed plasma was pre-treated using 25% polyethylene glycol to precipitate antibodies.

2.5. Faecal Microbiota Analysis

Participants provided a faecal sample at their study appointment, which they had collected at home in a sterile collection bottle no more than 24 h prior to their study visit. The sample was either stored in an insulated bag with an ice pack or in a home refrigerator. Samples were transported in a coolie bag with an ice pack to their study appointment. All samples were processed within 24 h of the patient collecting their sample. The samples were processed in a microbiological sterile hood into four aliquots of 0.5–1.0 g of faeces and stored in sterile 1.5 mL Eppendorf tubes at −80 °C for batched analyses. Faecal sample collection methodology was adapted from the International Human Microbiome standard operating procedures and with the Human Microbiome Project Methodology (www.ncbi.nlm.nih.gov/projects/gap/cgi-bin/document.cgi?study_id=phs000228.v3.p1&phd=3190#sec114).

2.5.1. DNA Extraction and Sequence Analysis

DNA was extracted from stool using the MoBio PowerSoil DNA Isolation kit according to the Human Microbiome Project standard operating procedures (www.ncbi.nlm.nih.gov/projects/gap/cgi-bin/document.cgi?study_id=phs000228.v3.p1&phd=3190#sec114). Genomic DNA was submitted to Argonne National Laboratories for barcoded amplification of the V4 region of the bacterial 16S rRNA gene and sequencing on a MiSeq (Illumina, San Diego, CA, USA) instrument. DNA sequences were processed using the QIIME v. 1.9.1 and vsearch v.2.0.2 suite of programs [32,33]. Genus level taxonomy was obtained by filtering Operational Taxonomic Unit (OTU) tables containing taxonomic data generated using the RDP classifier, extracting representative sequences and using BLAST to identify genus level matches, where possible, within the NCBI database. Alpha- and beta-diversity analysis of phylogenetic data compared the coverage and richness (number of phylotypes) and similarity or difference in the composition of the stool microbiota between subjects and treatment groups.

2.5.2. Faecal Water Content

Water content of faeces reflects gut transit time. Shorter transit time means more water in faeces. Shorter transit time means less time for bacterial replication and might favour species with shorter doubling times. For each faecal sample, approximately 200 mg of faeces was placed in a pre-weighed microfuge tube, the weight was recorded and the tube with cap open was placed in a 37 °C incubator. The tubes were dried until a constant dry weight was obtained and percentage water content was then calculated.

2.6. Questionnaires

2.6.1. Demographic Information

Participants recorded their date of birth, sex, ethnicity and qualification. Information on medical history, alcohol consumption and smoking status was also collected.

2.6.2. Medication and Supplement Use

At baseline participants were asked to record any medications (prescription or non-prescription) they were currently taking, the dose, the number per day and the length of time they had been taking the medication. They were also asked if they were taking any dietary supplements, how frequently they took the supplement and when their last dose was. At weeks 6 and 12 they were asked if they had stopped taking any medications/supplements or if they had started taking a new medication or supplement and if so the details were recorded.

2.6.3. Dietary Intake

Participants completed a three day (two weekdays and one weekend day) estimated food diary during their lead-in week and during their final week of consuming the SunGold kiwifruit (week 12). Participants' daily dietary intake was calculated as an average over the three days. Participants were asked to record everything they ate or drank over the three days; describing each item in detail, including cooking details and any salt, sugar, spices and sauces they may have added before eating. They were also asked to record the brand name of each food, drink or cooking ingredient and also if possible to attach the wrappers of foods to provide the nutrition information. Tips were provided to assist with estimation of portion sizes such as using household measures, for example, two rounded teaspoons of sugar. A book with photos of commonly eaten foods of different portion sizes was also provided. Participants were also encouraged to take photos of their meals in addition to completing the food diary with estimated portions. Once completed the diary was reviewed during their study appointment to add any missing information if necessary.

The food diaries were entered into Kaiculator (version 1.08d), a nutrient analysing programme developed by the Department of Human Nutrition at the University of Otago, New Zealand. Kaiculator uses the 2014 version of the New Zealand food composition database, NZ FOODfiles. The methodology for entering the food diaries has been described for our previous observational study [34]. Average total daily energy and fibre were calculated along with percent energy values for total fat, carbohydrate and protein. Dietary vitamin C was also analysed. Food groups for fresh fruit and total fruit were created and calculated for comparison of fruit intake prior to (lead-in phase) and when consuming the two SunGold kiwifruit daily (week 12). At week 12 both fresh and total fruit, with and without the SunGold kiwifruit, were created for comparison with baseline fruit intake. Kiwifruit consumption recorded in the week 12 food diary was used as an indication of compliance.

Percent energy from macronutrients per day was calculated from the average total daily dietary intake as follows [35]:

- percent energy from fat = (fat (g/day) × 37.7 kJ/g)/energy (kJ/day)
- percent energy from carbohydrate = (carbohydrate (g/day) × 16.7 kJ/g)/energy (kJ/day)
- percent energy from protein = (protein (g/day) × 16.7 kJ/g)/energy (kJ/day)

2.6.4. Physical Activity

A physical activity questionnaire was collected to monitor that participants maintained their usual activity levels. Participants completed the self-administered International Physical Activity Questionnaire (IPAQ) short form. The questionnaire asks about physical activity over the previous seven days. Participants were scored as MET-minutes per week using the IPAQ scoring protocol [36].

2.7. Statistical Analysis

Standard descriptive statistics including means, medians, standard deviations, interquartile ranges, frequencies and percentages were used to describe the baseline demographic, anthropometric, laboratory and questionnaire data. The changes in these measures over time were compared by paired t-tests and Wilcoxon Signed rank tests as appropriate. Changes in taxonomic relative abundance (RA) and diversity data was statistically analysed using Wilcoxon signed rank tests and are presented as medians and interquartile ranges. The association between vitamin C concentrations and intakes and demographic, dietary, laboratory and anthropometric measures were tested by Pearson's correlation coefficients. Changes in anthropometric and laboratory measures were compared between the two vitamin C adequacy groups by one-way ANOVA. A two-tailed $p < 0.05$ was taken to indicate statistical significance.

3. Results

The average age of the participants was 66 years and ranged from 44 to 85 years old. There was an equal number of male and female participants and the majority of participants were European (81%) (Table 2). There was a mix of educational qualifications, which is expected given the age range of the participants. There were fewer participants currently smoking (15%) compared to the number of participants who reported being ex- (39%) or non-smokers (46%). The majority of participants reported consuming alcohol (73%) (Table 2).

Table 2. General characteristics of study participants.

Characteristics	$n = 26$
Age (years) (mean $\pm$ SD)	66 $\pm$ 9
Gender	
Female % (n)	50 (13)
Male % (n)	50 (13)
Ethnicity	
European % (n)	81 (21)
Māori % (n)	8 (2)
Samoan % (n)	4 (1)
Asian/Chinese % (n)	4 (1)
Other % (n)	4 (1)
Qualification	
No qualification % (n)	27 (7)

Table 2. General characteristics of study participants.

Characteristics	$n = 26$
Secondary school % (n)	19 (5)
Post-secondary certificate, diploma or trade diploma % (n)	42 (11)
University % (n)	12 (3)
Smoking Status	
Current smoker % (n)	15 (4)
Ex-smoker % (n)	39 (10)
Non-smoker % (n)	46 (12)
Alcohol Status	
Current drinker % (n)	73 (19)
Ex-drinker % (n)	12 (3)
Non-drinker % (n)	15 (4)

3.1. Dietary Intakes: Macronutrients, Micronutrients, Fruit Intake

There were no significant differences in daily energy, fibre, protein, total fat and total available carbohydrate when week 12 was compared to baseline (Table 3). There was a non-significant trend towards an increase in total available sugars and when investigated further results showed the daily intake of fructose and glucose to be significantly higher at week 12 compared to baseline ($p < 0.001$) and the intake of sucrose to be significantly lower at week 12 compared to baseline ($p = 0.018$). Starch intake was not significantly different at week 12 compared to baseline. Significant changes in micronutrient intake are included in Table 3. There was a significant increase in vitamin C ($p < 0.001$) and E ($p = 0.037$) intakes (Table 3). There was a significantly higher intake of folate at week 12 compared to baseline ($p = 0.012$) and when investigated further this was attributed to folate naturally occurring in foods ($p = 0.002$).

At baseline the amount of fruit eaten (fresh and total) is the same whether or not kiwifruit is excluded, as participants were instructed not to eat any kiwifruit during the lead-in phase of the trial, during which time the baseline food diaries were completed (Table 3). Analysis of total and fresh fruit intake including and excluding kiwifruit consumption showed that participants were substituting some of their usual fruit intake for kiwifruit during the study (Table 3). At week 12 compliance with the intervention was calculated from the food diary data to be 91%. This was calculated for every individual as the percentage of the six kiwifruit consumed over three days.

Table 3. Dietary Intake of participants at week 0 and week 12.

Daily Dietary Intake	Week 0 ($n = 26$)	Week 12 ($n = 24$)
Macronutrients		
Energy (KJ)	7407 ± 2759	7176 ± 1683
Fibre (g)	23 ± 8	23 ± 8
Protein (g)	81 ± 24	80 ± 22
Protein (% of energy)	19 ± 4	19 ± 4
Total fat (g)	72 ± 35	68 ± 18
Total fat (% of energy)	35 ± 6	36 ± 6
Total carbohydrate (g)	190 ± 71	184 ± 49
Total carbohydrate (% of energy)	43 ± 5	43 ± 6
Total available sugars (g)	82 ± 33	86 ± 23
Fructose (g)	16 ± 8	22 ± 6 ***
Glucose (g)	14 ± 6	20 ± 5 ***
Sucrose (g)	35 ± 25	29 ± 16 *
Lactose (g)	14 ± 8	20 ± 5
Maltose (g)	3.0 ± 1.8	2.8 ± 1.5
Total starch (g)	108 ± 43	97 ± 34
Micronutrients †		

Table 3. *Cont.*

Daily Dietary Intake	Week 0 (*n* = 26)	Week 12 (*n* = 24)
vitamin C (mg)	79 ± 35	347 ± 70 ***
vitamin E (mg)	8.5 ± 3.9	10.3 ± 3.3 *
Total folate (µg)	271 ± 126	337 ± 119 *
Folate (naturally occurring) (µg)	236 ± 105	291 ± 98 **
Food Groups		
Fresh fruit including kiwifruit (g)	131 ± 91	237 ± 68 ***
Fresh fruit excluding kiwifruit (g)	131 ± 91	72 ± 55 ***
Total fruit including kiwifruit (g)	184 ± 101	274 ± 104 **
Total fruit excluding kiwifruit (g)	184 ± 101	108 ± 94 **

Values presented as mean ± SD. Paired sample t-tests were used to compare dietary data between times. * Significant at the 0.05 level, ** significant at the 0.01 level, *** significant at the 0.001 level. † Micronutrients that were significantly different when week 12 concentrations were compared to baseline.

3.2. Dietary Vitamin C Intakes

At baseline the majority of participants (*n* = 20) met the New Zealand RDI for vitamin C of 45 mg/day (Figure 2). There was only one participant who had a dietary intake below the New Zealand Estimated Average Requirement (EAR) (30 mg/day) and there were no participants reaching the New Zealand Ministry of Health suggested dietary target (SDT) to reduce chronic disease risk, that is, 220 mg/day for men and 190 mg/day for women (Figure 2). At the end of the study the majority of participants (*n* = 22) had dietary intakes reaching the SDT and the other participants had intakes above the Recommended Dietary Intake (RDI) (*n* = 2) (Figure 2).

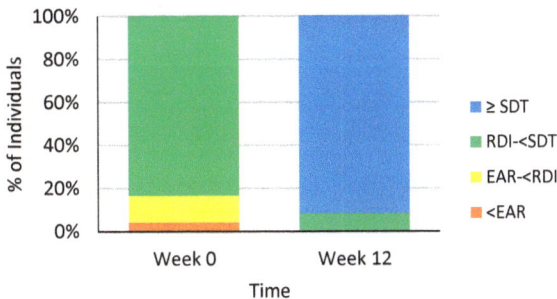

Figure 2. Dietary vitamin C intake of individuals at weeks 0 and week 12 meeting the estimated average requirement (EAR) (30 mg/day), recommended dietary intake (RDI) (45 mg/day) and suggested dietary target (SDT) to reduce chronic disease risk (220 mg/day for men and 190 mg/day for women) [36].

3.3. Anthropometry and Blood Pressure

From baseline to the end of the study there were no significant changes in weight, BMI or fat mass. There was a significant decrease in waist circumference at week 6 of 0.9 cm ($p = 0.019$) and 3.1 cm at week 12 ($p = 0.001$) compared to baseline (Table 4). Although waist-to-hip ratio was significantly lower at week 12 compared to baseline ($p = 0.032$), the difference was small and not clinically significant (Table 4). Blood pressure also decreased over the duration of the study (Table 3). At week 6 diastolic and systolic blood pressure had decreased from baseline by 3 mmHg ($p = 0.040$) and 5 mmHg ($p = 0.026$) respectively (Table 4). At week 12 systolic and diastolic blood pressure were 4 mmHg ($p = 0.029$) and 6 mmHg ($p = 0.003$) lower than baseline (Table 4). At baseline 42% (*n* = 11) of participants recorded taking medication that lowers blood pressure. There were changes to blood pressure medication for only two of these participants during the trial. One participant had their blood pressure medication dose reduced by half from week 6 to 12 and another participant had it increased between baseline and week 6 but then reduced back to the baseline dose between week 6 and 12.

Table 4. Anthropometric, blood pressure and physical activity measures.

Characteristics	Week 0 (*n* = 26)	Week 6 (*n* = 26)	Week 12 (*n* = 24)
Anthropometry			
Weight (kg)	80.2 ± 19.8	80.1 ± 20.0	77.9 ± 18.6
BMI (kg/m²)	29.4 ± 7.3	29.4 ± 7.4	28.6 ± 7.0
Fat mass (%)	34.3 ± 6.6	34.4 ± 6.6	34.0 ± 6.9
Waist circumference (cm)	98.6 ± 15.3	97.7 ± 15.2 *	95.5 ± 14.6 ***
Waist-to-hip ratio	0.90 ± 0.09	0.90 ± 0.09	0.89 ± 0.09 *
Blood Pressure			
Diastolic (mmHg)	76 ± 8	73 ± 9 *	72 ± 10 *
Systolic (mmHg)	129 ± 14	124 ± 17 *	123 ± 18 **
Physical Activity			
(met-minutes/week)	3598 ± 5273		

Values presented as mean ± SD. Wilcoxon Signed Ranks tests were used to compare physical activity between times. Paired sample t-tests were used for all other variables. * Significant at the 0.05 level, ** significant at the 0.01 level, *** significant at the 0.001 level. In addition to the missing data for the two participants who did not complete week 12 there were missing data at baseline and week 6 for fat mass (one participant) and for physical activity at week 12 (one participant).

3.4. Biochemical Indices

There was a small but statistically significant decrease in HbA1c of 1 mmol/mol at week 12 compared to baseline (*p* = 0.005) (Table 5). This decrease, however, would not be considered clinically significant. Although fasting glucose significantly increased by 0.2 mmol/L at week 6 (*p* = 0.001), it was only 0.1 mmol/L higher than baseline at week 12 (*p* = 0.046), which is not clinically significant (Table 5).

Table 5. Laboratory measures of participants at week 0 and week 12.

Biochemical Indices	Week 0 (*n* = 26)	Week 12 (*n* = 24)
HbA1c (mmol/mol)	43 ± 2	42 ± 2 **
Fasting Glucose (mmol/L)	5.4 ± 0.7	5.5 ± 0.8 *
Plasma vitamin C (μmol/L)	50 ± 19	64 ± 13 ***
Total cholesterol (mmol/L)	5.2 ± 1.3	5.1 ± 1.3
HDL cholesterol (mmol/L)	1.35 ± 0.23	1.35 ± 0.23
LDL cholesterol (mmol/L)	3.3 ± 1.0	3.3 ± 1.1
Triglycerides (mmol/L)	1.1 ± 0.5	1.1 ± 0.4
Cholesterol (total/HDL) ratio	3.9 ± 0.9	3.8 ± 0.9
hs-CRP (mg/L)	1.8 (0.6–3.2)	0.9 (0.5–2.2)
Insulin (pmol/L)	51 (31–73)	42 (31–67)
Ghrelin (pmol/L)	162 (110–204)	154 (119–206)
Leptin (ng/mL)	38 (27–71)	35 (25–75)
Adiponectin (μg/mL)	9 (6–11)	10 (7–12)

Values presented as mean ± SD or median and interquartile range (25th to 75th percentiles). Wilcoxon Signed Ranks tests were used to compare hs-CRP and hormones (insulin, ghrelin, leptin and adiponectin) between times. Paired sample t-tests were used for all other variables. * Significant at the 0.05 level, ** significant at the 0.01 level, *** significant at the 0.001 level. In addition to the two participants who did not complete the trial there was missing data at baseline and week 6 for fasting glucose (one participant), plasma vitamin C (one participant), and insulin at week 12 (one participant).

3.5. Plasma Vitamin C Levels

At baseline, none of the participants met the criteria for plasma vitamin C deficiency (<11 μmol/L). There were three participants (13%) with marginal (11–23 μmol/L) and seven (29%) with inadequate (24–49 μmol/L) plasma vitamin C concentrations (Figure 3). Over half of the cohort (*n* = 14) had either adequate (42%, 50–69 μmol/L) or saturating (17%, ≥70 μmol/L) plasma vitamin C concentrations at baseline (Figure 3). Consistent with a previous observational study [37], baseline fasting glucose

($r = -0.450$, $p = 0.024$), insulin ($r = -0.520$, $p = 0.008$) and waist circumference ($r = -0.399$, $p = 0.048$) were inversely associated with plasma vitamin C concentrations.

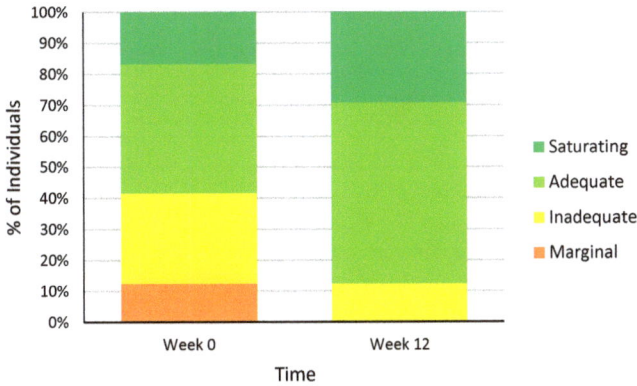

Figure 3. Plasma vitamin C status of individuals at weeks 0 and 12 classified as having saturating ($\geq$70 µmol/L), adequate (50–69 µmol/L), inadequate (24–49 µmol/L) and marginal (11–23 µmol/L) plasma vitamin C. There were no participants classified as having deficient (<11 µmol/L) plasma vitamin C concentrations [38].

After 12 weeks supplementation, plasma vitamin C concentrations were significantly higher compared to baseline (mean increase of 14 µmol/L, $p < 0.001$) indicating compliance with kiwifruit consumption (Table 5). The increase in plasma vitamin C concentrations was greatest in those who had started the trial with inadequate plasma vitamin C concentration (increase of 22 µmol/L, $p = 0.004$), compared to those who already had adequate plasma vitamin C concentrations at baseline (increase of 7 µmol/L, $p = 0.029$). At the end of the study, there were no participants with marginal plasma vitamin C and only three participants (13%) had inadequate plasma vitamin C concentrations. Fourteen (58%) of the participants had adequate and 7 (29%) of the participants had saturating plasma vitamin C concentrations at week 12 (Figure 3).

3.6. Faecal Microbiota

The faecal samples of four participants (one of whom did not complete the trial) were excluded from analysis due to starting a course of antibiotics during the trial. For this analysis, there were 22 participants at week 6 and 21 participants at week 12, due to another participant not completing the trial.

All DNA samples passed quality check and each sample was amplified and barcoded twice to reduce the possibility of losing a sample to sequence failure. Only a single amplification product failed to sequence (1/152 = 0.7%; well within accepted rate of 4%), however the duplicate reaction from this sample sequenced well. Thus, all submitted samples generated good sequence data. A total of 5,527,067 sequences were available for further analysis following quality checking procedures. Each sample generated an average of 72,725 sequences (range 39,216–117,799).

Rarefaction curves showed good coverage of microbiota composition (Figure 4A). Comparison of study time points at a rarefaction level of 35,000 sequences per sample did not show a statistically significant difference in alpha diversity (the complexity in composition of the microbiota) using a variety of metrics (Table 6).

Table 6. Diversity (at 35,000 sequences/sample) of participants at week 0, 6 and 12.

Diversity Measure	Week 0 (*n* = 22)	Week 6 (*n* = 22)	Week 12 (*n* = 21)
Observed species	250 (213–316)	279 (232–306)	241 (217–283)
Whole tree (PD)	19 (17–23)	21 (18–22)	20 (17–22)
Shannon index	5.1 (4.6–5.4)	5.4 (4.7–5.8)	5.0 (4.9–5.3)
Simpson's diversity	0.95 (0.91–0.96)	0.96 (0.93–0.97)	0.94 (0.93–0.95)
Chao index	318 (257–377)	367 (288–396)	338 (307–389)

Values presented as median and interquartile range (25th to 75th percentiles). Wilcoxon Signed Ranks tests were used to compare the diversity between times. There were no significant differences.

Beta-diversity (unique fraction metric (Unifrac) weighted and unweighted) was used to compare similarities in microbiota composition over time. A comparison of distances within and between time points did not reveal significant changes in community structure with time (Figure 4B,C). Unweighted unifrac distances (kinds of bacteria and phylogenetic relationships) indicated that the microbiotas of the participants tended to be more similar to each other after 12 weeks intervention than at baseline or 6 weeks (Figure 4B). Applying a weighting (based on the relative abundance of OTUs) suggested that the microbiota of participants are more similar to each other at both 6 and 12 weeks than at baseline (Figure 4C).

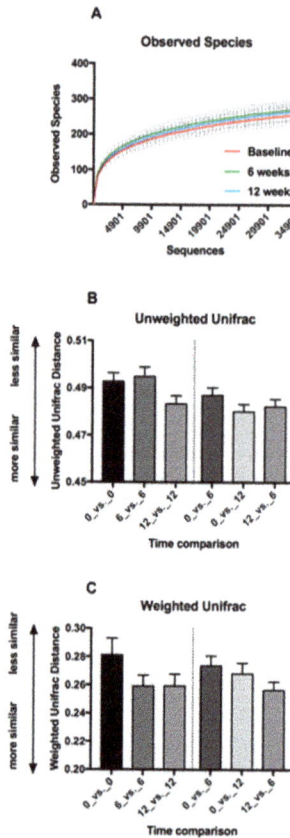

Figure 4. Faecal microbiota diversity metrics. (**A**) Rarefaction curves based on Observed Species metric of alpha diversity, showing coverage of DNA sequences obtained from faecal DNA. Means and 95% CI are shown. (**B,C**) Beta diversity metrics comparing microbiota similarity distances within and between groups. Means and SEM are shown. (**B**) Unweighted Unifrac (kinds of bacteria and phylogenetic relatedness). (**C**) Weighted Unifrac (kinds of bacteria, phylogenetic relatedness and relative abundances).

The complete results of taxonomic analysis of the faecal microbiota at the Family level are supplied in Supplementary Material Table S1. Sequences from members of the bacterial phylum *Actinobacteria* and a bacterial family within this taxon, *Coriobacteriaceae*, were more abundant in faecal samples collected during the kiwifruit intervention compared to baseline (Figure 5A,B). The original OTU table contained 10 clusters identified as *Coriobacteriacae*, including one OTU each in the genera; *Atopobium*, *Collinsella*, *Eggerthella*, *Gordonibacter* and *Senegalimassilia*. The other five OTUs were 'unidentified' (i.e., never cultured and characterised). Combining the abundances from these OTUs replicated the significant increase in relative abundance of the Family *Coriobacteriaceae* observed with time (Figure 5C). Thus, it appears that as yet uncultivated member(s) of the *Coriobacteriaceae* contributed to a significant increase in relative abundance during the intervention.

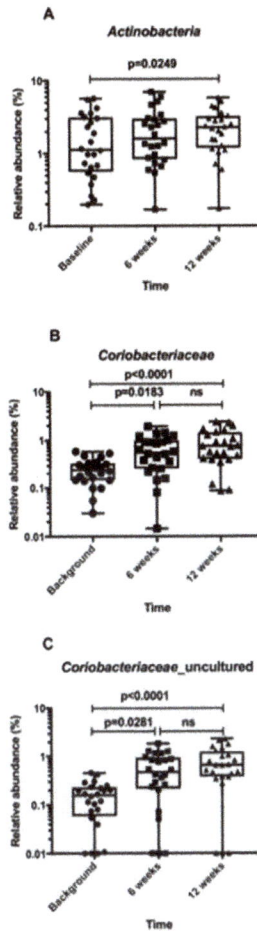

Figure 5. Relative abundances of bacterial groups in faeces of participants at baseline and during supplementation of the diet with kiwifruit. Box and whiskers plots showing individual values and means as horizontal lines. (**A**) Phylum *Actinobacteria*. (**B**) Family *Coriobacteriaceae*. (**C**) OTUs of uncharacterized bacteria of the Family *Coriobacteriaceae*. Statistical evaluation by Wilcoxon matched pairs test using Prism 7.

Dietary intervention of two SunGold kiwifruit per day resulted in significantly greater faecal water content at weeks 6 (76%, $p < 0.001$) and 12 (74%, $p = 0.01$) compared to baseline (68%).

4. Discussion

In this study, consuming two SunGold kiwifruit per day was associated with a significant increase in plasma vitamin C and fasting glucose, and a decrease in HbA1c, however, these latter two changes were small and, although statistically significant, were not clinically significant. There was a significant reduction in both diastolic and systolic blood pressure. A significant reduction in waist circumference and waist-to-hip ratio was also seen, despite small and non-significant reductions in average BMI and fat mass.

Consumption of two SunGold kiwifruit per day (total of 190 g flesh) for three months provided approximately 300 mg of vitamin C daily from the kiwifruit alone. This increase in dietary vitamin C from the SunGold kiwifruit resulted in most participants meeting the New Zealand Ministry of Health's suggested dietary target to reduce chronic disease risk [35]. This increase in dietary vitamin C resulted in a significant increase in plasma vitamin C concentrations (mean increase of 14 μmol/L). The increase in plasma vitamin C concentrations was greatest in those who had started the trial with inadequate plasma vitamin C concentration (i.e., <50 μmol/L), compared to those who already had adequate plasma vitamin C concentrations at baseline. This result is consistent with findings from an earlier kiwifruit trial where those with lower baseline plasma vitamin C concentrations showed an earlier and greater response to supplementation, compared to those with adequate plasma vitamin C concentrations at baseline, who showed little effect from supplementation [17]. Three participants (13%) had only adequate plasma vitamin C concentrations at week 12 which may indicate non-compliance or be related to some lifestyle factor, such as smoking, or chronic disease [39].

While all participants met the ADA criteria for prediabetes using HbA1c (39–46 mmol/mol) at baseline, there was still a range of anthropometric and laboratory measures for participants. For example, fasting glucose ranged from 3.9 to 7.5 mmol/L, insulin ranged from 15 to 220 pmol/L and waist circumference ranged from 70 to 125 cm. Fasting glucose, insulin and waist circumference were all inversely associated with plasma vitamin C concentrations at baseline. This result is consistent with previous research [6–10,37,38].

It has been suggested that vitamin C concentrations at baseline may represent a critical factor in predicting the metabolic responses to nutritional interventions tackling oxidative stress and may in part explain why there have been inconsistent findings in RCTs investigating supplementation with vitamin C and glycaemic control [17,39]. Individuals in this study were supplemented with vitamin C-rich kiwifruit; however, there were only three participants with marginal vitamin C levels and no participants with deficient levels at baseline. This may explain why no clinically significant differences in metabolic markers were observed between baseline and week 12. Furthermore, the length of the intervention may need to be longer than 12 weeks to see biological changes [14].

There was a small statistically significant reduction in both diastolic and systolic blood pressure over the duration of the study. This result is unlikely to be due to changes in blood pressure medication as only two participants reported changes to the dose of their blood pressure medication during the study. One of these participants actually had their blood pressure medication dose reduced by half between week 6 and 12 and the other participant was taking the same dose at week 12 as they were at baseline despite having it increased earlier in the study. Those with inadequate vitamin C levels at baseline (i.e., <50 μmol/L) had a greater reduction in blood pressure (decrease of 7 ± 9 mmHg diastolic and 10 ± 11 mmHg systolic) compared to those who had adequate levels (decrease of 2 ± 8 mmHg diastolic and 5 ± 10 mmHg systolic) when week 12 was compared to baseline. This may be related to their level of oxidative stress as hypertension has been related to increased oxidative stress and reduced antioxidant status [40]. Kiwifruit contain a wide range of natural antioxidants; they are rich in vitamin C and also contain vitamin E, polyphenols and flavonoids which are all potent antioxidants [41]. This result is consistent with a RCT of smokers, who are also known to have lower vitamin C concentrations, which showed three kiwifruit per day for eight weeks was associated with reductions of 10 mmHg in systolic blood pressure and 9 mmHg in diastolic blood pressure [42].

Despite the small increase in fruit intake at week 12, there were no significant differences in energy, fibre, protein, total fat and total carbohydrate intake when dietary data at week 12 was compared to baseline. This result suggests participants did not make major changes to their diet during the trial. The addition of the SunGold kiwifruit also had no significant impact on their macronutrient intake as it is relatively low in calories (63 kcal/100 g), protein (1.0 g/100 g), fat (0.3 g/100 g) and carbohydrate (16 g/100 g) [16]. However, SunGold kiwifruit does contain 12 g/100 g of sugar [16], which may have contributed to the significantly higher intake of fructose (increase of 6 g) and glucose (increase of 6 g) at week 12 compared to baseline. SunGold kiwifruit also contains vitamin E (1.4 mg/100 g) and folate (31 μg/100 g), so would have contributed to the higher intake of these vitamins at week 12 compared to baseline.

Although faecal microbiota diversity was stable across the 12-week intervention when viewing the cohort as a whole, *Coriobacteriaceae* family members showed a significant increase in relative abundance during the course of the study. The assignment of these bacteria to uncharacterised bacterial species was particularly interesting because it suggests that as yet uncultivated bacteria that use substrates associated with kiwifruit (such as pectins) exist in the human faecal microbiota. Future work should include efforts to cultivate these bacteria and to determine their functional characteristics. The *Coriobacteriaceae* are in general a poorly studied bacterial family, however they can chemically transform plant polyphenols [43] and thus their activities may be of interest in promoting human health [44]. Certainly, future work should investigate the potential link between *Coriobacteriaceae* and polyphenolic compounds in the faeces of kiwifruit-fed subjects and chemical derivatives of these substances in the blood circulation. While the increased relative abundances of *Coriobacteriaceae* were small, this does not preclude an important role for the bacteria in bowel ecology because low abundance bacteria in microbial communities can have a disproportionally large effect relative to abundance [45].

Our human intervention trial did not confirm the reported in vitro effect of kiwifruit fermentation [25]. In the vitro study, *Bacteroides* spp., *Parabacteroides* spp. and *Bifidobacterium* spp. were reported to increase in cultures containing kiwifruit and inoculated with human faeces. Increased *Coriobacteriaceae* relative abundances were the only impact of dietary modification seen in the participants in our study.

Dietary intervention in the form of two gold kiwifruit per day led to an increase in stool water content at both 6 and 12 weeks. This indicates a shortened gut transit time (laxative effect) and has been linked to decreases in community diversity in other studies. Stool consistency is strongly associated with gut microbiota richness and composition, enterotypes and bacteria growth rates [46]. In our study, the observation may be confounded by the fact that kiwifruit contains 1.4 g/100 g of fibre [16], which is comprised of both soluble and insoluble components at a ratio of approximately 1:3 [19]. The soluble fibre is made up almost exclusively of pectic polysaccharides that have the ability to retain water and form gels, which increases the size and softness of the faeces and aids stimulation of peristaltic movements [19]. The soluble fibre may be the cause of the increase in faecal water seen in this study. Results from several clinical trials also show that kiwifruit promotes laxation [47–50].

This was the first study to measure changes in the gut microbiota and vitamin C status associated with a whole fruit (SunGold kiwifruit) in people with prediabetes. The participants were free-living representing a realistic intervention for the general population. The use of a whole food rather than an extract/supplement in this study also makes it more affordable and available for people. Although there was no control group in this study, participants acted as their own control with baseline measurements for comparison and dietary intake was consistent over time. In this study plasma vitamin C status corroborated the food diaries as an objective measure of compliance. The study duration of three months enabled the use of HbA1c as a measure of glycaemic control and allowed us to investigate temporary and longer-term shifts in the microbiota.

As this was a pilot exploratory study with a limited number of participants it may not have been sufficient to identify some clinically relevant associations. Additionally, we did not pre-screen participants for vitamin C intake or status and, as a result, half the study cohort already had adequate plasma vitamin C status at baseline. Furthermore, because we did not include an arm with vitamin C supplementation alone, it is difficult to ascertain the contribution of the vitamin C content of the fruit to the observed effects. When assessing dietary intakes there are also limitations around misreporting and a potential bias in recording "good/bad" foods.

5. Conclusions

Supplementation with two SunGold kiwifruit per day significantly increased plasma vitamin C concentrations and provided small improvements in several markers of metabolic and cardiovascular health. The results of faecal microbiota analysis point to the need for novel bacteriological investigations of *Coriobacteriaceae* in order to explain their faecal abundances and to investigate mechanistic relationships with regard to kiwifruit polysaccharides and polyphenols. Due to the small sample size of this pilot study a larger study is indicated, particularly focusing on recruiting participants with low vitamin C status at baseline and determinations of polyphenol derivatives in faeces and blood.

Supplementary Materials: The following is available online at http://www.mdpi.com/2072-6643/10/7/895/s1. Supplementary Table S1. OTU table collapsed to family level, showing number of curated sequences 1 per family per sample.

Author Contributions: R.W. conducted participant recruitment and study visits, administration of questionnaires, collection of clinical data; R.W., P.S., E.F., A.A. and L.J. dietary analysis; A.C.C., vitamin C analysis; B.L., A.H. and G.W.T. microbiota analysis; C.F. statistical analysis; R.W., G.T., A.C., J.W. and R.B.G. undertook the conception and writing of the paper.

Funding: This research was funded by Zespri International Ltd.

Acknowledgments: We would like to thank all participants for volunteering their time to take part in the study. We would also like to thank Sharon Berry for helping take blood samples and Philippa Wadsworth for delivering the kiwifruit. R.W., J.W., R.B.G., P.S. and G.T. are the recipients of a Zespri International Ltd. grant. A.C. is supported by a Health Research Council of New Zealand Sir Charles Hercus Health Research Fellowship.

Conflicts of Interest: The authors declare no conflict of interest.

References

1. International Diabetes Federation. IDF Diabetes Atlas 2015. Available online: www.diabetesatlas.org (accessed on 12 June 2017).
2. World Health Organization, Diabetes Fact Sheet N°312 [Internet], World Health Organization Media Centre. Available online: http://www.who.int/mediacentre/factsheets/fs312/en/index.html (accessed on 12 June 2017).
3. Coppell, K.J.; Mann, J.I.; Williams, S.M.; Jo, E.; Drury, P.L.; Miller, J.C.; Parnell, W.R. Prevalence of diagnosed and undiagnosed diabetes and prediabetes in New Zealand: Findings from the 2008/09 Adult Nutrition Survey. *N. Z. Med. J.* **2013**, *126*, 23–42. [PubMed]
4. Brownlee, M. Biochemistry and molecular cell biology of diabetic complications. *Nature* **2001**, *414*, 813. [CrossRef] [PubMed]
5. Evert, A.B.; Boucher, J.L.; Cypress, M.; Dunbar, S.A.; Franz, M.J.; Mayer-Davis, E.J.; Neumiller, J.J.; Nwankwo, R.; Verdi, C.L.; Urbanski, P.; et al. Nutrition therapy recommendations for the management of adults with diabetes. *Diabetes Care* **2014**, *37*, S120–S143. [CrossRef] [PubMed]
6. Sargeant, L.; Wareham, N.; Bingham, S.; Day, N. Vitamin C and hyperglycemia in the European prospective investigation into cancer-Norfolk (EPIC-Norfolk) study: A population-based study. *Diabetes Care* **2000**, *23*, 726–732. [CrossRef] [PubMed]
7. Feskens, E.J.M.; Virtanen, S.M.; Räsänen, L.; Tuomilehto, J.; Stengård, J.; Pekkanen, J.; Nissinen, A.; Kromhout, D. Dietary factors determining diabetes and impaired glucose tolerance: A 20-year follow-up of the Finnish and Dutch cohorts of the Seven Countries Study. *Diabetes Care* **1995**, *18*, 1104–1112. [CrossRef] [PubMed]
8. Will, J.; Ford, E.; Bowman, B. Serum vitamin C concentrations and diabetes: Findings from the third National Health and Nutrition Examination Survey, 1988–1994. *Am. J. Clin. Nutr.* **1999**, *70*, 49–52. [CrossRef] [PubMed]
9. Harding, A.-H.; Wareham, N.J.; Bingham, S.A.; Khaw, K.; Luben, R.; Welch, A.; Forouhiet, N.G. Plasma vitamin C level, fruit and vegetable consumption and the risk of new-onset type 2 diabetes mellitus: The European prospective investigation of cancer-Norfolk prospective study. *Arch. Intern. Med.* **2008**, *168*, 1493–1499. [CrossRef] [PubMed]

10. Zhou, C.; Na, L.; Shan, R.; Cheng, Y.; Li, Y.; Wu, X.; Sun, C. Dietary Vitamin C Intake Reduces the Risk of Type 2 Diabetes in Chinese Adults: HOMA-IR and T-AOC as Potential Mediators. *PLoS ONE* **2016**, *11*, e0163571. Available online: https://www.ncbi.nlm.nih.gov/pmc/articles/PMC5042374/ (accessed on 12 June 2017). [CrossRef] [PubMed]

11. Ellulu, M.S.; Rahmat, A.; Patimah, I.; Khaza'ai, H.; Abed, Y. Effect of vitamin C on inflammation and metabolic markers in hypertensive and/or diabetic obese adults: A randomized controlled trial. *Drug Des. Dev. Ther.* **2015**, *9*, 3405–3412. [CrossRef] [PubMed]

12. Gutierrez, A.; Duran-Valdez, E.; Robinson, I.; De Serna, D.; Schade, D. Does Short-term Vitamin C Reduce Cardiovascular Risk in Type 2 Diabetes? *Endocr. Pract.* **2013**, *19*, 785–791. [CrossRef] [PubMed]

13. Dakhale, G.N.; Chaudhari, H.V.; Shrivastava, M. Supplementation of vitamin C reduces blood glucose and improves glycosylated hemoglobin in type 2 diabetes mellitus: A randomized, double-blind study. *Adv. Pharmacol. Sci.* **2011**, *2011*, 195271. [CrossRef] [PubMed]

14. Ashor, A.W.; Werner, A.D.; Lara, J.; Willis, N.D.; Mathers, J.C.; Siervo, M. Effects of vitamin C supplementation on glycaemic control: A systematic review and meta-analysis of randomised controlled trials. *Eur. J. Clin. Nutr.* **2017**, *71*, 1371–1380. [CrossRef] [PubMed]

15. Gillani, S.W.; Sulaiman, S.A.S.; Abdul, M.I.M.; Baig, M.R. Combined effect of metformin with ascorbic acid versus acetyl salicylic acid on diabetes-related cardiovascular complication: A 12-month single blind multicenter randomized control trial. *Cardiovasc. Diabetol.* **2017**, *16*, 103. [CrossRef] [PubMed]

16. Sivakumaran, S.; Huffman, L.; Sivakumaran, S.; Drummond, L. The nutritional composition of Zespri SunGold Kiwifruit and Zespri Sweet Green Kiwifruit. *Food Chem.* **2018**, *238*, 195–202. [CrossRef] [PubMed]

17. Carr, A.C.; Pullar, J.M.; Moran, S.; Vissers, M.C. Bioavailability of vitamin C from kiwifruit in non-smoking males: Determination of 'healthy' and 'optimal' intakes. *J. Nutr. Sci.* **2012**, *1*, e14. [CrossRef] [PubMed]

18. Monro, J.A. Kiwifruit, Carbohydrate Availability and the Glycemic Response. *Adv. Food Nutr. Res.* **2013**, *68*, 257–271. [PubMed]

19. Sims, I.M.; Monro, J.A. Fiber: Composition, structures and functional properties. *Adv. Food Nutr. Res.* **2013**, *68*, 81–99. [PubMed]

20. Qin, J.; Li, Y.; Cai, Z.; Li, S.; Zhu, J.; Zhang, F.; Liang, S.; Zhang, W.; Guan, Y.; Shen, D.; et al. A Metagenome-wide association study of gut microbiota in type 2 diabetes. *Nature* **2012**, *490*, 55–60. [CrossRef] [PubMed]

21. Larsen, N.; Vogensen, F.K.; Van den Berg, F.W.J.; Nielsen, D.S.; Andreasen, A.S.; Pedersen, B.K.; Al-Soud, W.A.; Sørensen, S.J.; Hansen, L.H.; Jakobsenet, M. Gut Microbiota in Human Adults with Type 2 Diabetes Differs from Non-Diabetic Adults. *PLoS ONE* **2010**, *5*, e9085. [CrossRef] [PubMed]

22. Karlsson, F.H.; Tremaroli, V.; Nookaew, I.; Bergström, G.; Behre, C.J.; Fagerberg, B.; Nielsen, J.; Bäckhed, F. Gut metagenome in European women with normal, impaired and diabetic glucose control. *Nature* **2013**, *498*, 99–103. [CrossRef] [PubMed]

23. Zhang, X.; Shen, D.; Fang, Z.; Jie, Z.; Qiu, X.; Zhang, C.; Chen, Y.; Ji, L. Human gut microbiota changes reveal the progression of glucose intolerance. *PLoS ONE* **2013**, *8*, e71108. [CrossRef] [PubMed]

24. Cani, P.D. The gut microbiota manages host metabolism. *Nat. Rev. Endocrinol.* **2014**, *10*, 74–76. [CrossRef] [PubMed]

25. Blatchford, P.; Bentley-Hewitt, K.L.; Stoklosinski, H.; McGhie, T.; Gearry, R.; Gibson, G.; Ansell, J. In vitro characterisation of the fermentation profile and prebiotic capacity of gold-fleshed kiwifruit. *Benef. Microbes* **2015**, *6*, 829–839. [CrossRef] [PubMed]

26. Braatvedt, G.D.; Cundy, T.; Crooke, M.; Florkowski, C.; Mann, J.I.; Lunt, H.; Rodney, J.; Orr-Walker, B.; Timothy, K.; Drury, P.L. Understanding the new HbA1c units for the diagnosis of Type 2 diabetes. *N. Z. Med. J.* **2012**, *125*, 70. [PubMed]

27. World Health Organization. Section 5: Collecting Step 2 Data: Physical Measurements. Available online: http://www.who.int/chp/steps/Part3_Section5.pdf?ua=1 (accessed on 19 June 2017).

28. Ricós, C.; Alvarez, V.; Cava, F.; García-Lario, J.V.; Hernández, A.; Jiménez, C.V.; Minchinela, J.; Perich, C.; Simón, M. Current databases on biological variation: Pros, cons and progress. *Scand. J. Clin. Lab. Investig.* **1999**, *59*, 491–500.

29. PullaR, J.M.; Bozonet, S.M.; Carr, A.C. Appropriate Handling, Processing and Analysis of Blood Samples Is Essential to Avoid Oxidation of Vitamin C to Dehydroascorbic Acid. *Antioxid* **2018**, *7*, 29. [CrossRef] [PubMed]

30. Bozkaya, G.; Uzuncan, N.; Bilgili, S.; Demirezen, O. Evaluation of analytical performance of Variant II turbo HbA1c analyzer according to sigma metrics. *J. Med. Biochem.* **2018**, *37*, 1–13. [CrossRef]

31. Bang, A.S.; Soule, S.G.; Yandle, T.G.; Richards, A.M.; Pemberton, C.J. Characterisation of proghrelin peptides in mammalian tissue and plasma. *J. Endocrinol.* **2007**, *192*, 313–323. [CrossRef] [PubMed]
32. Caporaso, J.G.; Kuczynski, J.; Stombaugh, J.; Bittinger, K.; Bushman, F.D.; Costello, E.K.; Fierer, N.; Peña, A.G.; Goodrich, J.K.; Gordonet, J.I.; et al. QIIME allows analysis of high-throughput community sequencing data. *Nat. Methods* **2010**, *7*, 335. [CrossRef] [PubMed]
33. Rognes, T.; Flouri, T.; Nichols, B.; Quince, C.; Mahé, F. VSEARCH: A versatile open source tool for metagenomics. *PeerJ* **2016**, *4*, e2584. [CrossRef] [PubMed]
34. Wilson, R.; Willis, J.; Gearry, R.; Skidmore, P.; Fleming, E.; Frampton, C.; Carr, A. Inadequate Vitamin C status in prediabetes and type 2 diabetes mellitus: Associations with glycaemic control, obesity, and smoking. *Nutrients* **2017**, *9*, 997. [CrossRef] [PubMed]
35. NHMRC. Nutrient Reference Values for Australia and New Zealand Including Recommended Dietary Intakes Canberra: ACT: National Health and Medical Research Council. 2006. Available online: https://www. nhmrc.gov.au/_files_nhmrc/file/publications/17122_nhmrc_nrv_update--dietary_intakes--web.pdf (accessed on 12 June 2017).
36. IPAQ. Guidelines for Data Processing and Analysis of the International Physical Activity Questionnaire (IPAQ): Short and Long Forms. 2005. Available online: https://sites.google.com/site/theipaq/ (accessed on 12 June 2017).
37. Will, J.C.; Byers, T. Does diabetes mellitus increase the requirement for vitamin C? *Nutr. Rev.* **1996**, *54*, 193–202. [CrossRef] [PubMed]
38. Kositsawat, J.; Freeman, V.L. Vitamin C and A1c relationship in the National Health and Nutrition Examination Survey (NHANES) 2003–2006. *J. Am. Coll. Nutr.* **2011**, *30*, 477–483. [CrossRef] [PubMed]
39. Lykkesfeldt, J.; Poulsen, H.E. Is vitamin C supplementation beneficial? Lessons learned from randomised controlled trials. *Br. J. Nutr.* **2010**, *103*, 1251–1259. [CrossRef] [PubMed]
40. Tandon, R.; Sinha, M.K.; Garg, H.; Khanna, R.; Khanna, H.D. Oxidative stress in patients with essential hypertension. *Natl. Med. J. India* **2005**, *18*, 297–299. [PubMed]
41. Boland, M. Advances in Food and Nutrition Research. In *Nutritional Benefits of Kiwifruit*; Moughan, P.J., Ed.; Elsevier Science: Burlington, MA, USA, 2013.
42. Karlsen, A.; Svendsen, M.; Seljeflot, I.; Laake, P.; Duttaroy, A.K.; Drevon, C.A.; Arnesen, H.; Tonstad, S.; Blomhoffet, R. Kiwifruit decreases blood pressure and whole-blood platelet aggregation in male smokers. *J. Hum. Hypertens.* **2012**, *27*, 126. [CrossRef] [PubMed]
43. Clavel, T.; Lepage, P.; Charrier, C. The family coriobacteriaceae. In *The Prokaryotes*, 4th ed.; Rosenberg, E., DeLong, E.F., Lory, S., Stackebrandt, E., Thompson, F., Eds.; Springer International Publishing: Berlin, Germany, 2014; pp. 201–238.
44. Del Rio, D.; Costa, L.G.; Lean, M.E.J.; Crozier, A. Polyphenols and health: What compounds are involved? *Nutr. Metab. Cardiovasc. Dis.* **2010**, *20*, 1–6. [CrossRef] [PubMed]
45. Power, M.E.; Tilman, D.; Estes, J.A.; Menge, B.A.; Bond, W.J.; Mills, L.S.; Daily, G.; Castilla, G.C.; Lubchenco, J.; Paine, R.T. Challenges in the Quest for Keystones. *BioScience* **1996**, *46*, 609–620. [CrossRef]
46. Tigchelaar, E.F.; Bonder, M.J.; Jankipersadsing, S.A.; Fu, J.; Wijmenga, C.; Zhernakova, A. Gut microbiota composition associated with stool consistency. *Gut* **2015**, *65*, 540–542. [CrossRef] [PubMed]
47. Rush, E.C.; Patel, M.; Plank, L.D.; Ferguson, L.R. Kiwifruit promotes laxation in the elderly. *Asia Pac. J. Clin. Nutr.* **2002**, *11*, 164–168. [CrossRef] [PubMed]
48. Chan, A.O.; Leung, G.; Tong, T.; Wong, N.Y. Increasing dietary fiber intake in terms of kiwifruit improves constipation in Chinese patients—Increasing dietary fiber intake in terms of kiwifruit improves constipation in Chinese patients. *World J. Gastroenterol.* **2007**, *13*, 4771–4775. [CrossRef] [PubMed]
49. Chang, C.-C.; Lin, Y.-T.; Lu, Y.-T.; Liu, Y.-S.; Liu, J.-F. Kiwifruit improves bowel function in patients with irritable bowel syndrome with constipation. *Asia Pac. J. Clin. Nutr.* **2010**, *19*, 451–457. [PubMed]
50. Cunillera, O.; Almeda, J.; Mascort, J.J.; Basora, J.; Marzo-Castillejo, M. Improvement of functional constipation with kiwifruit intake in a Mediterranean patient population: An open, non-randomized pilot study. *Revista Española de Nutrición Humana y Dietética* **2015**, *19*, 58–67. [CrossRef]

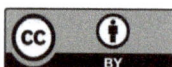

nutrients

MDPI

Review

Nutritional Interventions as Beneficial Strategies to Delay Cognitive Decline in Healthy Older Individuals

Blanka Klímová [1,*] and Martin Vališ [2]

[1] Department of Applied Linguistics, University of Hradec Kralove, Rokitanskeho 62,
   Hradec Kralove 500 03, Czech Republic
[2] Department of Neurology, University Hospital Hradec Kralove, Sokolska 581,
   Hradec Kralove 500 05, Czech Republic; martin.valis@fnhk.cz
* Correspondence: blanka.klimova@uhk.cz; Tel.: +420-604-737-645

Received: 22 June 2018; Accepted: 13 July 2018; Published: 15 July 2018

Abstract: Current demographic trends indicate that the population is aging. The aging process is inevitably connected with cognitive decline, which manifests itself in worsening working memory, processing speed, and attention. Therefore, apart from pharmacological therapies, non-pharmacological approaches which can influence cognitive performance (such as physical activities or healthy diet), are being investigated. The purpose of this study is to explore the types of nutritional interventions and their benefits in the prevention and delay of cognitive delay in healthy older individuals. The methods used in this study include a literature review of the available studies on the research topic found in Web of Science, Scopus, and MEDLINE. The findings show that nutritional intervention has a positive impact on cognitive function in healthy older people. However, it seems that the interactions between more than one nutrient are most effective. The results reveal that specifically the Mediterranean diet appears to be effective in this respect. Moreover, the findings also indicate that multi-domain interventions including diet, exercise, cognitive training, and vascular risk monitoring have a far more significant effect on the enhancement of cognitive functions among healthy older individuals.

Keywords: nutrition; healthy older individuals; cognitive decline; intervention; prevention; randomized clinical trials

---

1. Introduction

Currently, the number of older people is rapidly increasing. For instance, in 2017 there were 962 million people aged 60+ years worldwide, with their number increasing by 3% every year. The largest proportion of the aging population can be found in Europe (25%). By 2050, all continents except Africa will have one quarter or more of their population aged over 60 years [1]. This demographic trend of aging population will cause significant social and economic problems [2]. Therefore, there are efforts to develop relevant strategies and guidelines both at national and international levels in order to delay this process of aging and prolong the active age of older individuals, as well as to maintain quality of life [3].

The aging process is inevitably connected with cognitive decline, which manifests itself in worsening working memory, processing speed, and attention [4], i.e., in so-called fluid intelligence, which deteriorates at different rate in each individual [5]. The rate and severity of cognitive decline varies from normal age-related change to chronic neurodegenerative diseases such as Alzheimer's disease for which at present there is no cure [6]. Therefore, non-pharmacological approaches which can influence fluid intelligence, such as physical activities or healthy diet, are being investigated [6–8].

Evidence-based studies [9,10] indicate that specifically the Mediterranean diet (MedDiet) rich in olive oil and nuts, seems to contribute to the prevention of cognitive impairment among healthy older people. However, other food products, for example, avocados [11], or nutritional supplements such as consumption of flavanone-rich 100% orange juice [12] or omega-3 fatty acid [13] also play an important role in the prevention of cognitive decline in healthy older individuals. In addition, nutritional interventions in comparison with the pharmacological treatment, are usually well-tolerated, easy-to-implement, cost-effective, and safe for long-term use [13].

The purpose of this study is to explore the types of nutrition intervention and its benefits in the prevention and delay of cognitive delay in healthy older individuals.

2. Methods

The authors conducted a literature review of the research studies on the basis of the key words in three acknowledged databases: Web of Science, Scopus, and MEDLINE. This review was performed over the period from 2014 to June 2018 since several review studies had been already written on this topic [14,15]. The key words were as follows: diet AND cognitive decline AND healthy older people, diet AND cognitive decline AND healthy elderly, nutrition intervention AND cognitive decline AND healthy older people, nutrition intervention AND cognitive decline AND healthy elderly, nutrition AND cognitive decline AND healthy older people, nutrition AND cognitive decline AND healthy elderly, diet AND dementia AND healthy older people, diet AND dementia AND healthy elderly, nutrition intervention AND dementia AND healthy older people, nutrition intervention AND dementia AND healthy elderly, nutrition AND dementia AND healthy older people, nutrition AND dementia AND healthy elderly.

The majority of the studies were detected in the Web of Science database (97 studies), followed by Scopus (66 studies) and MEDLINE (45 studies). However, in MEDLINE it is possible to look only for clinical trials, and therefore the selection was easier. Altogether, 208 studies were found via the database search and 11 from other available sources (i.e., web pages, conference proceedings and books outside the scope of the databases described above). The titles of all studies were then checked in order to discover whether they focused on the research topic or not and irrelevant studies were excluded. In addition, the duplicate studies were also excluded. Afterwards, the authors checked the content of the abstracts whether the study examined the research topic. Thirty-two studies/articles were selected for the full-text analysis. Only 12 studies were then able to be used for detailed analysis of the research topic. The selection of these studies is described below (Figure 1).

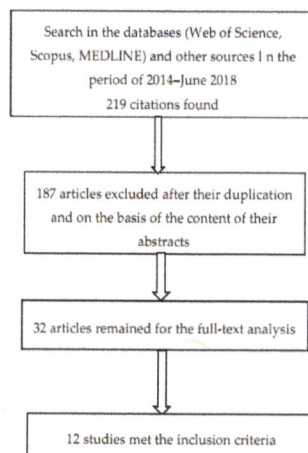

Figure 1. An overview of the selection procedure.

The study was included if it was a randomized controlled trial, and matched the corresponding period, i.e., from 2014 up to June 2018. Furthermore, the study was included if it involved healthy older people, i.e., those without any cognitive impairment or dementia aged 50+ years, and focused on the research topic, i.e., nutritional intervention in the delay and prevention of cognitive decline in healthy older individuals. All studies had to be written in English. Thus, studies such as [5] were excluded, as well as cross-sectional descriptive and cohort studies, for example [16–18].

3. Results

Altogether 12 randomized controlled trials (RCT) were found. The majority of were from Europe (i.e., Finland, Germany, Italy, Spain, and the UK) [10,12,13,19–24] and the rest from the USA and Australia [11,25,26]. The nutrition intervention involved dietary supplements (i.e., cocoa flavanols, *Vitis vinifera*, docosahexaenoic acid (DHA)-rich fish oil, or omega-3 fatty acid), vegetable (e.g., avocado), berry and orange beverages, and the MedDiet. Two of the studies were multidomain lifestyle intervention studies including, apart from healthy diet, physical exercises, social activities, cognitive training, and vascular risk management [20,24]. The intervention period in the studies ranged from five weeks to five years. The subject samples also varied; the smallest sample of subjects consisted of 37 healthy older individuals and the largest included 775 healthy older people. The efficacy of the nutrition intervention focused on the prevention and delay of cognitive decline in the studies was measured with available validated cognitive assessment tools such as a battery of cognitive tests aimed at assessing working memory, attention, or processing speed. Table 1 below provides an overview of the main findings of these studies. They are summarized in alphabetical order of their first author.

Table 1. Overview of the twelve selected studies focused on cognitive decline and its prevention by nutrition intervention.

Author	Objective	Type of The Nutrition Intervention And Its Frequency	Intervention Period	Number of Subjects	Main Outcome Assessments	Main Findings
Brickman et al. [25] RCT (USA)	To investigate whether the enhancement of dentate gyrus (DG) function with dietary flavanols improves cognition in older adults.	Daily intake of 900 mg cocoa flavanols in the intervention vs. 10 mg cocoa flavanols in the control group.	Three months.	37 healthy older individuals, age: 50–69 years.	Functional magnetic resonance imaging (fMRI), a battery of cognitive tests, statistical analysis.	The results indicate that DG dysfunction is a driver of age-related cognitive decline and suggest non-pharmacological means for its amelioration such as the daily high flavanol intake.
Calapai et al. [19] RCT (Italy)	To investigate the potential beneficial effects of a *Vitis vinifera*-based dietary supplement on cognitive function and neuropsychological status in healthy older adults.	Cognigrape® (250 mg/day) in the intervention group and placebo in the control group.	12 weeks.	57 subjects in the intervention group and 54 subjects in the control group; age: 55–75 years.	A battery of cognitive and neuropsychological tests, statistical analysis.	The findings reveal that 12 weeks of Cognigrape® supplementation is safe, can improve physiological cognitive profiles, and can concurrently ameliorate negative neuropsychological status in healthy older adults.
Clare et al. [20] RCT (UK)	To evaluate a goal-setting intervention aimed at promoting increased cognitive and physical activity and improving mental and physical fitness, diet and health.	Three groups: control (IC)—an interview in which information about activities and health was discussed; goal-setting (GS)—an interview in which they set behaviour change goals relating to physical, cognitive and social activity, health and nutrition; and goal-setting with mentoring (GM)—the goal-setting interview followed by bi-monthly telephone mentoring. The one-to-one interviews lasted for 90 min.	12 months.	75 healthy elderly (IC—27 subjects; GS—24 subjects; GM—24 subjects); age: 50+ years.	The Lifetime of Experiences Questionnaire (LEQ), Physical Activities Scale for the Elderly (PASE), a battery of cognitive tests, audio-recordings of the interviews, statistical analysis.	The results show that at 12-month follow-up, the two goal-setting groups increased their level of physical (effect size 0.37) and cognitive (effect size 0.15) activity relative to controls.

Table 1. *Cont.*

Author	Objective	Type of The Nutrition Intervention And Its Frequency	Intervention Period	Number of Subjects	Main Outcome Assessments	Main Findings
Danthiir et al. [26] RCT (Australia)	To test whether docosahexaenoic acid (DHA)-rich fish oil slows 18-month cognitive decline in cognitively healthy individuals.	1720 mg DHA and 600 mg eicosapentaenoic acid or low-polyphenolic olive oil daily, as capsules in the intervention group and placebo in the control group.	18 months.	194 subjects in the intervention group and 196 in the control group; age: 65–90 years.	A battery of cognitive tests, statistical analysis.	The results show that supplementing older adults with fish oil does not prevent cognitive decline.
Kean et al. [12] RCT (UK)	To examine whether eight weeks of daily flavanone-rich orange juice consumption was beneficial for cognitive performance in healthy older people.	Daily 350 mg consumption of flavanone-rich 100% orange juice and equicaloric low-flavone (37 mg) orange flavoured cordial (500 mL).	Eight weeks	37 healthy subjects, mean age: 67 years.	A battery of cognitive, executive function and episodic memory tests, statistical analysis.	The results indicate that after the 8-week consumption of flavanone rich 100% orange juice, the global cognitive performance was significantly improved ($p < 0.05$).
Kulzow et al. [13] RCT (Germany)	To investigate the impact of omega-3 fatty acid supplementation on memory functions in healthy older adults.	Daily intake of 2200 mg long-chain polyunsaturated omega-3 fatty acids (LC-n3-FA) in the intervention group and placebo in the control group.	26 weeks.	22 healthy older subjects in the intervention group and 22 in the control group, age: 50–75 years.	Visuospatial object-location-memory task (LOCATO), standard neuropsychological tests, statistical analysis.	The findings reveal that the daily intake of LC-n3-FA has a positive impact on memory functions in healthy older people ($p = 0.049$).
Lehtisalo et al. [21] RCT (Finland)	To discuss the success of dietary counselling intervention among healthy older individuals.	Dietary intervention counselling: 3 individual and 8 group sessions.	Two years.	631 healthy older subjects in the intervention group and 629 in the control group, age: 60–77 years.	Food records, statistical analysis.	The findings show that the intake of several vitamins and minerals remained unchanged or increased in the intervention group and that the dietary counselling may have a positive impact on age-related diet quality and cognitive performance.
Mastroiacovo et al. [22] RCT (Italy)	To evaluate the effect of flavanol consumption on cognitive performance in cognitively intact elderly people.	A drink containing 993 mg high flavanol (HF), 520 mg intermediate flavanol (IF), or 48 mg low flavanol (LF) cocoa flavanols (CFs).	Eight weeks.	90 cognitively intact elderly subjects divided into three groups (HF; IF; LF); age: 61–85 years.	A battery of neuropsychological tests, blood pressure measures, statistical analysis.	The results reveal that regular CF consumption can reduce some measures of age-related cognitive dysfunction, possibly through an improvement in insulin sensitivity.

Table 1. *Cont.*

Author	Objective	Type of The Nutrition Intervention And Its Frequency	Intervention Period	Number of Subjects	Main Outcome Assessments	Main Findings
Nilsson et al. [23] RCT (Spain)	To evaluate effects on cognitive functions and cardiometabolic risk markers with a mixture of berries intervention in healthy older individuals.	Daily intake of 795 mg berry beverage with polyphenols or dietary fibre or 11 mg berry control beverage with no poly phenols or dietary fibre.	Five weeks.	20 healthy subjects in the intervention group and 20 healthy subjects in the control group, mean age: 50–70 years.	A battery of cognitive tests, cardiometabolic tests and statistical analysis.	The results indicate that the subjects performed better in the working memory test after the berry beverage compared to after the control beverage ($p < 0.05$).
Scott et al. [11] RCT (USA)	To explore the effect of the daily consumption of one avocado on cognition.	1 avocado daily in the intervention group and 1 potato or 1 cup of chickpeas in the control group.	Six months.	20 healthy subjects in the intervention group and 20 healthy subjects in the control group, mean age: 63 years.	A battery of cognitive tests, statistical analysis.	The results show that including the daily intake of one avocado may have a positive impact on cognitive performance in healthy older individuals, specifically on their working memory ($p = 0.036$) or sustained attention ($p = 0.033$).
Sindi et al. [24] RCT (Finland)	To assess whether baseline leukocyte telomere length (LTL) modified the cognitive benefits of a 2-year multidomain lifestyle intervention.	Participants were randomly assigned to the lifestyle intervention (diet, exercise, cognitive training, and vascular risk management) and control (general health advice) groups.	Two years.	775 healthy subjects (392 control, 383 intervention), at the age of 30–77 years.	A battery of neuropsychological tests, blood samples, statistical analysis.	The findings of the intervention reveal that cognitive benefits were more pronounced with shorter baseline LTL, particularly for executive functioning, indicating that the multi-domain lifestyle intervention was especially beneficial among higher-risk individuals.
Valls-Pedret et al. [10] RCT (Spain)	To investigate whether a Mediterranean diet supplemented with antioxidant-rich foods influences cognitive function compared with a control diet.	Participants were randomly assigned to a Mediterranean diet supplemented with extra virgin olive oil (1 L/week), a Mediterranean diet supplemented with mixed nuts (30 g/day), or a control diet (advice to reduce dietary fat).	Five years.	447 cognitively healthy volunteers (233 women (52.1%); mean age, 66.9 years); three groups: two intervention groups and one control group.	A neuropsychological test battery, statistical analysis.	In an older population, a Mediterranean diet supplemented with olive oil or nuts is associated with improved cognitive function.

RCT: randomized controlled trial.

Apart from one study [26], results of all RCTs indicate that the nutritional interventions had a positive impact on the cognitive performance of healthy older individuals, specifically on their working memory and attention [10,11,23]. Moreover, the findings of the multidomain lifestyle intervention studies reveal that such interventions exhibit significant impacts on cognitive functioning in later life [20,24]. The results also show that the change in the cognitive performance can be already detected after five weeks of intervention [23]. However, this is questionable because according to Kurz and van Baelen [27], the relevant period for medication assessment by regulatory authorities is 24 weeks at a minimum.

4. Discussion

The findings described in Table 1 show that nutrition intervention has a positive impact on cognitive functioning of healthy older people. The trials with the exception of four RCTs [10,19,23,26], concentrated only on one type of nutritional supplement (i.e., *Vitis vinifera*, docosahexaenoic acid (DHA)-rich fish oil, omega-3 fatty acid, avocado, and berry). Three RCTs [12,22,25] focused on high flavanol-rich drinks, which appeared to have quite a positive effect on cognitive performance among healthy older individuals. In fact, all nutrients described in Table 1 are part of the traditional multi-nutrient MedDiet pattern, and the research [28] indicates that the interaction of specific foods and nutrients, especially in the MedDiet, is more powerful on the aging brain than individual nutrients or a low-fat diet. In fact, the MedDiet seems to be a nutritional model for healthy dietary habits since it contains all the needed nutrients: monounsaturated fatty acids, polyunsaturated fatty acids, antioxidants (e.g., allium sulphur compounds, anthocyanins, beta-carotene-flavonoids, catechins, carotenoids, indoles, or lutein), vitamins (A, B1, 6, 9, 12, D, E), and minerals (magnesium, potassium, calcium, iodine, zinc, selenium) [28]. In addition, the combination of these nutrients positively affects pathological neurodegenerative processes such as oxidative stress, neuroinflammation, insulin resistance, and reduced cerebral blood flow [29]. Nevertheless, the MedDiet appears to improve cognitive performance in case there is a high adherence to this diet [30–32]. Furthermore, the MedDiet has a positive impact on neuropsychological [19] and physical state of older people [16] and on vascular diseases and diabetes [22–24,33]. Although the results mainly concerned western developed countries, similar research (however, non-RCT) was conducted among healthy older adults in Asian countries such as Taiwan [34] and Japan [35]. The findings of these studies also show a positive correlation between the healthy diet rich in vegetables, soy products, fruit, and fish and the prevention and delay of cognitive decline in older age. Wright et al. [36] in their study carried out among 2090 African Americans and whites emphasized that higher diet quality was associated with higher performance on tests of attention and cognitive flexibility, visuospatial ability, and perceptual speed. This was also evidenced by Smyth et al. [18] who in their cohort study claimed that higher diet quality is associated with a reduced risk of cognitive decline. Hosking et al. [37] report that adequate nutrition is essential for cognitive development in childhood and cognitive ability in childhood is strongly associated with cognitive performance across the lifetime.

Moreover, it seems that multi-nutrient dietary intervention should be implemented in the delay of cognitive decline among healthy older individuals. The multi-nutrient intervention is also one of the priorities discussed at the First WHO Ministerial Conference on Global Action against Dementia in March 2015 [38]. Furthermore, Shilsky et al. [39] suggest in their study that healthcare systems should play a more significant role in integrating nutrition care for healthy older individuals and that the nutrition assessment should be incorporated in the medical records. This was also confirmed by the discussed study [21], for which findings revealed that the dietary counselling had a positive impact on age-related diet quality and cognitive performance.

The findings of the reviewed RCTs [20,24] indicate that the multi-domain interventions including healthy diet, physical exercises, cognitive training, and vascular risk monitoring have a far more significant effect on the enhancement of cognitive functions among healthy older individuals [40]. In fact, these non-pharmacological strategies (healthy diet, physical exercises and cognitive training) have been confirmed by other research studies [7,8] and they should be all integrated at an optimal level into daily regime of healthy older individuals in order to prolong their active and quality life. This was also proposed at the International Conference on Nutrition and the Brain in Washington in 2013 [41].

On the contrary, research implies that dietary patterns rich in fat and sugar, with high intake of meat/poultry or eggs, have negative, harmful effects on cognitive functioning in older age [34,35,37].

The limitations of the reviewed studies consist in the small sample sizes, different types of nutrition interventions and outcome measures, and a lack of follow-up assessments, as well as the fact that not all studies were specifically designed to examine cognitive performance. All these insufficiencies might generate overestimated conclusions in this review study [42,43]. Therefore, more RCTs should be conducted to prove the efficacy of nutritional interventions on the prevention and delay of cognitive decline.

Author Contributions: Conceptualization, B.K. and M.V.; Methodology, M.V.; Software, B.K.; Validation, B.K. and M.V.; Formal Analysis, B.K.; Investigation, B.K.; Resources, B.K.; Data Curation, B.K.; Writing—Original Draft Preparation, B.K.; Writing—Review and Editing, M.V.; Visualization, M.V.; Supervision, M.V.; Project Administration, M.V.; Funding Acquisition, M.V.

Funding: This research received no external funding.

Acknowledgments: This paper was supported by the research project Excellence 2018, Faculty of Informatics and Management, University of Hradec Kralove, Czech Republic, as well as by MH CZ – DRO (UHHK 00179906) and PROGRES Q40 run at the Medical Faculty Charles University, Czech Republic.

Conflicts of Interest: The authors declare no conflicts of interest.

References

1. United Nations. Ageing. Available online: http://www.un.org/en/sections/issues-depth/ageing/ (accessed on 17 June 2018).
2. Klimova, B.; Maresova, P.; Valis, M.; Hort, J.; Kuca, K. Alzheimer's disease and language impairments: Social intervention and medical treatment. *Clin. Interv. Aging* **2015**, *10*, 1401–1408. [PubMed]
3. Marešová, P.; Klímová, B.; Kuča, K. Alzheimer's disease: Cost cuts call for novel drugs development and national strategy. *Čes. Slov. Farm.* **2015**, *64*, 25–30.
4. Klimova, B. Computer-Based Cognitive Training in Aging. *Front. Aging Neurosci.* **2016**, *8*, 313. [CrossRef] [PubMed]
5. Hardman, R.J.; Kennedy, G.; Macpherson, H.; Scholey, A.B.; Pipingas, A. A randomised controlled trial investigating the effects of Mediterranean diet and aerobic exercise on cognition in cognitively healthy older people living independently within aged care facilities: The Lifestyle Intervention in Independent Living Aged Care (LIILAC) study protocol [ACTRN12614001133628]. *Nutr. J.* **2015**, *14*, 53. [PubMed]
6. Knight, A.; Bryan, J.; Wilson, C.; Hodgson, J.; Murphy, K. A randomised controlled intervention trial evaluating the efficacy of a Mediterranean dietary pattern on cognitive function and psychological wellbeing in healthy older adults: The MedLey study. *BMC Geriatr.* **2015**, *15*, 55. [CrossRef] [PubMed]
7. Klimova, B.; Maresova, P.; Kuca, K. Non-pharmacological approaches to the prevention and treatment of Alzheimer's disease with respect to the rising treatment costs. *Curr. Alzheimer Res.* **2016**, *13*, 1249–1258. [CrossRef] [PubMed]
8. Klimova, B.; Valis, M.; Kuca, K. Cognitive decline in normal aging and its prevention: A review on non-pharmacological lifestyle strategies. *Clin. Interv. Aging* **2017**, *12*, 903–910. [CrossRef] [PubMed]
9. Martinez-Lapiscina, E.H.; Clavero, P.; Toledo, E.; San Julian, B.; Sanchez-Tainta, A.; Corella, D.; Lamuela-Raventos, R.M.; Martinez, J.A.; Martinez-Gonzalez, M.A. Virgin olive oil supplementation and long-term cognition: The PREDIMED-NAVARRA randomized, trial. *J. Nutr. Health Aging* **2013**, *17*, 544–552. [CrossRef] [PubMed]
10. Valls-Pedret, C.; Sala-Vila, A.; Serra-Mir, M.; Corella, D.; de la Torre, R.; Martínez-González, M.A.; Martínez-Lapiscina, E.H.; Fitó, M.; Pérez-Heras, A.; Salas-Salvadó, J.; et al. Mediterranean Diet and Age-Related Cognitive Decline: A Randomized Clinical Trial. *JAMA Intern. Med.* **2015**, *175*, 1094–1103. [CrossRef] [PubMed]

11. Scott, T.M.; Rasmussen, H.M.; Chen, O.; Johnson, E.J. Avocado consumption increases macular pigment density in older adults: A randomized, controlled trial. *Nutrients* **2016**, *9*, 919. [CrossRef] [PubMed]
12. Kean, R.J.; Lamport, D.J.; Dodd, G.F.; Freeman, J.E.; Williams, C.M.; Ellis, J.A.; Butler, L.T.; Spencer, J.P. Chronic consumption of flavanone-rich orange juice is associated with cognitive benefits: An 8-wk, randomized, double-blind, placebo-controlled trial in healthy older adults. *Am. J. Clin. Nutr.* **2015**, *101*, 506–514. [CrossRef] [PubMed]
13. Külzow, N.; Witte, A.V.; Kerti, L.; Grittner, U.; Schuchardt, J.P.; Hahn, A.; Flöel, A. Impact of omega-3 fatty acid supplementation on memory functions in healthy older adults. *J. Alzheimers Dis.* **2016**, *51*, 713–725. [CrossRef] [PubMed]
14. Swaminathan, A.; Jicha, G.A. Nutrition and prevention of Alzheimer's dementia. *Front. Aging Neurosci.* **2014**, *6*, 282. [CrossRef] [PubMed]
15. Hardman, R.J.; Kennedy, G.; Macpherson, H.; Scholey, A.B.; Pipingas, A. Adherence to a Mediterranean-style diet and effects on cognition in adults: A qualitative evaluation and systematic review of longitudinal and prospective trials. *Front. Nutr.* **2016**, *3*, 22. [CrossRef] [PubMed]
16. Zaragoza-Marti, A.; Ferrer-Cascales, R.; Hurtado-Sanchez, J.A.; Laguna-Perez, A.; Cabanero-Martinez, M.J. Relationship between adherence to the Mediterranean diet and health-related quality of life and life satisfaction among older adults. *J. Nutr. Health Aging* **2018**, *22*, 89–96. [CrossRef] [PubMed]
17. Clare, L.; Wu, Y.T.; Teale, J.C.; MacLeod, C.; Matthews, F.; Brayne, C.; Woods, B.; CFAS-Wales Study Team. Potentially modifiable lifestyle factors, cognitive reserve, and cognitive function in later life: A cross-sectional study. *PLoS Med.* **2017**, *14*, e1002259. [CrossRef] [PubMed]
18. Smyth, A.; Dehghan, M.; O'Donnell, M.; Anderson, C.; Teo, K.; Gao, P.; Sleight, P.; Dagenais, G.; Probstfield, J.L.; Mente, A.; et al. Healthy eating and reduced risk of cognitive decline: A cohort from 40 countries. *Neurology* **2015**, *84*, 2258–2265. [CrossRef] [PubMed]
19. Calapai, G.; Bonina, F.; Bonina, A.; Rizza, L.; Mannucci, C.; Arcoraci, V.; Laganà, G.; Alibrandi, A.; Pollicino, C.; Inferrera, S.; et al. A Randomized, double-blinded, clinical trial on effects of a *Vitis vinifera* extract on cognitive function in healthy older adults. *Front. Pharmacol.* **2017**, *8*, 776. [CrossRef] [PubMed]
20. Clare, L.; Nelis, S.M.; Jones, I.R.; Hindle, J.V.; Thom, J.M.; Nixon, J.A.; Cooney, J.; Jones, C.L.; Edwards, R.T.; Whitaker, C.J. The Agewell trial: A pilot randomised controlled trial of a behaviour change intervention to promote healthy ageing and reduce risk of dementia in later life. *BMC Psychiatry* **2015**, *15*, 25. [CrossRef] [PubMed]
21. Lehtisalo, J.; Ngandu, T.; Valve, P.; Antikainen, R.; Laatikainen, T.; Strandberg, T.; Soininen, H.; Tuomilehto, J.; Kivipelto, M.; Lindström, J. Nutrient intake and dietary changes during a 2-year multi-domain lifestyle intervention among older adults: Secondary analysis of the Finnish Geriatric Intervention Study to Prevent Cognitive Impairment and Disability (FINGER) randomised controlled trial. *Br. J. Nutr.* **2017**, *118*, 291–302. [CrossRef] [PubMed]
22. Mastroiacovo, D.; Kwik-Uribe, C.; Grassi, D.; Necozione, S.; Raffaele, A.; Pistacchio, L.; Righetti, R.; Bocale, R.; Lechiara, M.C.; Marini, C.; et al. Cocoa flavanol consumption improves cognitive function, blood pressure control, and metabolic profile in elderly subjects: The Cocoa, Cognition, and Aging (CoCoA) Study—A randomized controlled trial. *Am. J. Clin. Nutr.* **2015**, *101*, 538–548. [CrossRef] [PubMed]
23. Nilsson, A.; Salo, I.; Plaza, M.; Björck, I. Effects of a mixed berry beverage on cognitive functions and cardiometabolic risk markers; A randomized cross-over study in healthy older adults. *PLoS ONE* **2017**, *12*, e0188173. [CrossRef] [PubMed]
24. Sindi, S.; Ngandu, T.; Hovatta, I.; Kåreholt, I.; Antikainen, R.; Hänninen, T.; Levälahti, E.; Laatikainen, T.; Lindström, J.; Paajanen, T.; et al. Baseline telomere length and effects of a multidomain lifestyle intervention on cognition: The FINGER randomized controlled trial. *J. Alzheimers Dis.* **2017**, *59*, 1459–1470. [CrossRef] [PubMed]
25. Brickman, A.M.; Khan, U.A.; Provenzano, F.A.; Yeung, L.K.; Suzuki, W.; Schroeter, H.; Wall, M.; Sloan, R.P.; Small, S.A. Enhancing dentate gyrus function with dietary flavanols improves cognition in older adults. *Nat. Neurosci.* **2014**, *17*, 1798–1803. [CrossRef] [PubMed]
26. Danthiir, V.; Hosking, D.E.; Nettelbeck, T.; Vincent, A.D.; Wilson, C.; O'Callaghan, N.; Calvaresi, E.; Clifton, P.; Wittert, G.A. An 18-mo randomized, double-blind, placebo-controlled trial of DHA-rich fish oil to prevent age-related cognitive decline in cognitively normal older adults. *Am. J. Clin. Nutr.* **2018**, *107*, 754–762. [CrossRef] [PubMed]

27. Kurz, A.; van Baelen, B. Ginkgo biloba compared with cholinesterase inhibitors in the treatment of dementia: A review based on meta-analyses by the Cochrane collaboration. *Dement. Geriatr. Cogn. Disord.* **2004**, *18*, 217–226. [CrossRef] [PubMed]

28. Knight, A.; Bryan, J.; Murphy, K. Is the Mediterranean diet a feasible approach to preserving cognitive function and reducing risk of dementia for older adults in Western countries: New insights and future directions. *Ageing Res. Rev.* **2016**, *25*, 85–101. [CrossRef] [PubMed]

29. Scarmeas, N.; Stern, N.; Tang, M.X.; Mayeux, R.; Luchsinger, J.A. Mediterranean diet and risk for Alzheimer's disease. *Ann. Neurol.* **2006**, *59*, 912–921. [CrossRef] [PubMed]

30. Tagney, C.C. DASH and Mediterranean-type dietary patterns to maintain cognitive health. *Curr. Nutr. Rep.* **2014**, *3*, 51–61. [CrossRef] [PubMed]

31. Mosconi, L.; Murray, J.; Tsui, W.H.; Li, Y.; Davis, M.; Williams, S.; Pirraglia, E.; Spector, N.; Osorio, R.S.; Glodzik, L.; et al. Mediterranean diet and magnetic resonance imaging-assessed brain atrophy in cognitively normal individuals at risk for Alzheimer's disease. *J. Prev. Alzheimers Dis.* **2014**, *1*, 23–32. [PubMed]

32. Frisardi, V.; Panza, F.; Seripa, D.; Imbimbo, B.P.; Vendemiale, G.; Pilotto, A.; Solfrizzi, V. Nutraceutical properties of Mediterranean diet and cognitive decline: Possible underlying mechanisms. *J. Alzheimers Dis.* **2010**, *22*, 715–740. [CrossRef] [PubMed]

33. Pope, S.K.; Shue, V.M.; Beck, C. Will a healthy lifestyle help prevent Alzheimer's disease? *Annu. Rev. Public Health* **2003**, *24*, 111–132. [CrossRef] [PubMed]

34. Tsai, H.J. Dietary patterns and cognitive decline in Taiwanese aged 65 years and older. *Int. J. Geriatr. Psychiatry* **2015**, *30*, 523–530. [CrossRef] [PubMed]

35. Okubo, H.; Inagaki, H.; Gondo, Y.; Kamide, K.; Ikebe, K.; Masui, Y.; Arai, Y.; Ishizaki, T.; Sasaki, S.; Nakagawa, T.; et al. Association between dietary patterns and cognitive function among 70-year-old Japanese elderly: A cross-sectional analysis of the SONIC study. *Nutr. J.* **2017**, *16*, 56. [CrossRef] [PubMed]

36. Wright, R.S.; Waldstein, S.R.; Kuczmarski, M.F.; Pohlig, R.T.; Gerassimakis, C.S.; Gaynor, B.; Evans, M.K.; Zonderman, A.B. Diet quality and cognitive function in an urban sample: Findings from the Healthy Aging in Neighborhoods of Diversity across the Life Span (HANDLS) study. *Public Health Nutr.* **2017**, *20*, 92–101. [CrossRef] [PubMed]

37. Hosking, D.E.; Nettelbeck, T.; Wilson, C.; Danthiir, V. Retrospective lifetime dietary patterns predict cognitive performance in community-dwelling older Australians. *Br. J. Nutr.* **2014**, *112*, 228–237. [CrossRef] [PubMed]

38. Shah, H.; Albanese, E.; Duggan, C.; Rudan, I.; Langa, K.M.; Carrillo, M.C.; Chan, K.Y.; Joanette, Y.; Prince, M.; Rossor, M.; et al. Research priorities to reduce the global burden of dementia by 2025. *Lancet Neurol.* **2016**, *15*, 1285–1294. [CrossRef]

39. Shlisky, J.; Bloom, D.E.; Beaudreault, A.R.; Tucker, K.L.; Keller, H.H.; Freund-Levi, Y.; Fielding, R.A.; Cheng, F.W.; Jensen, G.L.; Wu, D.; et al. Nutritional considerations for healthy aging and reduction in age-related chronic disease. *Adv. Nutr.* **2017**, *8*, 17–26. [CrossRef] [PubMed]

40. Ngandu, T.; Lehtisalo, J.; Solomon, A.; Levalahti, E.; Ahtiluoto, S.; Antikainen, R.; Bäckman, L.; Hänninen, T.; Jula, A.; Laatikainen, T.; et al. A 2 year multidomain intervention of diet, exercise, cognitive training, and vascular risk monitoring versus control to prevent cognitive decline in at-risk people (FINGER): A randomised controlled trial. *Lancet* **2015**, *385*, 2255–2263. [CrossRef]

41. Barnard, N.D.; Bush, A.I.; Ceccarelli, A.; Cooper, J.; de Jager, C.A.; Fraser, G.; Fraser, G.; Kesler, S.; Levin, S.M.; Lucey, B.; et al. Dietary and lifestyle guidelines for the prevention of Alzheimer's disease. *Neurobiol. Aging* **2014**, *35*, S74–S78. [CrossRef] [PubMed]

42. Melby-Lervag, M.; Hulme, C. There is no convincing evidence that working memory training is effective: A reply to Au et al. (2014) and Karbach and Verhaeghen (2014). *Psychon. Bull. Rev.* **2016**, *23*, 324–330. [CrossRef] [PubMed]

43. Melby-Lervag, M.; Hulme, C. Is working memory training effective? A meta-analytic review. *Dev. Psychol.* **2013**, *49*, 270–291. [CrossRef] [PubMed]

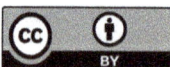

nutrients

MDPI

Article

Food Consumption, Knowledge, Attitudes, and Practices Related to Salt in Urban Areas in Five Sub-Saharan African Countries

Magali Leyvraz [1], Carmelle Mizéhoun-Adissoda [2], Dismand Houinato [3], Naby Moussa Baldé [4], Albertino Damasceno [5], Bharathi Viswanathan [6], Mary Amyunzu-Nyamongo [7], Jared Owuor [7], Arnaud Chiolero [1,8] and Pascal Bovet [1,6,*]

[1]   Institute of Social and Preventive Medicine (IUMSP), Canton University Hospital (CHUV), 1010 Lausanne, Switzerland; magali.leyvraz@chuv.ch (M.L.); arnaud.chiolero@chuv.ch (A.C.)
[2]   School of Nutrition and Dietetics, Faculty of Health Science, University of Abomey-Calavi, Cotonou 01 BP 526, Benin; carmelle.mizehoun@gmail.com
[3]   Laboratory of Noncommunicable and Neurologic Diseases Epidemiology, Faculty of Health Science, University of Abomey-Calavi, Cotonou 01 BP 526, Benin; dshouinato@gmail.com
[4]   Department of Endocrinology and Diabetes, Donka University Hospital, Conakry, Guinea; naby.balde@gmail.com or naby@afribone.net.gn
[5]   Department of Medicine, Eduardo Mondlane University, Maputo, Mozambique; tino_7117@hotmail.com
[6]   Ministry of Health, Victoria, Republic of Seychelles; barathi.viswanathan@health.gov.sc
[7]   African Institute for Health and Development (AIHD), Nairobi 00100, Kenya; mnyamongo@aihdint.org (M.A.-N.); jowuor@aihdint.org (J.O.)
[8]   Institute of Primary Health Care (BIHAM), University of Bern, 3012 Bern, Switzerland
*   Correspondence: pascal.bovet@chuv.ch; Tel.: +41-21-314-72-72

Received: 28 June 2018; Accepted: 3 August 2018; Published: 7 August 2018

Abstract: High salt intake is a major risk factor of hypertension and cardiovascular disease. Improving knowledge, attitudes, and practices (KAP) related to salt intake in the general population is a key component of salt reduction strategies. The objective of this study was to describe and compare the KAP of adults related to salt in urban areas of five countries in sub-Saharan Africa. The survey included 588 participants aged 25 to 65 years who were selected using convenience samples in the urban areas of Benin, Guinea, Kenya, Mozambique, and Seychelles. Socio-demographic and food consumption were assessed using a structured closed-ended questionnaire administered by survey officers. Height, weight, and blood pressure were measured. Food consumption varied largely between countries. Processed foods high in salt, such as processed meat, cheese, pizzas, and savory snacks were consumed rather infrequently in all the countries, but salt-rich foods, such as soups or bread and salty condiments, were consumed frequently in all countries. The majority of the participants knew that high salt intake can cause health problems (85%) and thought that it is important to limit salt intake (91%). However, slightly over half (56%) of the respondents regularly tried to limit their salt intake while only 8% of the respondents thought that they consumed too much salt. Salt and salty condiments were added most of the time during cooking (92% and 64%, respectively) but rarely at the table (11%). These findings support the need for education campaigns to reduce salt added during cooking and for strategies to reduce salt content in selected manufactured foods in the region.

Keywords: salt; sodium; hypertension; knowledge; attitudes; practices; diet; Africa; Benin; Guinea; Mozambique; Kenya; Seychelles

---

1. Introduction

Cardiovascular disease (CVD) is the leading cause of deaths worldwide including in low-income and middle-income countries (LMICs) [1]. It is estimated that high salt intake accounts for 9.5% of all CVD deaths globally due to its effect on blood pressure [2]. In sub-Saharan Africa (SSA), approximately 800,000 deaths per year are due to CVD and 6% of these deaths are attributable to high salt intake [2]. The disease burden related to elevated salt intake is expected to further increase over the next decade in LMICs [3] due to the growing and aging populations and trends towards urbanization and westernization of the diet in these countries.

Reducing dietary salt intake in the population is a key strategy to reduce the CVD burden [4]. Strategies to reduce salt intake at the population level include awareness campaigns advising individuals to reduce their salt consumption, food labeling, and reformulation of selected industrially produced foods [5]. Improving knowledge, attitudes, and practices (KAP) related to salt intake in the population is an important part of any salt reduction strategy [6]. In particular, dietary advice can reduce salt intake, blood pressure, and other CVD risk factors [7,8]. In 2015, 40 countries worldwide were implementing some organized policy or program to reduce salt consumption in the population but only one program was implemented in SSA (i.e., in South Africa) [9].

Only a few studies have examined KAP related to salt intake in SSA countries [10–14]. These studies have generally found low levels of KAP related to salt intake. However, most of these studies were conducted in specific population groups (e.g., hypertensive patients) and in selected settings. Given the scarcity of data on KAP related to salt intake and the high burden of CVD in LMICs [15], it was recently recommended that more studies should be conducted to assess dietary patterns and key sources of sodium in these countries [16].

The objective of this study was to describe and compare the food consumption, KAP related to salt intake, and associated factors in adults from the general population in urban areas of five SSA countries. This information is expected to be useful for guiding the development of salt reduction programs and policies in SSA.

2. Materials and Methods

Cross-sectional surveys were conducted in a main city in each of the five countries (Bohicon in Benin, Conakry in Guinea, Mombasa in Kenya, Maputo in Mozambique, and Victoria in Seychelles) between January 2012 and April 2013. The countries were selected based on the geographical diversity and the presence of investigators who expressed interest in examining these issues in the countries.

For four countries, participant selection was based on the convenience of a three-stage sampling strategy. The first stage was the selection of two areas in the selected cities. The second stage was the selection of households within each area and the third stage was the selection of one person within a household. The person was chosen to ensure similar numbers of participants from 25 to 44 years of age and from 45 to 65 years of age and similar numbers of men and women. Pregnant women and adults unable to understand the questionnaire were excluded. In Seychelles, participants were selected from an electronic register of all inhabitants living around Victoria while ensuring similar numbers of participants 25–44 years of age and 45–65 years of age and similar numbers of men and women.

Survey officers administered a structured closed-ended questionnaire and performed anthropometric measurements. In view of the lack of a standardized dietary questionnaire in SSA and the large variety of diets across countries in the region, a questionnaire was developed during a two-day meeting with the main investigators of each country with several questions being adapted from World Health Organization (WHO) instruments [17]. Questions assessed household characteristics, socio-demographic characteristics, health-related behaviors, and frequency of selected common food items including food items rich in salt (e.g., processed meats, cheeses, pizzas, savory snacks, bread, soups, and relevant local dishes). The questionnaire also included questions on KAP related to salt intake. Height, weight, and three blood pressure readings were measured. Informed consent was obtained from each participant. In each country, the study was approved by the locally relevant institutional ethical review boards.

Weight was measured with an electronic weighing scale to the nearest 0.1 kg. Height was measured with a fixed height rod to the nearest 0.1 cm in all countries. Overweight and obesity were defined for body mass index (BMI) between 25 and 29 or $\geq$30 kg/m^2, respectively. Blood pressure was measured with an electronic blood pressure device and high blood pressure defined as systolic/diastolic blood pressure $\geq$140/90 mmHg or taking treatment for hypertension.

We assessed associations between KAP variables and selected predictors using Spearman correlation coefficients and using stratified analysis. We used the chi-square test to test for differences between categories. Means for all countries were weighted so that each country had the same weight. The level of significance was set at 0.05. Analyses were conducted using Stata 14.1 (StataCorp, College Station, TX, USA).

Publication of data on KAP from this study was delayed because the assessment of salt excretion, which was originally another goal of this study in addition to KAP, had to be cancelled due to funding and other issues. Moreover, sample size was limited when compared to the initially four-time larger anticipated sample size due to discontinued funding by the donor.

3. Results

3.1. Sample Characteristics

A total of 588 adults between 25 and 65 years old participated in the survey. The characteristics of the participants and their households are described in Table 1. The country samples included similar proportions of men versus women and younger persons (25–44 years of age) versus older person (45–65 years of age). This was consistent with the selection strategy of the participants. Slightly more than half of the participants (54%) were overweight or obese and approximately one-fourth (26%) had high blood pressure. Nearly all households had electricity (90%), a television set (87%), or a radio (89%). Women cooked food more often than men with 60% of the women cooking food every day versus 36% of the men. In addition, 5.4% of the women never cooked versus 20% of the men.

Table 1. Socio-demographic characteristics of the participants [1].

Characteristics	All [2]	Benin	Guinea	Kenya	Mozambique	Seychelles
Participant characteristics						
Total sample size (*n*)	588	140	119	102	77	150
Female (%)	54 (50–58)	51 (43–60)	52 (43–61)	49 (39–59)	61 (50–71)	58 (50–66)
Age (mean)	42 (41–43)	42 (41–44)	43 (41–45)	43 (41–45)	41 (39–43)	42 (40–44)
25–44 years (%)	57 (53–61)	54 (45–62)	59 (50–67)	54 (44–63)	61 (50–71)	56 (48–64)
45–65 years (%)	43 (39–47)	46 (38–55)	41 (33–50)	46 (37–56)	39 (29–50)	44 (36–52)
Completed primary school (%)	80 (76–83)	56 (47–64)	78 (70–85)	88 (80–93)	77 (66–85)	99 (95–100)
Overweight (%)	30 (26–34)	31 (24–39)	24 (17–32)	24 (16–33)	32 (22–43)	40 (32–48)
Obese (%)	24 (21–28)	24 (17–31)	16 (10–24)	23 (16–32)	29 (20–41)	29 (23–37)
High blood pressure or treatment for hypertension (%)	26 (22–30)	26 (20–34)	18 (12–26)	25 (18–35)	26 (17–37)	37 (29–45)
Treatment for hypertension (%)	15 (12–18)	9 (5–15)	13 (8–21)	17 (11–25)	17 (10–27)	19 (13–26)
Household assets						
Running water (%)	74 (70–78)	68 (60–75)	83 (75–89)	30 (22–40)	90 (80–95)	99 (95–100)
Electricity (%)	90 (87–92)	86 (80–91)	99 (94–100)	70 (60–78)	96 (89–99)	100 (100–100)
Fridge (%)	59 (55–63)	19 (13–26)	71 (62–78)	30 (22–40)	77 (66–85)	100 (100–100)
Radio (%)	89 (86–92)	87 (80–92)	80 (72–87)	86 (78–92)	94 (85–97)	99 (95–100)
Television (%)	87 (84–89)	77 (69–83)	92 (86–96)	66 (56–74)	99 (91–100)	100 (100–100)
Cable television (%)	47 (43–51)	48 (40–56)	79 (71–85)	29 (21–39)	16 (9–26)	65 (57–72)
Bicycle or motorcycle (%)	28 (25–32)	64 (55–71)	29 (21–37)	30 (22–40)	5 (2–13)	13 (8–19)
Car or truck (%)	24 (21–28)	6 (3–12)	40 (32–49)	8 (4–15)	22 (14–33)	43 (36–51)

[1] Values are means (95% confidence intervals). [2] Estimates for all were weighted so that data from each country had the same weight.

3.2. Food Consumption

The usual consumption of foods in each country is shown in Table 2. The most frequently consumed staple foods were maize in Benin, rice and bread in Guinea, Mozambique, and Seychelles, and maize and bread in Kenya. Fish was the most frequent source of animal protein in all countries. The most frequently consumed beverages were tea in Kenya, Mozambique, and Seychelles, coffee in Guinea, and fruit juices in Benin. Participants consumed on average 2.7 meals (95% confidence interval (CI) 2.6–2.7) and 1.2 snacks (95% CI 1.2–1.3) per day and ate 3.0 meals (95% CI 2.8–3.3) outside the home on a weekly basis.

Table 2. Consumption of selected food items according to country [1].

Food item	Benin	Guinea	Kenya	Mozambique	Seychelles
Staple foods					
Rice					
Maize					
Potato					
Yam					
Bread					
Fruits and vegetables					
Salad					
Vegetables					
Fruits					
Animal products					
Chicken					
Red meat					
Processed meat					
Fish					
Eggs					
Cheese					
Other foods					
Soup					
Pizza					
Breakfast cereals					
Savory snacks					
Sweets and pastries					
Supplements or vitamins					
Non-alcoholic beverages					
Tea					
Coffee					
Commercial soft drink					
Locally made lemonade					
Fresh fruit juice					
Non-fresh fruit juice					
Milk					

[1] ☐: <1 times/week, ☐: 1–3 times/week, ▬: 4–6 times/week, ▬: every day.

A number of processed food items with known high salt content including processed meat, cheese, pizzas, breakfast cereals, and savory snacks were consumed rather infrequently in all the countries. However, soup and bread, which often contain high amounts of salt, were consumed frequently in all countries. As mentioned in the next paragraph, salt-rich condiments (e.g., Maggi cubes and food spreads such as Marmite/Vegemite), which are often added in soups and other dishes, were also used frequently in all countries.

3.3. Knowledge, Attitudes, and Practices (KAP) Related to Salt

Levels of KAP related to salt intake are shown in Table 3. The majority of the participants knew that high salt intake can cause health problems (85%) and could name at least one adequate health problem that can arise from high salt intake (66%). Most of the participants thought it was important to limit salt intake (91% 'very important' and 'somehow important'). However, only 56% of the respondents often tried to limit their salt intake. Moreover, only a small proportion of respondents thought that they consumed too much salt (8%), while a substantial proportion of the respondents thought they consumed too little salt (26%).

Table 3. Knowledge, attitudes, and practices related to salt intake according to country (in %).

Knowledge, Attitudes, and Practices	All [1]	Benin	Guinea	Kenya	Mozambique	Seychelles
Knowledge						
High salt intake can cause serious health problems						
Yes	85 (82–88)	93 (88–97)	66 (57–74)	87 (79–92)	88 (78–93)	92 (86–95)
No	5 (3–7)	2 (1–7)	5 (2–11)	6 (3–13)	4 (1–12)	6 (3–11)
Don't know	10 (8–13)	4 (2–9)	28 (21–37)	7 (3–14)	8 (4–17)	2 (1–6)
Health problems are associated with high salt intake						
≥1 problem known	66 (61–70)	87 (78–92)	64 (52–74)	48 (38–59)	93 (81–98)	50 (41–59)
None known	34 (30–39)	13 (8–22)	36 (26–48)	52 (41–62)	7 (2–19)	50 (41–59)
It is important to limit salt intake						
Very important	9 (7–12)	7 (4–13)	20 (13–28)	7 (3–14)	7 (3–15)	5 (2–10)
Somehow important	12 (9–14)	4 (1–8)	23 (16–32)	14 (9–23)	0 (0–0)	17 (12–24)
Not really important	79 (76–82)	89 (83–93)	57 (48–66)	79 (70–86)	93 (85–97)	78 (70–84)
Attitudes						
Try to limit salt						
Often	55 (51–59)	76 (68–82)	47 (38–57)	54 (44–63)	66 (54–76)	32 (25–40)
Sometimes	16 (13–19)	11 (7–18)	18 (12–26)	26 (18–36)	3 (1–11)	22 (16–29)
Not really	29 (25–33)	13 (8–20)	35 (26–44)	20 (13–29)	31 (21–43)	46 (38–54)
Perceived amount of salt consumed						
Too little	26 (22–30)	2 (1–6)	55 (46–64)	36 (27–45)	30 (21–41)	7 (4–12)
About right	59 (55–63)	96 (92–99)	20 (14–28)	52 (43–62)	60 (48–70)	67 (59–74)
Too much	8 (6–10)	1 (0–5)	5 (2–11)	12 (7–20)	10 (5–20)	11 (7–17)
Don't know	7 (5–9)	1 (0–5)	19 (13–27)	0 (0–0)	0 (0–0)	16 (11–23)
Practices						
Salt is added during cooking						
Never	2 (1–3)	2 (1–6)	3 (1–8)	2 (0–8)	0 (0–0)	1 (0–5)
Sometimes (1–2 times/week)	7 (5–9)	1 (0–5)	27 (20–36)	3 (1–9)	3 (1–10)	0 (0–0)
Often (most meals)	19 (16–22)	5 (2–10)	18 (12–26)	30 (22–39)	27 (18–38)	15 (10–21)
Always (all meals)	73 (69–76)	92 (86–96)	52 (43–61)	65 (56–74)	70 (59–79)	84 (77–89)
Salty condiments are used during cooking [2]						
Never	9 (6–11)	6 (3–12)	8 (4–14)	21 (14–31)	4 (1–11)	4 (2–9)
Sometimes (1–2 times/week)	26 (23–30)	7 (4–13)	29 (22–38)	32 (23–42)	25 (16–36)	38 (30–46)
Often (most meals)	22 (18–25)	9 (5–15)	11 (6–18)	24 (17–34)	25 (16–36)	40 (32–48)
Always (all meals)	42 (38–47)	78 (70–84)	50 (41–59)	17 (11–26)	47 (36–58)	18 (13–25)
Salt is added to food at the table						
Never	66 (62–70)	71 (63–78)	46 (37–55)	46 (36–56)	82 (72–89)	87 (80–91)
Sometimes (1–2 times/week)	23 (20–27)	24 (17–31)	33 (25–42)	37 (28–47)	12 (6–21)	9 (6–15)
Often (most meals)	6 (4–8)	2 (1–6)	14 (8–21)	8 (4–15)	4 (1–11)	2 (1–6)
Always (all meals)	5 (3–7)	3 (1–7)	8 (4–14)	9 (5–16)	3 (1–10)	2 (1–6)
Consumption of foods high in salt [3]						
Never	34 (30–38)	1 (0–6)	41 (32–50)	16 (10–24)	83 (73–90)	28 (21–36)
1–2 times/week	15 (13–18)	7 (4–13)	38 (30–48)	18 (11–27)	1 (0–9)	12 (8–18)
3–4 times/week	29 (25–32)	5 (2–10)	9 (5–16)	54 (45–64)	16 (9–26)	58 (50–66)
Every day/almost every day	21 (18–25)	86 (79–91)	6 (3–12)	12 (7–20)	0 (0–0)	2 (1–6)

[1] Estimates for all were weighted so that data from each country had the same weight. [2] These condiments included bouillon cubes, Aromat powder, soy sauce, food spreads (e.g., Vegemite, Marmite), and similar items. [3] These foods included salted fish, salted meat, salami, salted peanuts, food spreads, pizza, and other typical local meals rich in salt.

Most participants reported that salt was added to the foods most of the time during cooking (92% 'often' and 'always'). Salty condiments such as bouillon cubes, aroma enhancing powders, and sauces were used frequently in all countries especially in Benin, Guinea, and Mozambique (87%, 61%, and 72% added 'often' and 'always'). In contrast, few participants reported adding salt to meals at the table (11% 'often' and 'always').

3.4. Associations between KAP Related to Salt and Socio-Demographic Characteristics

The distribution of several KAP variables was significantly different between countries ($p < 0.001$), but not consistent with sex, age, education, and hypertension treatment (see Supplemental Table S1). Women added salt and other salty condiments during cooking more often than men ($p = 0.045$ and $p = 0.006$, respectively) and added salt less often at the table ($p = 0.043$). KAP levels did not differ significantly between participants who completed primary school vs. those who did not, except for the use of salty condiments (such as bouillon cubes), which were used more frequently among persons with lower education levels ($p < 0.001$). KAP levels did not differ according to anti-hypertensive treatment, except that salty condiments were used less frequently by treated persons ($p < 0.05$) and treated persons thought more often that they consumed too little salt ($p < 0.05$).

Most of the KAP variables were not associated with each other (data not shown). The small sample sizes in several categories precluded meaningful statistical analyses. However, lower discretionary use of salt was associated with higher levels of knowledge related to salt intake ("thinks high salt intake can cause serious health problems": $\rho = -0.23$, $p < 0.001$, "knows at least one correct salt-related health problem": $\rho = -0.09$, $p < 0.05$, "thinks it is important to limit salt intake": $\rho = -0.20$, $p < 0.001$).

4. Discussion

Overall, the study shows that the distribution of intake of food items varied widely between countries. Several processed food items with known or presumably high salt content (such as pizzas and savory snacks) were consumed rather infrequently (<3 times/week), but soups and bread were consumed frequently in all countries (>3 times/week), which may suggest substantial salt intake. The study also shows a fairly good level of KAP in relation to salt intake in urban settings among five countries in Africa. However, there were some gaps. A fairly modest proportion of persons added salt at the table. The large majority of participants were aware of health risks related to salt intake and recognized the importance of limiting dietary salt intake. Yet, less than one in ten participants believed they consumed too much salt. We did not find substantial associations within KAP variables or between KAP variables and socio-demographic characteristics, except for an inverse association between the knowledge of the need to restrict salt intake and the discretionary use of salt at the table.

Food consumption differed largely between countries, which underlies the difficulty of developing dietary questionnaires and nutritional guidelines that could apply to all countries. However, certain processed foods such as soups and bread were consumed frequently in all countries. These findings suggest the need for voluntary or mandatory reformulation strategies to reduce the salt content of selected manufactured foods that are both commonly consumed and have high salt content. A study conducted in the early 2000s in South Africa reported that bread was a main source of dietary salt in this country [18]. As a result, the South African government regulated the maximum levels of salt permitted in a wide range of industrially processed food categories, including breads, in order to reduce salt intake in the population [19,20]. Reformulation policies aimed at reducing salt in manufactured foods can be highly cost-effective [21] and are recommended by the WHO's Global Action Plan for the Prevention and Control of Non-Communicable Diseases [4]. Several countries have implemented policies to reformulate selected manufactured foods with subsequent reductions of the salt intake at the population level [22–24]. However, none of the five countries included in this survey have implemented such reformulation strategies [9]. South Africa is the only country in the African region that has taken regulatory steps to mandatorily reduce the salt content of selected foods [9]. Findings of our study also emphasize the need for continued education campaigns in order to encourage people to limit dietary salt intake. Such campaigns are also useful when advocating for studies assessing sources of salt intake in a particular population and when advocating for corresponding reformulation strategies. Policy aimed at reformulating foods frequently consumed and high in salt is a cornerstone strategy for effective reduction of salt intake in the population.

Knowledge on the detrimental effect of high salt intake was fairly high and higher than could have been anticipated from previous research [10–14]. However, fairly good knowledge about health effects of salt did not seem to have translated into strong attitudes and practices with regards to salt intake reduction. For example, knowledge that salt could be detrimental for health was associated with only one salt-related practice, i.e., low discretionary use of salt. A study conducted in 2014–2015 in Mozambique also found participants high in knowledge but low in attitudes and practices, in which is similar to our study [25]. This suggests that campaigns aimed at raising awareness about the detrimental impact of salt intake on health might better translate in actual salt reduction if structural measures are also implemented, e.g., programs to reduce salt in the food served in work or school canteens and measures to limit salt intake in selected manufactured foods (e.g., bread). This is consistent with a review showing that the implementation of education and awareness-raising interventions alone is unlikely to be adequate in reducing population salt intake to the recommended levels, which suggests that behavior change might better occur when combining health education and public awareness campaigns [26]. The quasi-ubiquitous presence of television and radio in the surveyed households suggests that these media could be the main instruments to relay such public awareness campaigns.

The main strengths of this study were the inclusion of population-based samples in five countries and the use of the same methodology, which allows direct comparison between countries. The study also has limitations. First, salt intake was not measured in all countries and we cannot report on the relation between salt-related behaviors and an objective measurement of salt intake. Moreover, our study did not allow for the quantification of salt added at the table or the contribution of salt in the form of processed versus non-processed foods. Second, a number of selection biases may have occurred in the sampling of participants. For example, persons present in a household at the time of the survey may have been different than persons absent. This may, however, have limited impact, since food consumption tends to be fairly homogenous at a household level. Individuals from a low socioeconomic status (e.g., the illiterate persons unable to understand questions) may also have been under-represented in this study. However, this proportion is likely small and has little overall impact on the results. Our survey was limited to urban areas and the generalization of the findings is, therefore, limited to such urban areas. Admittedly, food consumption may differ largely in rural areas and further studies need to be conducted in these different areas. Yet, urbanization is rapidly increasing in SSA and findings in this study may reflect dietary habits among large segments of the population on the continent. Third, the study relied on reported information, which is prone to recall and other biases that can lead to under-reporting or over-reporting of certain foods and practices. Fourth, the fairly low numbers of participants precluded meaningful statistical analyses of associations between KAP variables and socio-demographic characteristics.

Very little data is available on actual salt intake, the sources of salt intake, and KAP related to salt in SSA. One systematic review aimed to identify all published studies reporting salt intake in countries of SSA until 2015 [27]. This review found that 81% of the adult populations consumed salt intake above the recommended maximum 5 g per day [27], which suggests overall high intake in the region. Intake was higher in urban than in rural populations [27]. With regard to countries included in this study, the review identified one study in children in Benin in 1996 [28] and one study in Kenya in 1986 in rural areas [29]. When looking for more recent studies, urinary excretion of salt was assessed in Benin based on the same study on KAP and in Mozambique using another study. Both studies found high salt intake (10.2 g and 10.5 g of salt per day in Benin and Mozambique, respectively) [30,31]. A global modelling study [32] estimated that mean salt intake in all of the five countries in our study, apart from Kenya, was above the maximum 5 g of salt recommend by the WHO [33].

Future research on KAP related to salt is recommended in these countries among others in the region. An objective measurement of the actual amount of salt consumed in these populations is needed to assess whether salt intake is above recommendations and in which population groups. In addition, further qualitative studies should examine specific practices that may favor salt intake. Lastly, analyses of salt intake of foods especially in bread, instant soups and selected local foods as well as market studies are needed to identify the main sources of dietary salt in these populations in order to guide reformulation guidelines.

5. Conclusions

In conclusion, our study among adults in urban settings found largely different food consumption patterns between countries but consumption of salt-rich bread, soup, and salty condiments was frequent in all countries, which suggests that the salt intake could be substantial in all countries. We found fairly good knowledge related to the detrimental effects of high salt intake, but mixed findings related to the attitudes and practices related to the reduction of salt intake. These findings support the need for both education campaigns to promote knowledge, attitudes, and behaviors for the control of dietary salt intake and reformulation strategies to reduce salt content of selected frequently eaten foods high in salt.

Supplementary Materials: The following are available online at http://www.mdpi.com/2072-6643/10/8/1028/s1, Table S1: Knowledge, attitudes, and practices related to salt intake according to sex, age, education, and hypertension treatment.

Author Contributions: Conceptualization, P.B. and M.A.-N. Study design and Methodology, P.B., D.H., A.D., N.M.B., and M.A.-N. Data Analysis, M.L. and P.B. Writing-Original Draft Preparation, M.L. and P.B. Writing-Review & Editing, C.M.-A., D.H., N.M.B., A.D., B.V., M.A.-N., J.O., and A.C. Supervision, P.B. and A.C. Project Administration, M.A.-N. and P.B. Funding Acquisition, M.A.-N. and P.B.

Funding: This research benefited partly from an unconditional seed grant by PepsiCo. M.L. led the analysis and writing of the manuscript during her PhD studies, which was funded by the Federal Food Safety and Veterinary Office.

Acknowledgments: The authors thank all the survey officers and collaborators involved in data collection as well as the participants.

Conflicts of Interest: The authors declare no conflict of interest. The funder had no role in the design of the study, in the collection, analyses, or interpretation of data, in the writing of the manuscript, or in the decision to publish the results.

References

1. World Health Organization. *Global Status Report on Noncommunicable Diseases*; World Health Organization: Geneva, Switzerland, 2014.
2. Mozaffarian, D.; Fahimi, S.; Singh, G.M.; Micha, R.; Khatibzadeh, S.; Engell, R.E.; Lim, S.; Danaei, G.; Ezzati, M.; Powles, J. Global Sodium Consumption and Death from Cardiovascular Causes. *N. Engl. J. Med.* **2014**, *371*, 624–634. [CrossRef] [PubMed]
3. Twagirumukiza, M.; Dirk, D.B.; Kips, J.G.; Guy, D.B.; Stichele, R.V.; Van Bortel, L.M. Current and Projected Prevalence of Arterial Hypertension in Sub-Saharan Africa by Sex, Age and Habitat: An Estimate from Population Studies. *J. Hypertens.* **2011**, *29*, 1243–1252. [CrossRef] [PubMed]
4. World Health Organization. *Global Action Plan for the Prevention and Control of Noncommunicable Diseases 2013–2020*; World Health Organization: Geneva, Switzerland, 2013.
5. The Shake Technical Package for Salt Reduction. Available online: http://apps.who.int/iris/bitstream/handle/10665/250135/9789241511346-eng.pdf;jsessionid=5BACD9B4917B297D370C440E99791E7A?sequence=1 (accessed on 6 August 2018).
6. He, F.J.; Macgregor, G.A. Salt and Sugar: Their Effects on Blood Pressure. *Pflugers Arch. Eur. J. Physiol.* **2015**, *467*, 577–586. [CrossRef] [PubMed]
7. Rees, K.; Dyakova, M.; Wilson, N.; Ward, K.; Thorogood, M.; Brunner, E. Dietary Advice for Reducing Cardiovascular Risk. *Cochrane Database Syst. Rev.* **2013**, *3*. [CrossRef]
8. Hooper, L.; Bartlett, C.; Davey, S.G.; Ebrahim, S. Advice to Reduce Dietary Salt for Prevention of Cardiovascular Disease. *Cochrane Database Syst. Rev.* **2004**, *3*. [CrossRef] [PubMed]

9.   World Health Organization. *Report of the 2015 Global NCD Survey*; World Health Organization: Geneva, Switzerland, 2016.

10.   Salaudeen, A.G.; Musa, O.I.; Babatunde, O.A.; Atoyebi, O.A.; Durowade, K.A.; Omokanye, L.O. Knowledge and Prevalence of Risk Factors for Arterial Hypertension and Blood Pressure Pattern among Bankers and Traffic Wardens in Ilorin, Nigeria. *Afr. Health Sci.* **2014**, *14*, 593–599. [CrossRef] [PubMed]

11.   Katibi, I.A.; Olarinoye, J.K.; Kuranga, S.A. Knowledge and Practice of Hypertensive Patients as Seen in a Tertiary Hospital in the Middle Belt of Nigeria. *Niger. J. Clin. Pract.* **2010**, *13*, 159–162. [PubMed]

12.   Becker, H.; Bester, M.; Reyneke, N.; Labadarios, D.; Monyeki, K.D.; Steyn, N.P. Nutrition Related Knowledge and Practices of Hypertensive Adults Attending Hypertensive Clinics at Day Hospitals in the Cape Metropole. *Curationis* **2004**, *27*, 63–69. [CrossRef] [PubMed]

13.   Aubert, L.; Bovet, P.; Gervasoni, J.P.; Rwebogora, A.; Waeber, B.; Paccaud, F. Knowledge, Attitudes, and Practices on Hypertension in a Country in Epidemiological Transition. *Hypertension* **1998**, *31*, 1136–1145. [CrossRef] [PubMed]

14.   Kaddumukasa, M.N.; Katabira, E.; Sajatovic, M.; Pundik, S.; Kaddumukasa, M.; Goldstein, L.B. Influence of Sodium Consumption and Associated Knowledge on Poststroke Hypertension in Uganda. *Neurology* **2016**, *87*, 1198–1205. [CrossRef] [PubMed]

15.   Olsen, M.H.; Angell, S.Y.; Asma, S.; Boutouyrie, P.; Burger, D.; Chirinos, J.A.; Damasceno, A.; Delles, C.; Gimenez-Roqueplo, A.P.; Hering, D.; et al. A Call to Action and a Lifecourse Strategy to Address the Global Burden of Raised Blood Pressure on Current and Future Generations: The Lancet Commission on Hypertension. *Lancet* **2016**, *388*, 2665–2712. [CrossRef]

16.   Mancia, G.; Oparil, S.; Whelton, P.K.; McKee, M.; Dominiczak, A.; Luft, F.C.; AlHabib, K.; Lanas, F.; Damasceno, A.; Prabhakaran, D.; et al. The Technical Report on Sodium Intake and Cardiovascular Disease in Low- and Middle-Income Countries by the Joint Working Group of the World Heart Federation, the European Society of Hypertension and the European Public Health Association. *Eur. Heart J.* **2017**, *38*, 712–719. [CrossRef] [PubMed]

17.   World Health Organization. *Who Steps Surveillance Manual*; World Health Organization: Geneva, Switzerland, 2008.

18.   Charlton, K.E.; Steyn, K.; Levitt, N.S.; Zulu, J.V.; Jonathan, D.; Veldman, F.J.; Nel, J.H. Diet and Blood Pressure in South Africa: Intake of Foods Containing Sodium, Potassium, Calcium, and Magnesium in Three Ethnic Groups. *Nutrition* **2005**, *21*, 39–50. [CrossRef] [PubMed]

19.   Department of Health. *Foodstuffs, Cosmetics and Disinfectants Act, 1972 (Act 54 of 1972): Regulations Relating to the Reduction in Certain Foodstuffs and Related Matters*; Government Gazette: Pretoria, South Africa, 2013.

20.   Charlton, K.; Webster, J.; Kowal, P. To Legislate or Not to Legislate? A Comparison of the UK and South African Approaches to the Development and Implementation of Salt Reduction Programs. *Nutrients* **2014**, *6*, 3672–3695. [CrossRef] [PubMed]

21.   Wang, G.; Labarthe, D. The Cost-Effectiveness of Interventions Designed to Reduce Sodium Intake. *J. Hypertens.* **2011**, *29*, 1693–1699. [CrossRef] [PubMed]

22.   Christoforou, A.; Trieu, K.; Land, M.A.; Bolam, B.; Webster, J. State-Level and Community-Level Salt Reduction Initiatives: A Systematic Review of Global Programmes and Their Impact. *J. Epidemiol. Public Health* **2016**, *70*, 1140–1150. [CrossRef] [PubMed]

23.   Trieu, K.; Neal, B.; Hawkes, C.; Dunford, E.; Campbell, N.; Rodriguez-Fernandez, R.; Legetic, B.; McLaren, L.; Barberio, A.; Webster, J. Salt Reduction Initiatives around the World—A Systematic Review of Progress Towards the Global Target. *PLoS ONE* **2015**, *10*, e0130247. [CrossRef] [PubMed]

24.   Webster, J.L.; Dunford, E.K.; Hawkes, C.; Neal, B.C. Salt Reduction Initiatives around the World. *J. Hypertens.* **2011**, *29*, 1043–1050. [CrossRef] [PubMed]

25.   Jessen, N.; Santos, A.; Damasceno, A.; Silva-Matos, C.; Severo, M.; Padrao, P.; Lunet, N. Knowledge and Behaviors Regarding Salt Intake in Mozambique. *Eur. J. Clin. Nutr.* **2018**, *1*. [CrossRef] [PubMed]

26.   Trieu, K.; McMahon, E.; Santos, J.A.; Bauman, A.; Jolly, K.A.; Bolam, B.; Webster, J. Review of Behaviour Change Interventions to Reduce Population Salt Intake. *Int. J. Behav. Nutr. Phys. Act.* **2017**, *14*. [CrossRef] [PubMed]

27.   Oyebode, O.; Oti, S.; Chen, Y.F.; Lilford, R.J. Salt Intakes in Sub-Saharan Africa: A Systematic Review and Meta-Regression. *Popul. Health Metr.* **2016**, *14*. [CrossRef] [PubMed]

28. Melse-Boonstra, A.; Rozendaal, M.; Rexwinkel, H.; Gerichhausen, M.J.; van den Briel, T.; Bulux, J.; Solomons, N.W.; West, C.E. Determination of Discretionary Salt Intake in Rural Guatemala and Benin to Determine the Iodine Fortification of Salt Required to Control Iodine Deficiency Disorders: Studies Using Lithium-Labeled Salt. *Am. J. Clin. Nutr.* **1998**, *68*, 636–641. [CrossRef] [PubMed]

29. Poulter, N.R.; Khaw, K.T.; Mugambi, M.; Peart, W.S.; Sever, P.S. Migration-Induced Changes in Blood Pressure: A Controlled Longitudinal Study. *Clin. Exp. Pharmacol. Physiol.* **1985**, *12*, 211–216. [CrossRef]

30. Mizehoun-Adissoda, C.; Houinato, D.; Houehanou, C.; Chianea, T.; Dalmay, F.; Bigot, A.; Aboyans, V.; Preux, P.M.; Bovet, P.; Desport, J.C. Dietary Sodium and Potassium Intakes: Data from Urban and Rural Areas. *Nutrition* **2017**, *33*, 35–41. [CrossRef] [PubMed]

31. Queiroz, A.; Damasceno, A.; Jessen, N.; Novela, C.; Moreira, P.; Lunet, N.; Padrao, P. Urinary Sodium and Potassium Excretion and Dietary Sources of Sodium in Maputo, Mozambique. *Nutrients* **2017**, *9*, 830. [CrossRef] [PubMed]

32. Powles, J.; Fahimi, S.; Micha, R.; Khatibzadeh, S.; Shi, P.; Ezzati, M.; Engell, R.E.; Lim, S.S.; Danaei, G.; Mozaffarian, D. Global, Regional and National Sodium Intakes in 1990 and 2010: A Systematic Analysis of 24 H Urinary Sodium Excretion and Dietary Surveys Worldwide. *BMJ Open* **2013**, *3*, e003733. [CrossRef] [PubMed]

33. World Health Organization. *Guideline: Sodium Intake for Adults and Children*; World Health Organization: Geneva, Switzerland, 2012.

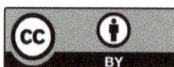

nutrients

MDPI

Article

Lactase Persistence, Milk Intake, and Adult Acne: A Mendelian Randomization Study of 20,416 Danish Adults

Christian R. Juhl [1], Helle K. M. Bergholdt [2], Iben M. Miller [3], Gregor B. E. Jemec [3], Jørgen K. Kanters [1,*]and Christina Ellervik [2,4,5,6,*]

[1] Department of Biomedical Sciences, Faculty of Health and Medical Sciences, University of Copenhagen, 2100 Copenhagen, Denmark; christian.r.juhl@gmail.com
[2] Department of Production, Research, and Innovation, Region Zealand, 4180 Sorø, Denmark; hellebergholdt@hotmail.com
[3] Department of Dermatology, Zealand University Hospital, 4000 Roskilde, Denmark; miller@dadlnet.dk (I.M.M.); gbj@regionsjaelland.dk (G.B.E.J.)
[4] Department of Clinical Medicine, Faculty of Health and Medical Sciences, University of Copenhagen, 2100 Copenhagen, Denmark
[5] Department of Laboratory Medicine, Boston Children's Hospital, 300 Longwood Avenue, Boston, MA 02115, USA
[6] Department of Pathology, Harvard Medical School, Boston, MA 02115, USA
* Correspondence: jkanters@sund.ku.dk (J.K.K.); christina@ellervik.dk or christina.ellervik@childrens.harvard.edu (C.E.)

Received: 15 July 2018; Accepted: 3 August 2018; Published: 8 August 2018

Abstract: Whether there is a causal relationship between milk intake and acne is unknown. We tested the hypothesis that genetically determined milk intake is associated with acne in adults using a Mendelian randomization design. *LCT-13910 C/T* (rs4988235) is associated with lactase persistence (*TT/TC*) in Northern Europeans. We investigated the association between milk intake, *LCT-13910 C/T* (rs4988235), and acne in 20,416 adults (age-range: 20–96) from The Danish General Suburban Population Study (GESUS). The adjusted observational odds ratio for acne in any milk intake vs. no milk intake was 0.93(95% confidence interval: 0.48–1.78) in females and 0.49(0.22–1.08) in males aged 20–39 years, and 1.15(95% confidence interval: 0.66–1.99) in females and 1.02(0.61–1.72) in males above 40 years. The unadjusted odds ratio for acne in TT+TC vs. CC was 0.84(0.43–1.62) in the age group 20–39 years, and 0.99(0.52–1.88) above 40 years. We did not find any observational or genetic association between milk intake and acne in our population of adults.

Keywords: acne; acne vulgaris; milk; dairy; diet; Mendelian randomization; adults

1. Introduction

Acne is a common chronic inflammatory skin disease, which is almost universal in adolescence, with rates up to 85% [1–4]. After adolescence the prevalence decreases but a significant number of patients are affected by persistent acne or develop new-onset adult acne [5]. Acne is overall characterized by open comedones, papules, pustules, and nodules [6], but the clinical appearance varies by age and lifestyle [5,7,8].

The genetic architecture of acne vulgaris is complex and multiple susceptible loci have been identified reflecting the multifactorial pathogenesis of acne involving the innate immune system, inflammation, modified lipogenesis, and androgens [9,10]. But there is likely also an environmental component in the development of acne vulgaris. Several observational studies have investigated the association of milk intake with acne in children, adolescents, and young adults [11–16]. However, no previous observational study has been performed in all adult ages.

In individuals of Northern European descent, the genetic variant *LCT-13910 C/T* (rs4988235) located 13,910 base pairs upstream of the lactase (*LCT*) gene on chromosome 2q21-22, within intron 13 of the adjacent *MCM6* gene, shows complete correlation with lactase persistence/non-persistence [17]. The T-allele is the lactase-persistent allele, whereas the C allele is the lactase non-persistent allele. The inheritance is autosomal recessive manner such that individuals homozygous for CC are unable to digest lactose, whereas individuals with TC or TT are able to digest lactose.

To investigate whether there is a causal relationship between milk intake and acne, large long-term randomized trials would be needed, but these are costly and it is difficult to uphold the randomization over time. Instead the epidemiological Mendelian randomization (MR) design offers a feasible alternative [18]. The underlying principle in the MR design is that genetic variants are randomly assorted during gamete formation, which is similar to the random assignment of patients to placebo or active treatment in a clinical intervention trial. In the MR design, confounders are, therefore, balanced across the genotypes, and the genotypes will serve as a proxy for lifelong exposure.

In this study, we used the Mendelian randomization design to investigate the long-term effect of milk intake on acne using the lactase persistent (TT + TC)/non-persistent(CC) *LCT-13910* C/T genotype in 20,416 adult individuals from The Danish General Population study (GESUS).

2. Materials and Methods

2.1. Participants

The cross-sectional population study The Danish General Population Study (GESUS) was conducted from January 2010 to October 2013 in Naestved Municipality, Denmark [19]. Criteria for invitation were age 20+, Danish citizenship and Danish Civil Registration number (CPR number).

All persons aged 30+ were invited and in the age group 20–30 years only a random 25% selection were invited. 21,205 adults were enrolled, with an overall participation rate of 43%.

In this present study, 20,850 persons was included of whom 98.9% were of Danish descent and the rest other Scandinavian or European descent. Individuals with missing values for acne diagnosis (*n* = 53) or *LCT-13910 C/T* genotyping (*n* = 381) were excluded, resulting in inclusion of 20,416 people.

A prerequisite for attending the health examination was a completed self-reported paper-questionnaire about demographic information, medical history, smoking, skin-condition, and food intake, among others. The health examination was performed by trained health professionals and took place at the department of clinical biochemistry at Naestved University Hospital, Denmark. Body mass index (BMI) was calculated as kg/m^2. Details about the study design of GESUS have been described elsewhere [19].

Written informed consent was obtained from all participants. The study conforms to the principles of the Declaration of Helsinki and is approved by the institutional review board, the ethical committee of Region Zealand (SJ-113, SJ-114, SJ-191) and the Danish Data Protection Agency.

2.2. Milk Intake

Intake of milk was reported in the questionnaire as: "How much milk do you averagely consume per week?" and the possible answers were glasses of whole milk (3.5% fat), semi-skimmed milk (0.5–1.5% fat), skimmed milk (0.1–0.3% fat), butter milk, and lactose free milk. A blank response in one variable was set as no intake, when any of the other variables were filled. Extreme values were confirmed/deferred by contacting the participants by phone [19]. Milk intake was divided into categorical variables, based on glasses of milk per day. Dichotomized variables for types of milk intake were performed to compare no milk intake with intake of low-fat (0.1–0.3%) and high-fat milk (0.5–3.5%).

2.3. Acne Diagnosis

The acne diagnosis was based on the self-reported questionnaire validated by Dalgard et al. [20] The questions in the questionnaire were as follows: "During the last week, have you had any of the following complaints?" one of the complaints was pimples and the possible answers were: No (0); Yes, a little (1); Yes, quite a lot (2) or Yes, very much (3). The criteria used for the diagnosis of acne was answering "Yes, quite a lot (2)" or "Yes, very much (3)". The validation study by Dalgard et al. showed a high specificity (96%) for a non-healthcare seeking population, but a low sensitivity (<50%) [20].

2.4. Genotyping

Every participant in the GESUS study was genotyped for *LCT-13910 C/T* variant (rs4988235). The genotyping was done by KASPar allelic discrimination (LGC Genomics) with a call rate of 99% [21]. The genotype *LCT-13910* TC and TT are lactase persistent and CC lactase non-persistent. The *LCT-13910* C/T genotype distribution, in the GESUS population, was in Hardy-Weinberg equilibrium (Supplementary Table S1).

2.5. Statistical Analyses

Statistical analyses were performed in SAS Enterprise Guide 7.1 (SAS institute Inc., Cary, NS, USA). The descriptive statistics of all the continuous variables showed normal distributions, except for milk intake. Transformation of the variable was performed, but this did not improve normal distribution substantially. Milk intake was instead categorized into quantiles (0, 1–3, 4–7, 8–14, >14 glasses/week) and dichotomized variables were performed for total milk, low-fat milk and high-fat milk. (any vs. none). Chi-square test and analysis of variance (ANOVA) was used to test relationships for categorical variables and differences in means. A p-value < 0.05 was considered significant. The Mendelian randomization design consisted of three analyses: First, logistic regressions were performed to test the observational associations of milk intake and acne. The logistic regressions were stratified by age, based on an empirical data description of milk intake and acne diagnosis (Supplementary Table S2). This resulted in the two age groups; 20–39 years and 40+ years. Furthermore, stratification by gender was performed, because of interaction with milk intake ($p = 0.003$) The logistic regressions were performed both unadjusted and adjusted for age, body mass index (BMI) and smoking, as BMI and smoking are related to acne in the literature [22,23]. Second, the median milk intake was studied for the *LCT-13910* C/T genotypes and the difference was tested with the Kruskal-Wallis test. Finally, logistic regressions were performed for the *LCT-13910* C/T genotypes and acne. An interaction test was performed for milk intake (no/yes) and lactase genotype in an additive (*TT; TC; CC*) and dominant (*TT/TC; CC*) model in both age groups.

2.6. Meta-Analysis of Acne in Adults

The aim was to meta-analyze the association between milk intake and acne in adults.

The search was performed on 11 December 2017 and included all studies up until that date. Studies were identified in the PubMed database using the search terms: ("Dairy products"[Mesh] OR "dairy"[All Fields] OR "milk"[Mesh] OR "milk"[All Fields] OR yogurt[All Fields] OR cheese[All Fields] OR lifestyle[All Fields]) AND ("Acne Vulgaris"[Mesh] OR "Acne"[All Fields]). We identified 241 records. Inclusion criteria was mean age ≥ 30 years, case (acne) and control (non-acne) groups, and information on odds ratio (95%CI) or raw numbers to calculate the odds ratio. Milk intake was defined as binary (yes, no), low-fat (yes/no), or high-fat (whole) milk (yes/no). We identified two studies of milk intake and adult acne [24,25], but only study met the inclusion criteria for case-control group design [25] which we meta-analyzed with our own results. We calculated pooled fixed and random effects odds ratios.

3. Results

3.1. Baseline Characteristics

Baseline characteristics of the 20,416 participants by acne, age group and *LCT-13910* genotype are presented in Table 1 and Supplementary Table S2. The acne group consisted of 303 participants, which were significantly younger, had a higher percentage of smokers, as well as a higher mean milk intake. The group aged 20–39 years had significantly fewer men, lower BMI, higher prevalence of acne, and a higher milk intake, compared to the group aged 40+. The lactase genotype groups were significantly different, with a higher BMI and milk intake in the lactase persistent TC/TT genotypes, compared to the lactase non-persistent genotype (CC).

3.2. Milk Intake and Acne

The adjusted observational odds ratio for acne in individuals with any milk intake vs. no milk intake was 0.93(95% confidence interval: 0.48–1.78) in females and 0.49(0.22–1.08) in males aged 20–39 years, and 1.15(95% confidence interval: 0.66–1.99) in females and 1.02(0.61–1.72) in males above 40 years (Tables 2 and 3). Results were similar for unadjusted analyses.

3.3. Lactase Genotype and Milk Intake

In the age group 20–39 years, the median milk intake (Table 4) for the lactase persistent genotypes was 10 glasses/week (inter-quantile range (IQR) [4:16]) for TT and 10 glasses/week [3:16] for TC compared to 7 glasses/week [2:14] for the non-persistent lactase genotype CC ($p = 6.32 \times 10^{-4}$). In the age group 40+ (Table 4), results were similar but attenuated with a median milk intake of 5 glasses/week [IQR: 0:10] for TT and 6 glasses/week [0:14] for TC compared to 3 glasses/week [0:14] for CC ($p = 3.78 \times 10^{-12}$).

3.4. Lactase Genotype and Acne

The unadjusted odds ratio for acne in individuals with the lactase persistent genotypes TC/TT vs. the lactase non-persistent genotype CC was 0.84 (0.43:1.62) in the age group 20–39 years, and 0.99 (0.52–1.88) above 40 years. (Table 5). No interactions were found for the lactase genotype and milk (no/yes) for both the additive and dominant model, in both age groups.

3.5. Meta-Analysis of Milk Intake and Adult Acne

Combining all age groups in our own study with the study by Landro [25], the pooled fixed effects odds ratios for acne was 1.04(0.79–1.37) for any milk intake (yes/no), 1.05(0.70–1.58) for whole milk, and 1.02(0.78–1.34) for low-fat milk intake (Table 6).

Table 1. Baseline characteristics for The Danish General Suburban Population study (GESUS) by acne, age groups, and *LCT-13910* genotype.

	All n = 20,416 100%	Acne n = 303 1.5%	Control n = 20,113 98.5%	p-Value *	Age 20–39 n = 2742 13.4%	Age > 40 n = 17,674 86.6%	p-Value *	LCT-13910 Genotype CC n = 1246 6.1%	TC n = 7377 36.1%	TT n = 11,793 57.8%	p-Value **
Acne, n (%)	303 (1.5)	-	-	-	141 (5.1)	162 (0.9)	<0.0001	20 (1.6)	119 (1.6)	164 (1.4)	0.4523
Age, mean (SD), years	56.3 (13.6)	44.2 (13.2)	56.5 (13.5)	<0.0001	35.0 (4.0)	59.7 (11.3)	<0.0001	55.7 (13.2)	56.4 (13.6)	56.4 (13.6)	0.1892
Age: 20–39, n (%)	2742 (13.4)	141 (46.5)	2601 (12.9)	<0.0001	-	-	-	166 (6.1)	955 (34.8)	1621 (59.1)	0.2851
Age: > 40, n (%)	17674 (86.6)	162 (53.5)	17512 (87.1)	<0.0001	-	-	-	1080 (6.1)	6422 (36.3)	10172 (57.6)	
Men, n (%)	9294 (45.5)	125 (41.3)	9169 (44.9)	0.1327	1193 (43.5)	8101 (45.8)	0.0228	540 (43.3)	3332 (45.2)	5422 (46.0)	0.1522
Body Mass Index, mean (SD), kg/m²	26.7 (4.7)	26.9 (5.6)	26.7 (4.7)	0.4549	25.9 (4.9)	26.9 (4.6)	<0.0001	26.5 (4.7)	26.6 (4.6)	26.8 (4.7)	0.0290
Current Smoker, n (%)	3632 (17.8)	75 (24.8)	3557 (17.7)	0.0014	490 (17.9)	3142 (17.8)	0.9060	233 (18.7)	1318 (17.9)	2081 (17.7)	0.6371
Milk Intake, mean (SD), glasses/week	8.1 (9.1)	10.2 (14.3)	8.1 (9.0)	<0.0001	11.0 (9.9)	7.7 (8.9)	<0.0001	6.1 (7.1)	8.2 (9.1)	8.3 (9.4)	<0.0001

* The chi-square test or the analysis of variance (ANOVA) test is used to calculate the p-value. ** Rao-Scott modified chi-square test is used for categorized variables and ANOVA for continuous variables. *LCT-13910* genotype (rs4988235): CC = the lactase non-persistent genotype, TC/TT = the lactase persistent genotype.

Table 2. Odds ratio for acne by milk intake in the age group 20–39 years.

Milk Intake (glasses/week)	Female						Male					
			Unadjusted		Adjusted *				Unadjusted		Adjusted *	
	n Total	n Acne	OR [95% CI]	p	OR [95% CI]	p	n Total	n Acne	OR [95% CI]	p	OR [95% CI]	p
0	172	11	1.00	-	1.00	-	122	8	1.00	-	1.00	-
1-3	274	19	1.09 [0.51:2.35]	0.82	0.98 [0.45:2.13]	0.96	147	4	0.40 [0.12:1.36]	0.14	0.43 [0.13:1.47]	0.18
4-7	375	25	1.05 [0.50:2.18]	0.91	0.98 [0.47:2.06]	0.96	186	11	0.90 [0.35:2.29]	0.82	0.93 [0.36:2.41]	0.89
8-14	397	25	0.98 [0.47:2.05]	0.96	0.90 [0.43:1.90]	0.79	322	7	0.32 [0.11:0.89]	0.03	0.36 [0.13:1.02]	0.06
>14	331	20	0.94 [0.44:2.01]	0.88	0.85 [0.39:1.83]	0.67	416	11	0.39 [0.15:0.98]	0.05	0.40 [0.16:1.02]	0.05
Any	1377	89	1.01 [0.53:1.93]	0.97	0.93 [0.48:1.78]	0.82	1071	33	0.45 [0.20:1.00]	0.05	0.49 [0.22:1.08]	0.08
Low-fat **	1348	85	0.83 [0.47:1.48]	0.53	0.84 [0.47:1.52]	0.57	1031	31	0.47 [0.23:0.98]	0.04	0.49 [0.23:1.03]	0.06
High-fat ***	58	7	2.06 [0.91:4.67]	0.08	1.42 [0.55:3.69]	0.47	82	5	1.94 [0.74:5.08]	0.18	2.01 [0.75:5.38]	0.17

* Adjusted for age, smoking and body mass index, ** Low-fat (0.1–0.3%), *** High-fat (0.5–3.5%). p-values are calculated as analysis of maximum likelihood estimates.

Table 3. Odds ratio for acne by milk intake for in the age group ≥40 years.

Milk Intake (glasses/week)	Female						Male					
			Unadjusted		Adjusted *				Unadjusted		Adjusted *	
	n Total	n Acne	OR [95% CI]	p	OR [95% CI]	p	n Total	n Acne	OR [95% CI]	p	OR [95% CI]	p
0	2802	17	1.00	-	1.00	-	2099	20	1.00	-	1.00	-
1-3	1564	16	1.69 [0.85:3.36]	0.13	1.30 [0.65:2.59]	0.46	1099	10	0.95 [0.45:2.05]	0.90	0.91 [0.42:1.96]	0.80
4-7	2129	22	1.71 [0.91:3.23]	0.10	1.40 [0.74:2.65]	0.31	1592	13	0.86 [0.42:1.73]	0.66	0.82 [0.40:1.68]	0.59
8-14	1816	11	1.00 [0.47:2.14]	1.00	0.76 [0.35:1.63]	0.48	1682	23	1.44 [0.79:2.63]	0.23	1.31 [0.71:2.43]	0.39
>14	1262	12	1.57 [0.75:3.30]	0.23	1.13 [0.53:2.40]	0.75	1629	18	1.16 [0.61:2.20]	0.65	0.99 [0.51:1.91]	0.97
Any	6771	61	1.49 [0.87:2.55]	0.15	1.15 [0.66:1.99]	0.62	6002	64	1.12 [0.68:1.86]	0.66	1.02 [0.61:1.72]	0.94
Low-fat **	6324	58	1.49 [0.90:2.49]	0.12	1.14 [0.68:1.91]	0.63	5268	57	1.14 [0.72:1.80]	0.59	0.98 [0.61:1.58]	0.94
High-fat ***	590	4	0.82 [0.30:2.26]	0.70	0.97 [0.35:2.68]	0.95	901	10	1.08 [0.56:2.10]	0.82	1.25 [0.64:2.46]	0.51

* Adjusted for age, smoking and body mass index, ** Low-fat (0.1–0.3%), *** High-fat (0.5–3.5%). p-values are calculated as analysis of maximum likelihood estimates.

Table 4. Differences in milk intake, glasses per week, by the *LCT-13910 C/T* genotype.

LCT-13910 Genotype	Lactase	n	%	Median	IQR	Kruskal-Wallis Test	
Age Group 20–39 Years							
CC	Non-persistent	166	6	7	[2:14]	Chi-Square	14.73
TC	Persistent	955	35	10	[3:16]	DF	2
TT	Persistent	1621	59	10	[4:16]	P	6.32×10^{-4}
Age Group ≥ 40 Years							
CC	Non-persistent	1080	6	3	[0:14]	Chi-Square	52.83
TC	Persistent	6422	36	6	[0:14]	DF	2
TT	Persistent	10,172	58	5	[0:10]	P	3.38×10^{-12}

IQR: Inter-quartile range.

Table 5. Odds ratio for acne by *LCT-13910 C/T* genotypes.

LCT-13910 C/T Genotype	Median Milk Intake [IQR]				
	Glasses/Week	*n* Total	*n* Acne	OR [95% CI]	*p*-Value
Age Group 20–39 Years					
CC	7 [2:14]	166	10	1	-
TC	10 [3:16]	955	50	0.86 [0.43:1.74]	0.68
TT	10 [4:16]	1621	81	0.82 [0.42:1.62]	0.57
TC/TT	10 [3:16]	2576	131	0.84 [0.43:1.62]	0.60
LCT gene (additive model) × milk (no/yes) interaction test					0.36
LCT gene (dominant model) × milk (no/yes) interaction test					0.15
Age Group ≥ 40 Years					
CC	3 [0:10]	1080	10	1	-
TC	6 [0:14]	6422	69	1.16 [0.60:2.26]	0.67
TT	5 [0:14]	10,172	83	0.88 [0.46:1.70]	0.70
TC/TT	5 [0:14]	16,594	152	0.99 [0.52:1.88]	0.97
LCT gene (additive model) × milk (no/yes) interaction test					0.32
LCT gene (dominant model) × milk (no/yes) interaction test					0.37

Table 6. Meta-analysis of milk intake and acne in adults.

Dairy	Author	Year	OR	Low 95% CI	Upper 95% CI	*p*-Value
Any intake	Di Landro [25]	2016	0.88	0.61	1.28	0.52
Any intake	Juhl	Current	1.27	0.84	1.92	0.26
Fixed effects pooled odds ratio			1.04	0.79	1.37	0.78
Random effects pooled odds ratio			1.05	0.74	1.49	0.80
Whole milk	Di Landro [25]	2016	0.84	0.49	1.44	0.53
Whole milk	Juhl	Current	1.43	0.76	2.70	0.27
Fixed effects pooled odds ratio			1.05	0.70	1.58	0.82
Random effects pooled odds ratio			1.07	0.64	1.79	0.81
Low-fat milk	Di Landro [25]	2016	0.90	0.61	1.32	0.59
Low-fat milk	Juhl	Current	1.15	0.79	1.68	0.47
Fixed effects pooled odds ratio			1.02	0.78	1.34	0.89
Random effects pooled odds ratio			1.02	0.78	1.34	0.89

4. Discussion

Among 20,419 adults from the Danish general population we found no association between milk intake and acne, observationally or genetically using the lactase persistent/non-persistent *LCT-13910 C/T* genotype in a Mendelian randomization design.

In the Mendelian randomization design the genetic variant is used as a proxy for the long-term differences in milk intake, thereby largely avoiding confounding and reverse causation, which can blur or distort the underlying true association in observational studies [18]. The *LCT-13910* fulfilled the requirements for using the Mendelian randomization design, as the variant is linked to the intermediate phenotype (milk intake) in a biologically explainable way [17], there is no known pleiotropic effects of the variant, and the variant was not associated with confounders. The Mendelian randomization design mimics a randomized clinical trial and takes advantage of the random assortment of alleles at conception which ensures random distribution of confounding factors thereby circumventing reverse causation and most confounding. Thus, the Mendelian randomization design provides an estimate of the long-term effect of milk intake on acne.

We showed that both the milk consumption and the acne diagnosis declined with age, and that fewer people drank milk as age increased. Nevertheless, we found a crude prevalence of self-reported acne of 6%. We also investigated milk intake and acne among adults by combining our current study with findings from Landro , but the associations were still null for any milk intake, whole milk, and low-fat milk. In contrast, observational studies of mostly childhood and adolescent acne have debated, but largely favored, the association between milk intake and acne [11–13,16,26–29]. These studies were heterogeneous with respect to geographical location, cultural dairy influence, gender, sample size, reporting of dairy frequency and type, and the ascertainment of participants (dermatology clinics, general population study, online questionnaire). Some of the studies did not run adjusted analyses [16,26,27], thus confounding may account for the associations. However, reasons for the discrepant findings between our study and the study by Landro [25] in adults versus the studies in adolescent acne [11–13,16,26–29] could also be related to different pathogenesis and the appearance of acne in different age groups. Milk intake increases levels of insulin-like growth factor-1 (IGF1), which is hypothesized to be a central link between milk intake and stimulation of the sebaceous gland [30]. Thus, as people age and drink less milk, they may be less exposed to IGF1 and, therefore, also less prone to the development of acne. The appearance of acne varies by age, such that acne precox and acne tarda are mostly variants with predominant inflammatory papules, pustules and nodules at the lower face half [5,31], while adolescent acne is mostly characterized by comedoes and papules/pustules at the entire face (chest and back) [7]. In contrast, acne in adult smokers is characterized by comedoes and scars [8] and acne fulminans exhibits a severe clinical picture [32]. Even though the acne diagnosis was questionnaire based as in many previous observational studies [16,28], it has been validated in a comparable setting with a high specificity but with a sensitivity of only 50% [20]. However, we did not have information on anatomical acne location or longer period of acne appearance. Additionally, our study spanned four years including all seasons, thereby compensating for seasonal variation in acne appearance [33].

The strength of our study is the homogenous population of largely Danish descent or other Scandinavian descent making confounding from population substructure less likely. Similarly, the rs4988235 variant is the most common lactase persistent variant in populations of Northern European descent, despite the many other lactase persistence haplotypes [34]. A limitation of our study included the low prevalence of lactase non-persistence (6%) and the fact that some of these individuals drank milk, which could offset and conceal a true association. Milk consumption was based on self-reported questionnaire data, with possible recall bias.

5. Conclusions

In conclusion, in the Danish General Suburban Population Study (GESUS) of adults we did not find any observational or genetic association between milk intake and acne using the lactase persistent/non-persistent *LCT-13910* C/T genotype in a Mendelian randomization design.

Supplementary Materials: The following are available online at http://www.mdpi.com/2072-6643/10/8/1041/s1, Table S1: Hardy-Weinberg equilibrium test; Table S2: Characteristics by age groups.

Author Contributions: Conceptualization, C.E., G.B.J., H.K.M.B., I.M.M., C.R.J., J.K.K.; Methodology, C.E., G.B.J., H.K.M.B., I.M.M., C.R.J., J.K.K.; Formal Analysis, C.R.J. , J.K.K., C.E.; Data Curation, C.E. and H.K.M.B.; Writing-Original Draft Preparation, C.R.J.; Writing-Review & Editing, C.E., G.B.J., H.K.M.B., I.M.M., C.R.J., J.K.K.; Visualization, C.R.J.; Supervision, C.E., G.B.J., H.K.M.B., I.M.M., C.R.J., J.K.K.; Project Administration, C.E., C.R.J., J.K.K.; Funding Acquisition, G.B.J., C.E., J.K.K.

Funding: C.R.J. was funded by Region Zealand. The Danish General Suburban Population Study was funded by the Region Zealand Foundation, Naestved Hospital Foundation, Edith and Henrik Henriksens Memorial Scholarship, Johan and Lise Boserup Foundation, TrygFonden, Johannes Fog's Foundation, Region Zealand, Naestved Hospital, The National Board of Health, and the Local Government Denmark Foundation.

Conflicts of Interest: The authors declare no conflict of interest. HKMB was partly funded by the Danish Dairy Research Foundation from 2012–2015; the foundation was not involved in this study.

References

1. White, G.M. Recent findings in the epidemiologic evidence, classification, and subtypes of acne vulgaris. *J. Am. Acad. Dermatol.* **1998**, *39*, S34–S37. [CrossRef]

2. Bhate, K.; Williams, H.C. Epidemiology of acne vulgaris. *Br. J. Dermatol.* **2013**, *168*, 474–485. [CrossRef] [PubMed]
3. Gollnick, H.; Cunliffe, W.; Berson, D.; Dreno, B.; Finlay, A.; Leyden, J.J.; Shalita, A.R.; Thiboutot, D. Management of acne: A report from a Global Alliance to Improve Outcomes in Acne. *J. Am. Acad. Dermatol.* **2003**, *49*, S1–S37. [CrossRef] [PubMed]
4. Ghodsi, S.Z.; Orawa, H.; Zouboulis, C.C. Prevalence, severity, and severity risk factors of acne in high school pupils: A community-based study. *J. Invest. Dermatol.* **2009**, *129*, 2136–2141. [CrossRef] [PubMed]
5. Perkins, A.C.; Maglione, J.; Hillebrand, G.G.; Miyamoto, K.; Kimball, A.B. Acne vulgaris in women: Prevalence across the life span. *J. Womens Health* **2012**, *21*, 223–230. [CrossRef] [PubMed]
6. Williams, H.C.; Dellavalle, R.P.; Garner, S. Acne vulgaris. *Lancet* **2012**, *379*, 361–372. [CrossRef]
7. Tuchayi, S.M.; Makrantonaki, E.; Ganceviciene, R.; Dessinioti, C.; Feldman, S.R.; Zouboulis, C.C. Acne vulgaris. *Nat. Rev. Dis. Primers* **2015**, *1*, 15029. [CrossRef] [PubMed]
8. Capitanio, B.; Sinagra, J.L.; Bordignon, V.; Fei, P.C.; Picardo, M.; Zouboulis, C.C. Underestimated clinical features of postadolescent acne. *J. Am. Acad. Dermatol.* **2010**, *63*, 782–788. [CrossRef] [PubMed]
9. Lichtenberger, R.; Simpson, M.A.; Smith, C.; Barker, J.; Navarini, A.A. Genetic architecture of acne vulgaris. *J. Eur. Acad. Dermatol. Venereol.* **2017**, *31*, 1978–1990. [CrossRef] [PubMed]
10. Zouboulis, C.C.; Jourdan, E.; Picardo, M. Acne is an inflammatory disease and alterations of sebum composition initiate acne lesions. *J. Eur. Acad. Dermatol. Venereol.* **2014**, *28*, 527–532. [CrossRef] [PubMed]
11. Adebamowo, C.A.; Spiegelman, D.; Danby, F.W.; Frazier, A.L.; Willett, W.C.; Holmes, M.D. High school dietary dairy intake and teenage acne. *J. Am. Acad. Dermatol.* **2005**, *52*, 207–214. [CrossRef] [PubMed]
12. Adebamowo, C.A.; Spiegelman, D.; Berkey, C.S.; Danby, F.W.; Rockett, H.H.; Colditz, G.A.; Walter, C.W.; Michelle, D.H. Milk consumption and acne in adolescent girls. *Dermatol. Online J.* **2006**, *12*, 1. [PubMed]
13. Adebamowo, C.A.; Spiegelman, D.; Berkey, C.S.; Danby, F.W.; Rockett, H.H.; Colditz, G.A.; Willett, W.C.; Holmes, M.D. Milk consumption and acne in teenaged boys. *J. Am. Acad. Dermatol.* **2008**, *58*, 787–793. [CrossRef] [PubMed]
14. Grossi, E.; Cazzaniga, S.; Crotti, S.; Naldi, L.; Di Landro, A.; Ingordo, V.; Cusano, F.; Atzori, L.; Tripodi Cutrì, F.; Musumeci, M.L.; et al. The constellation of dietary factors in adolescent acne: A semantic connectivity map approach. *J. Eur. Acad. Dermatol. Venereol.* **2016**, *30*, 96–100. [CrossRef] [PubMed]
15. Karadag, A.S.; Balta, I.; Saricaoglu, H.; Kilic, S.; Kelekci, K.H.; Yildirim, M.; Arica, D.A.; Öztürk, S.; Karaman, G.; Çerman, A.A.; et al. The effect of personal, familial, and environmental characteristics on acne vulgaris: A prospective, multicenter, case controlled study from Turkey. *G. Ital. Dermatol. Venereol.* **2017**. [CrossRef]
16. Wolkenstein, P.; Machovcova, A.; Szepietowski, J.C.; Tennstedt, D.; Veraldi, S.; Delarue, A. Acne prevalence and associations with lifestyle: A cross-sectional online survey of adolescents/young adults in 7 European countries. *J. Eur. Acad. Dermatol. Venereol.* **2017**. [CrossRef] [PubMed]
17. Enattah, N.S.; Sahi, T.; Savilahti, E.; Terwilliger, J.D.; Peltonen, L.; Järvelä, I. Identification of a variant associated with adult-type hypolactasia. *Nat. Genet.* **2002**, *30*, 233–247. [CrossRef] [PubMed]
18. Smith, G.D.; Ebrahim, S. Mendelian randomization: Prospects, potentials, and limitations. *Int. J. Epidemiol.* **2004**, *33*, 30–42. [CrossRef] [PubMed]
19. Bergholdt, H.K.M.; Bathum, L.; Kvetny, J.; Rasmussen, D.B.; Moldow, B.; Hoeg, T.; Jemec, G.B.E.; Berner-Nielsen, H.; Nordestgaard, B.G.; Ellervik, C. Study design, participation and characteristics of the Danish General Suburban Population Study. *Dan. Med. J.* **2013**, *60*, A4693. [PubMed]
20. Dalgard, F.; Svensson, A.; Holm, J.O.; Sundby, J. Self-reported skin complaints: validation of a questionnaire for population surveys. *Br. J. Dermatol.* **2003**, *149*, 794–810. [CrossRef] [PubMed]
21. Bergholdt, H.K.M.; Nordestgaard, B.G.; Varbo, A.; Ellervik, C. Milk intake is not associated with ischaemic heart disease in observational or Mendelian randomization analyses in 98 529 Danish adults. *Int. J. Epidemiol.* **2015**, *44*, 587–603. [CrossRef] [PubMed]
22. Jemec, G.B.; Linneberg, A.; Nielsen, N.H.; Frolund, L.; Madsen, F.; Jorgensen, T. Have oral contraceptives reduced the prevalence of acne? A population-based study of acne vulgaris, tobacco smoking and oral contraceptives. *Dermatology* **2002**, *204*, 179–184. [CrossRef] [PubMed]
23. Alan, S.; Cenesizoglu, E. Effects of hyperandrogenism and high body mass index on acne severity in women. *Saudi Med. J.* **2014**, *35*, 886–889. [PubMed]

24. Dreno, B.; Thiboutot, D.; Layton, A.M.; Berson, D.; Perez, M.; Kang, S. Large-scale international study enhances understanding of an emerging acne population: Adult females. *J. Eur. Acad. Dermatol. Venereol.* **2015**, *29*, 1096–1106. [CrossRef] [PubMed]

25. Di Landro, A.; Cazzaniga, S.; Cusano, F.; Bonci, A.; Carla, C.; Musumeci, M.L.; Patrizi, A.; Bettoli, V.; Pezzarossa, E.; Caproni, M.; et al. Adult female acne and associated risk factors: Results of a multicenter case-control study in Italy. *J. Am. Acad. Dermatol.* **2016**, *75*, 1134–1141. [CrossRef] [PubMed]

26. Wolkenstein, P.; Misery, L.; Amici, J.M.; Maghia, R.; Branchoux, S.; Cazeau, C.; Voisard, J.-J.; Taïeb, C. Smoking and dietary factors associated with moderate-to-severe acne in French adolescents and young adults: results of a survey using a representative sample. *Dermatology* **2015**, *230*, 34–39. [CrossRef] [PubMed]

27. Di Landro, A.; Cazzaniga, S.; Parazzini, F.; Ingordo, V.; Cusano, F.; Atzori, L.; Cutrì, F.T.; Musumeci, M.L.; Zinetti, C.; Pezzarossa, E.; et al. Family history, body mass index, selected dietary factors, menstrual history, and risk of moderate to severe acne in adolescents and young adults. *J. Am. Acad. Dermatol.* **2012**, *67*, 1129–1135. [CrossRef] [PubMed]

28. Ulvestad, M.; Bjertness, E.; Dalgard, F.; Halvorsen, J.A. Acne and dairy products in adolescence: Results from a Norwegian longitudinal study. *J. Eur. Acad. Dermatol. Venereol.* **2017**, *31*, 530–545. [CrossRef] [PubMed]

29. Juhl, C.R.; Berholdt, H.K.M.; Miller, I.M.; Jemec, G.B.; Kanters, J.K.; Ellervik, C. Dietary intake and acne vulgaris: a systematic review and meta-analysis of 78,529 children, adolescents, and young adults. *Nutrients* **2018**, in press.

30. Mirdamadi, Y.; Thielitz, A.; Wiede, A.; Goihl, A.; Papakonstantinou, E.; Hartig, R.; Zouboulis, C.C.; Reinhold, D.; Simeoni, L.; Bommhardt, U.; et al. Insulin and insulin-like growth factor-1 can modulate the phosphoinositide-3-kinase/Akt/FoxO1 pathway in SZ95 sebocytes in vitro. *Mol. Cell Endocrinol.* **2015**, *415*, 32–44. [CrossRef] [PubMed]

31. Jansen, T.; Janssen, O.E.; Plewig, G. [Acne tarda. Acne in adults]. *Hautarzt* **2013**, *64*, 241–251. [CrossRef] [PubMed]

32. Massa, A.F.; Burmeister, L.; Bass, D.; Zouboulis, C.C. Acne Fulminans: Treatment Experience from 26 Patients. *Dermatology* **2017**, *233*, 136–150. [CrossRef] [PubMed]

33. Pascoe, V.L.; Kimball, A.B. Seasonal variation of acne and psoriasis: A 3-year study using the Physician Global Assessment severity scale. *J. Am. Acad. Dermatol.* **2015**, *73*, 523–535. [CrossRef] [PubMed]

34. Itan, Y.; Jones, B.L.; Ingram, C.J.; Swallow, D.M.; Thomas, M.G. A worldwide correlation of lactase persistence phenotype and genotypes. *BMC Evol. Biol.* **2010**, *10*, 36. [CrossRef] [PubMed]

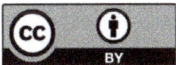

nutrients

MDPI

Article

Dairy Intake and Acne Vulgaris: A Systematic Review and Meta-Analysis of 78,529 Children, Adolescents, and Young Adults

Christian R. Juhl [1], Helle K. M. Bergholdt [2], Iben M. Miller [3], Gregor B. E. Jemec [3,4], Jørgen K. Kanters [1,*] and Christina Ellervik [2,4,5,6,*]

[1] Department of Biomedical Sciences, Faculty of Health and Medical Sciences, University of Copenhagen, 2100 Copenhagen, Denmark; christian.r.juhl@gmail.com
[2] Department of Production, Research, and Innovation, Region Zealand, 4180 Sorø, Denmark; hellebergholdt@hotmail.com
[3] Department of Dermatology, Zealand University Hospital, 4000 Roskilde, Denmark; miller@dadlnet.dk (I.M.M.); gbj@regionsjaelland.dk (G.B.E.J.)
[4] Department of Clinical Medicine, Faculty of Health and Medical Sciences, University of Copenhagen, 2100 Copenhagen, Denmark
[5] Department of Laboratory Medicine, Boston Children's Hospital, 300 Longwood Avenue, Boston, MA 02115, USA
[6] Department of Pathology, Harvard Medical School, Boston, MA 02115, USA
* Corresponding Authors: jkanters@sund.ku.dk (J.K.K.); christina@ellervik.dk or christina.ellervik@childrens.harvard.edu (C.E.)

Received: 15 July 2018; Accepted: 7 August 2018; Published: 9 August 2018

Abstract: A meta-analysis can help inform the debate about the epidemiological evidence on dairy intake and development of acne. A systematic literature search of PubMed from inception to 11 December 2017 was performed to estimate the association of dairy intake and acne in children, adolescents, and young adults in observational studies. We estimated the pooled random effects odds ratio (OR) (95% CI), heterogeneity (I^2-statistics, Q-statistics), and publication bias. We included 14 studies (n = 78,529; 23,046 acne-cases/55,483 controls) aged 7–30 years. ORs for acne were 1.25 (95% CI: 1.15–1.36; $p = 6.13 \times 10^{-8}$) for any dairy, 1.22 (1.08–1.38; $p = 1.62 \times 10^{-3}$) for full-fat dairy, 1.28 (1.13–1.44; $p = 8.23 \times 10^{-5}$) for any milk, 1.22 (1.06–1.41; $p = 6.66 \times 10^{-3}$) for whole milk, 1.32 (1.16–1.52; $p = 4.33 \times 10^{-5}$) for low-fat/skim milk, 1.22 (1.00–1.50; $p = 5.21 \times 10^{-2}$) for cheese, and 1.36 (1.05–1.77; $p = 2.21 \times 10^{-2}$) for yogurt compared to no intake. ORs per frequency of any milk intake were 1.24 (0.95–1.62) by 2–6 glasses per week, 1.41 (1.05–1.90) by 1 glass per day, and 1.43 (1.09–1.88) by ≥ 2 glasses per day compared to intake less than weekly. Adjusted results were attenuated and compared unadjusted. There was publication bias ($p = 4.71 \times 10^{-3}$), and heterogeneity in the meta-analyses were explained by dairy and study characteristics. In conclusion, any dairy, such as milk, yogurt, and cheese, was associated with an increased OR for acne in individuals aged 7–30 years. However, results should be interpreted with caution due to heterogeneity and bias across studies.

Keywords: meta-analysis; dairy; milk; acne; yogurt

1. Introduction

Acne is a common chronic inflammatory skin disease of sebaceous follicles [1,2]. Clinically, acne is characterized by the presence of open and closed comedones, papules, pustules, and dermal tissue damage with eventually heavy scar formation. Follicular hyperkeratosis, modifications of the sebofollicular microbiome, increase production of sebum with increased amounts of pro-inflammatory monounsaturated fatty acids, and Th17-cell-mediated inflammatory responses are all involved in acne pathogenesis. Sebum production can be induced by insulin-like growth factor-1 (IGF-1) and androgens, whose adrenal and gonadal synthesis is stimulated by IGF-1 [3]. Although prevalence varies across studies, acne is common in children and adolescents aged 12–24 years and is moderate to severe in 15–20% of cases [1,4–6].

Heritability of acne alone does not explain high acne prevalence rates of over 80% in western countries [5,7]. It has long been debated if a Western diet *per se* or specific dietary components contribute to the prevalence and severity of acne [4,8]. This has predominantly been investigated in observational studies and only a few trials exist [9]. In particular, dairy products have been incriminated. Milk-derived amino acids promote insulin secretion and induce hepatic insulin-like growth factor-1 (IGF-1) synthesis [10]. IGF-1 has been suggested as the pivotal driver of acne and stimulates follicular epithelial growth and keratinization [11–13]. IGF-1 gene polymorphism has been shown to increase susceptibility to acne [14] and IGF-1 plasma levels correlate with acne severity [12].

Several worldwide observational studies have been published on dairy intake and acne in children, adolescents, and young adults (7–30 years) in various countries [15–27]. Some narrative and systematic reviews about dairy intake and acne have been published [4,9,28]. Recently, a meta-analysis of dairy and acne was published [29] but with several methodological flaws, including lack of bias assessment and inadvertent double-counting of studies due to duplicate publications [19,23,30,31] that caused inappropriate weighting of results and skewed pooled estimates. So far, no previous meta-analysis has statistically combined the observational studies in an attempt to estimate the effect of the association of dairy intake and acne with the heterogeneity across studies, a bias assessment, a stratified analysis by study characteristics, and publication bias.

The primary objective of this study was therefore to perform a meta-analysis to estimate the association of acne in children, adolescents, and young adults consuming any dairy products. Furthermore, our aim was to explore the association between acne and intake of varies types of dairy (milk, yogurt, cheese), dairy subgroups (full fat, low fat, skim), and various amounts and frequencies of dairy intake (times per week or day).

2. Methods

This systematic review and meta-analysis was undertaken according to Meta-analysis of Observational Studies in Epidemiology (MOOSE) guidelines and according to a specified protocol (Supplementary Materials). The search, selection of studies, full-text reading, and data extraction were performed by CRJ and verified by CE.

2.1. Search Strategy

The search was performed on 11 December 2017 and included all studies up until that date. Studies were identified in the PubMed database using the search terms: ("Dairy products"[Mesh] OR dairy[All Fields] OR milk[Mesh] OR milk[All Fields] OR yogurt[All Fields] OR cheese[All Fields] OR lifestyle[All Fields]) AND ("Acne Vulgaris"[Mesh] OR Acne[All Fields]). We identified 241 records.

2.2. Eligibility Criteria

All observational studies (case-control, cross-sectional, population-based, retrospective) on childhood, adolescent, or young adult acne (max age of 30 years) were eligible if they reported a risk estimate and a 95% confidence interval for acne in a dairy group vs. a non-dairy group, or the raw numbers from 2 by 2 tables of dairy intake and acne.

2.3. Procedure for Selection of Studies

We screened the title and abstracts of 241 articles (Figure 1). If relevant, we retrieved the full-text articles. We identified 25 full-text articles, but excluded the following 11 studies: duplicate [19] (there was a statement in the article by Grossi that it was the same cohort and results as [23]), beliefs/opinions about acne aggravating food items [32,33], semi-fat/whole milk vs. skim milk/no milk drinkers [34], Chinese ying-yang medicine [35], no control group [36], adult acne (mean age ≥ 30 years) [37,38], milk as part of a Mediterranean diet [39], milk only as a continuous variable in acne and non-acne groups [40], and poorly defined intake [41]. In total, we included 14 studies. Two other studies were identified outside the search, but these studies were duplicates and published simultaneously without a clear statement of which one was the original; therefore, we did not include these papers [30,31]. The study selection process is shown in a flow diagram (Figure 1).

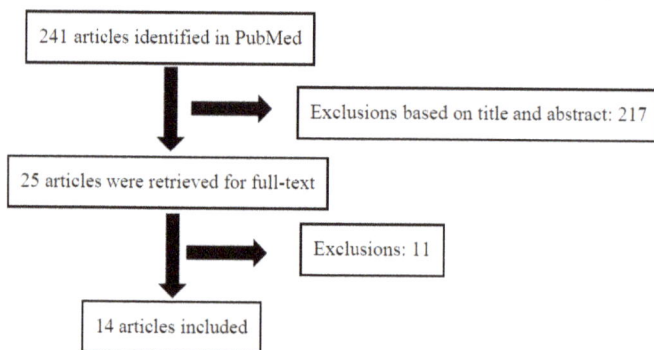

Figure 1. Flow diagram for meta-analysis.

2.4. Data Extraction and Management

We extracted the following data for each study and entered the information in an excel spreadsheet: author, year, population, country, age, gender, study design, how outcome was estimated, dairy type (dairy, milk, yogurt, cheese), dairy subtype (whole (full-fat), low-fat, skim), dairy amount, frequency of intake (times per day or week), numbers of acne patients and controls subjects in each category of dairy intake, crude and/or adjusted odds ratio (OR) or prevalence ratio with 95% confidence interval (CI), raw numbers to calculate crude OR (95% CI).

2.5. Overall and Subgroup Analyses

The primary objective was to perform a meta-analysis to estimate the odds ratio of acne in children, adolescents, and young adults consuming any dairy compared to those who do not. The secondary objective was to estimate the odds ratio of acne associated with intake of varies types of dairy (milk, yogurt, cheese), dairy subgroups (full-fat, low-fat, skim), and various amounts and frequencies of dairy intake (times per week or day) compared to those who did not consume any dairy/milk.

2.6. Risk of Bias and Study Quality Assessment

The quality of each study was evaluated and scored using the nine-star Newcastle-Ottawa Scale (NOS), a tool used for quality assessment of nonrandomized studies [42]. Studies were evaluated based on selection, comparability, exposure, and outcome, and scored by a maximum of nine points. Scores above five indicate moderate to high study quality. The NOS for cohort and case-control studies was retrieved from [43].

2.7. Statistical Analyses

The meta-analyses were performed with STATA SE 14.0 (Stata Corp., College Station, TX, USA). Using raw numbers, we calculated the crude odds ratios OR (95% CI). Analyses were performed for any dairy intake, any milk intake, full-fat dairy, whole milk, and low-fat/skim milk compared to those who did not consume any dairy/milk (study specific definitions). For any milk intake, whole milk and low-fat/skim milk, analyses of frequencies (times per week or day) were performed using studies by Adebamowo et al. [15–17], as these studies had identical ascertainment of the frequency of milk intake. DerSimonian and Laird (D + L) pooled random effects estimates were used. We also present inverse variance (I-V) fixed effects in supplementary Figures. Heterogeneity was assessed by Cochrane Q statistic test and I^2-statistical analysis. The I^2-statistical analysis assess what proportion of the observed variance reflects variance in true effect sizes rather than sampling error [44]. Publication bias was examined visually by funnel plots and statistically using Egger's test (one-sided) [45] and by using the Duval and Tweedie's Trim and Fill to simulate where potential unpublished studies would belong in the funnel plot and to calculate a hypothetical new pooled odds ratio based on the added simulated studies. Robustness of the meta-analysis was examined by "leaving-one-out" analysis. Publication bias and robustness were carried out by use of the statistical program Comprehensive Meta-Analysis (CMA) version 3 (Biostat, Englewood, NJ, USA) for any dairy intake vs. no dairy intake and any milk intake vs. no milk intake. Four studies provided adjusted estimates for milk intake, with one study providing them as odds ratios [46], and three studies as prevalence ratios [15–17]. In a sensitivity analysis, we used only adjusted prevalence ratios from the studies by Adebamowo et al. [15–17]. Stratification on acne severity was not possible because of too few studies.

3. Results

3.1. Description of the Studies

In total, 14 studies were eligible. Figure 1 shows the flow diagram of the selection of articles for the meta-analysis. The studies were published in 2005–2017 and included a total of 78,529 individuals of which 23,046 had acne and 55,483 were controls (Table 1). The prevalence of acne ranged from 7–89% in population studies and 36–83% in case-control studies. Two studies used non-acne dermatological controls [23,26] and the rest used healthy controls. Five studies were cross-sectional [20,21,27,46,47], five studies were case-control [18,22–24,26], one study was retrospective [15], and three studies were longitudinal [16,17,25]. The age-group ranged from 7–30 years. Two studies were only in females [15,17], three studies only in males [16,26,46], and the rest included both males and females. The studies covered five continents: Africa [21], Asia [18,24,47], Europe [20,22,23,25–27], North America [15–17], and South America [46]. Four studies included less than 1000 individuals in total [18,21–23,47], whereas the rest ranged from 1285 to 46,879 individuals (Table 1). Four studies used the Willet food frequency questionnaire [15–17,21]. In six studies, acne was self-reported in a questionnaire [15–17,20,25,27], and in eight studies, acne was a physician verified diagnosis [18,21–24,26,46,47]. Five studies provided adjusted estimates, including four on milk intake and one on dairy, two of the studies reported odds ratios, and three studies reported prevalence ratios [15–17,25,46]. The reference group varied among the articles and included not weekly [15–18,25], not daily [20,21,46], never [23,27], and unclear [24,26,47].

3.2. Findings

Random effects pooled unadjusted odds ratios for acne were 1.25 (95% CI: 1.15–1.36; $p = 6.13 \times 10^{-8}$) for any dairy (Figure 2), 1.22 (1.08–1.38; $p = 1.62 \times 10^{-3}$) for full-fat dairy, 1.28 (1.13–1.44; $p = 8.23 \times 10^{-5}$) for any milk, 1.22 (1.06–1.41; $p = 6.66 \times 10^{-3}$) for whole milk, 1.32 (1.16–1.52; $p = 4.33 \times 10^{-5}$) for low-fat/skim milk, 1.22 (1.00–1.50; $p = 5.21 \times 10^{-2}$) for cheese, and 1.36 (1.05–1.77; $p = 2.21 \times 10^{-2}$) for yogurt compared to those who did not consume these food items (Figure 3 and Supplementary Figures S1–S6).

Random effects meta-analyses for acne by frequency of any milk intake compared to an intake of ≤1 glass of milk per week showed an odds ratio of 1.24 (0.95–1.62) by 2–6 glasses per week, 1.41 (1.05–1.90) by 1 glass per day, and 1.43 (1.09–1.88) by ≥2 glasses per day for any milk; results for whole milk and low-fat/skim milk were close (Supplementary Figures S7–S10).

Table 1. Characteristics of included studies for the association of dairy intake with acne in children, adolescents, and young adults.

First Author	Year	Study Population	Design	Age, Year	Gender	Country	Total n	Acne n	Acne (%)	No Acne n	Milk Variables	Acne Diagnosis
Adebamowo [15]	2005	Population cohort (Nurses' Health Study II)	Retrospective	13–18	F	USA	46,879	3412	7.28	43,467	Any milk, whole milk, low-fat milk, skim milk	Q
Adebamowo [17]	2006	Population cohort (GUTS)—offspring of women in the Nurses' Health Study II	Follow-up	9–15	F	USA	3756	2588	68.9	1168	Any milk, whole milk, low-fat milk, skim milk	Q
Adebamowo [16]	2008	Population cohort (GUTS)—offspring of women in the Nurses' Health Study II	Follow-up	9–15	M	USA	2759	1856	67.3	903	Any milk, whole milk, low-fat milk, skim milk	Q
Cerman [22]	2016	Acne patients and healthy controls	Case-control	19	F/M	Turkey	86	50	58.1	36	Any milk	D
Duquia [46]	2017	Acne patients vs. healthy controls in the army	Cross-sectional	18	M	Brasil	2201	1960	89.1	241	Whole milk, low-fat milk, cheese, yogurt	P
Grossi [23]	2016	Acne patients and non-acne dermatology patient controls	Case-control	10–24	F/M	Italy	563	205	36.4	358	Any milk, whole milk, skim milk, cheese/yogurt combined	D
Ismail [18]	2012	Acne patients and healthy controls	Case-control	18–30	F/M	Malaysia	88	44	50	44	Any milk, yogurt, cheese	D
Karadag [26]	2017	Acne patients and non-acne dermatology patient controls	Case-control	21	M	Turkey	4595	3836	83.5	759	Milk/cheese combined	D
Jung [24]	2010	Acne patients and age-matched healthy controls	Case-control	24	F/M	South Korea	1285	783	60.9	502	Cheese	D
Okoro [21]	2016	Population cohort	Cross-sectional	11–30	F/M	Nigeria	450	292	64.9	158	Any milk	D
Park [47]	2015	Population cohort	Cross-sectional	7–12	F/M	South Korea	693	251	36.2	442	Any milk, cheese, yogurt	D
Ulvestad [25]	2016	Population cohort	Follow-up	15–19	F/M	Norway	2387	331	13.9	2056	Any milk, full-fat milk	Q
Wolkenstein [20]	2015	Population cohort	Cross-sectional	15–24	F/M	France	2266	1375	60.7	891	Any milk	Q
Wolkenstein [27]	2017	Population cohort	Cross-sectional	15–24	F/M	Europe *	10521	6063	57.6	4458	Whole milk, semi-skimmed milk, low-fat milk, dairy	Q

Age: mean or range. Q: Questionnaire. D: Dermatologist verified. GUTS: Growing Up Today Study. P: Physician verified. USA: United States of America. * 7 countries: Belgium, Czech and Slovak Republics, France, Italy, Poland, and Spain.

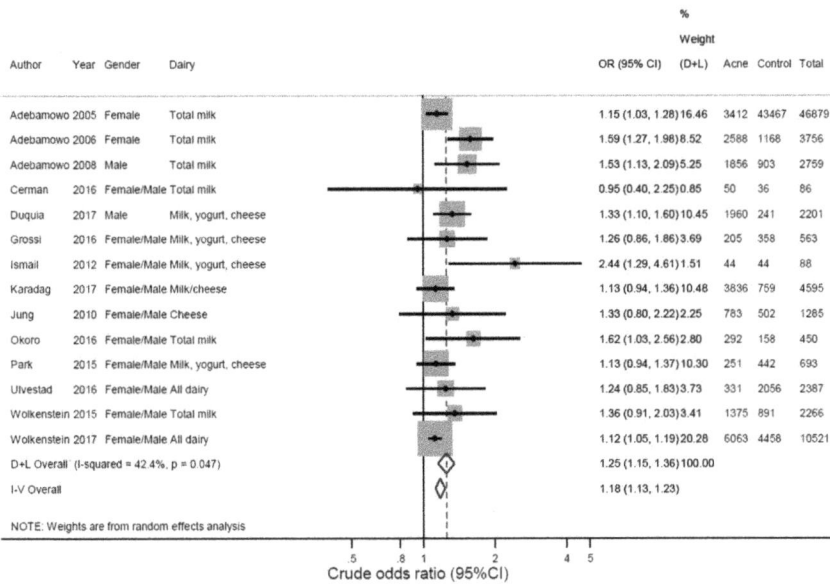

Figure 2. Meta-analysis of dairy intake and acne vulgaris: individual studies. The figure shows the individual studies and the unadjusted pooled random effect estimate from the meta-analysis of dairy intake and acne vulgaris. I^2(%): I-square heterogeneity expressed as percentage. p-value(het): p-value from Cochran's Q-statistic assessing heterogeneity. D + L: DerSimonian and Laird pooled random effects estimates. See Table 1 for references.

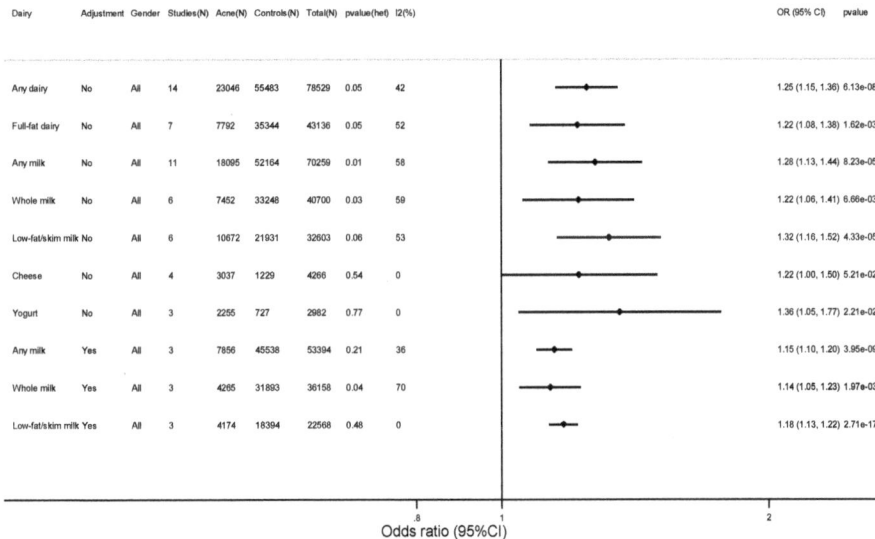

Figure 3. Meta-analyses of dairy intake and acne vulgaris: summary estimates. The figure shows the unadjusted pooled random effects estimates from each of the meta-analyses, which can be found in the supplementary material. I^2(%): I-square heterogeneity expressed as percentage. p-value(het): p-value from Cochran's Q-statistic assessing heterogeneity.

3.3. Sensitivity Analyses, Heterogeneity, Publication Bias, and Qualitative Bias Assessment

The I^2 heterogeneity ranged from 0–70% (Figure 2). To explore heterogeneity, we stratified the analysis for any dairy intake and acne by age, gender, number of cases, continent, design, acne diagnosis, and reference group (Supplementary Table S1, Supplementary Figures S11–S17). Stratifying by age did not show any differences. Stratifying by gender showed similar odds ratios in males and females, but meta-analyses of females had higher heterogeneity. Stratifying by the number of acne cases showed that larger studies had smaller odds ratios with more narrow confidence intervals, but higher heterogeneity compared to those of the smaller studies, but the confidence intervals were overlapping. Stratifying analyses by continent showed that studies from Europe had the smallest odds ratios, followed by North and South American studies, and with Asian and African studies with the largest odds ratios. Stratifying by design removed heterogeneity and showed that prospective studies had the largest odds ratios. Stratifying by ascertainment of acne diagnosis showed that studies using self-reported acne as an outcome had higher heterogeneity compared to studies with physician verified diagnoses of acne. Stratifying by reference group showed overall similar summary estimates, but with the highest heterogeneity in studies with "less than weekly" being the reference group. The Newcastle-Ottawa qualitative assessment scale of bias with similar items as in the statistical heterogeneity assessments revealed scores of 2–5 in case-control studies [18,22–24,26] and 2–6 in cohort studies [15–17,20,21,25,27,46,47] out of a potential max of 9 points (Supplementary Table S2).

Random effects pooled adjusted estimates for any milk, whole milk, and low-fat/skim milk were similar but attenuated compared to their unadjusted estimates (Supplementary Figures S18–S20).

Leave-one-out analyses for any dairy or any milk intake did not show any gross deviations, but the retrospective study by Adebamowo [15] influenced the summary estimates the most (Supplementary Figures S21–S22). Funnel plot and *p*-value for Egger's test revealed publication bias for any dairy (p-Egger $= 4.71 \times 10^{-3}$) (Supplementary Figure S23); Duval and Tweedie's Trim and Fill method estimated that five studies were missing for "any dairy", and the imputed point estimate would be 1.16 (1.06–1.28) had these five studies been added. Funnel plot and *p*-value for Egger's test revealed publication bias for any milk (p-Egger $= 2.73 \times 10^{-2}$) (Supplementary Figure S24); Duval and Tweedie's Trim and Fill method estimated that one study was missing for "any milk", and the imputed point estimate would be 1.26 (1.11–1.44) had this study been added.

The New-Castle Ottawa qualitative assessment scale of bias revealed a scores of 2–5 in case-control studies [18,22–24,26] and 2–6 in cohort studies [15–17,20,21,25,27,46,47].

4. Discussion

Intake of any dairy, any milk, full-fat dairy, whole milk, low-fat/skim milk, and yogurt regardless of amount or frequency were associated with a higher odds ratio for acne compared to no intake in individuals aged 7–30 years. Intake of cheese was associated with a borderline higher odds ratio for acne compared to no intake. Stratifying the association of any milk by frequency of intake revealed that intake of 1 glass of milk or more per day was associated with a higher odds ratio for acne, whereas 2–6 glasses per week was not, compared to intake less than weekly. Stratified analyses for any dairy intake and acne fat content demonstrated that full-fat dairy and whole milk had lower odds ratios, whereas low-fat/skim milk had higher odds ratios than the overall summary estimates; a likely explanation for this observation could be that the amount of milk consumed for low-fat/skim milk is higher than that for whole milk. However, results should be interpreted with caution due to heterogeneity and bias across studies.

The meta-analyses showed considerable heterogeneity reflecting the heterogeneous age and gender of the participants, various study characteristics, ascertainment of information about milk intake and acne, reporting of milk intake, and acne severity across the studies. In general, stratifying on subgroups in sensitivity analyses revealed that heterogeneity diminished for most subgroups, but also revealed that especially meta-analyses conducted on females, whole milk, North America, and questionnaire ascertained acne diagnosis demonstrated high heterogeneity. Prospective studies and studies with physician-verified diagnosis of acne had low heterogeneity.

Despite the stratifications, confidence intervals were overlapping.

Stratifying on age and gender demonstrated similar odds ratios; however, the gender stratified analyses had higher odds ratios than in the gender combined analyses. Smaller studies had higher odds ratios than large studies, African and Asian studies had higher odds ratios than other studies, and prospective designs had higher odds ratios than other designs. A recent multinational European online questionnaire study in adolescents showed that acne prevalence did not differ by gender but differed by country, and acne was more prevalent in younger people and obese people [27]. Intake of milk varies globally and is largely dependent on genetically determined lactase persistency, which is high in people of Northern European descent, but lower in people of Southern European descent, patchy in Africa, and low in the Middle East and Asia [48]. The weaning of the lactase enzyme activity usually happens in childhood and early adolescent years. How the age of weaning of the lactase enzyme activity impacts acne development is not known.

We used random effects method in all meta-analyses, which includes between-study variance and has a higher degree of statistical uncertainty built into the model. Thus, 95% confidence intervals are wider compared to fixed effects models. Even in these models, the results of the meta-analyses were significant. There was evidence of publication bias with Egger's test with an overweight of smaller studies overestimating the odds ratio compared to the pooled summary estimate. If the meta-analyses had captured all the relevant studies, we would expect the funnel plots to be symmetric. The selective reporting may be explained by studies with null-findings or negative results being deliberately not published because of authors not submitting or editors rejecting them or authors not finding enough merit in a potential publishable study [49]. Furthermore, some studies reported only the pooled exposures for different dairy groups rather than showing the stratified results for each of the dairy groups and/or for each reported frequency of intake [23,25,26], and some studies had only collected an overall dairy or milk variable with no possibility for stratification [20,22]. However, the trim and fill method did not change the overall estimates for "any dairy" or "any milk" remarkably.

There are many limitations of the included studies [4]. Self-reported acne with lack of a physician verified diagnosis of acne [15–17,20,25] may lead to misclassification bias as validity of self-reported acne is at best only moderate, with sensitivity of 55%, specificity of 72%, positive predictive value of 70%, and negative predictive value of 57% [50]. Including other dermatology patients as controls [26] may attenuate associations, as seborrhea may play a role in several diseases. The observational studies were cross-sectional [20,21,46,47], case-control [18,22–24,26], retrospective [15], or longitudinal [16,17,25]; thus, in most studies we cannot rule out reverse causation. Questionnaire ascertainment of dairy intake varied between the articles and only a few studies used validated food frequency questionnaires [15–17,21]. Despite the food questionnaire used, participants may deliberately over- or underestimate (information bias) or not accurately remember (recall bias) when filling out questionnaires about dairy intake and acne. Furthermore, it was not possible to differentiate acne development, acne triggers, and severity of acne in the meta-analyses. Only a few studies provided adjusted results [15–17,25] so we based most of the analyses on raw numbers, which makes it difficult to rule out confounding from other dietary factors (e.g., glycemic index or calorie intake) or other lifestyle factors previously associated with acne [4,9,28].

Acne prevalence varied remarkably across the included studies, between 7–89%. The retrospective study by Adebamowo in 2005 with 7.3% acne cases focused on recall data provided by subjects in the Nurses' Health Study II (NHS), which were aged 25–42 years old in 1989 when information on teenage acne was collected [15]; thus, the acne prevalence is likely underestimated and the results from this study may not be representative. Furthermore, the studies from 2006 and 2008 were offspring studies from the NHS in girls and boys [16,17]; however, leave-one-out analyses revealed that only the Adebamowo 2005 study was an outlier [15].

The observational studies may suffer from bias from confounding and reverse causation [9], are unable to indicate causality of the relationship between dairy and acne, and unable to prove preventive effects of abstaining from dairy. Only one study exists on milk intake and acne. The study is uncontrolled and unblinded and is based on medical students who drank milk or consumed other potential acne provoking foods. In addition, the total number of people with and without acne lesions were counted for all foods combined, but with no formal statistical testing [51]. Thus, there is still a knowledge gap with respect to whether dairy intake is causally associated with acne, acne flare, or acne severity and to what extent. To answer this question, we would ideally need results from large clinical randomized double-blind placebo-controlled trials (RCT); however, the question is whether this is realistically possible ethically, clinically, and/or operationally. Another approach (which no previous studies have yet undertaken) would be to perform a Mendelian Randomization study of lactase persistence, dairy intake, and acne using genetic lactase persistence as a proxy for lifetime dairy intake under the assumption that alleles are randomly distributed at conception [52,53]. Such a study design mimics an RCT and allows for the causal estimate of dairy intake and acne.

The observational studies all assessed dairy intake as an isolated factor. However, dairy is part of various individual and cultural specific diets and not a single factor with a single factor prediction ("reductionist approach" [54]). Instead, other factors which can affect the bioactive properties of nutrients in dairy and milk intake should be taken into consideration, such as macro- and micronutrients (fat, protein, carbohydrates, vitamins, sodium, and minerals), the dairy structure (liquid or solid), fermentation, and processing (holistic approach [55]). Only two studies in the meta-analysis also reported the glycemic load and glycemic indices of food consumed in conjunction with milk/dairy products [18,22], but did not report the glycemic load from the dairy consumption specifically. Hyperglycemic carbohydrates enhance insulin signaling, which promotes insulin and IGF-1 signaling, which in a synergistic fashion with milk stimulate mTORC1(mammalian target of rapamycin complex 1) signal transduction [56]. There is accumulating evidence that acne belongs to the spectrum of mTORC1-driven diseases of civilization including metabolic syndrome, obesity, insulin resistance, and cancer [57]. A randomized trial has shown that a low-glycemic-load diet improves symptoms in acne vulgaris patients [58]. Interestingly, no acne was observed in the Kitavan Islanders (Pacific Ocean) and in the Ache Hunter-Gatherers from Paraguay, who live under Paleolithic conditions without milk/dairy and hyperglycemic food, although it should be acknowledged that many other differences exist to Western societies [59]. To present the pathological effects of milk in the Western diet it is therefore important to provide controlled studies that consider milk consumption in association with glycemic load and index as part of a mixed diet [60].

Recently, a meta-analysis of dairy and acne was published [29] but with several methodological flaws, including the inadvertent double-counting of studies (Landro [19]/Grossi [23], and Tsoy [30]/Tsoy [31]) due to duplicate publications, which caused inappropriate weighting of results and skewed pooled estimates. Using the double-counted studies by Tsoy, the authors also only used the most severe category of acne, which caused extremely high odds ratios of 10 and 12 to be included in the meta-analysis, further skewing the pooled estimates. Furthermore, the meta-analysis included a study by Agamia [41], which we decided to exclude as the intake of "milk and dairy produce" was poorly defined as "low" and "high" intake but not defined with any frequency, type, or amount of milk. The previous meta-analysis also did not provide evidence for the exact search strategy to be replicated, for the bias assessment using the Newcastle Ottawa scale, for leave-one-out analyses, or funnel plots of publication bias. As a comparison, in our meta-analysis, we included the exact search string so it can be replicated, the heterogeneity across studies, a bias assessment using the Newcastle-Ottawa scale presented with a table, a stratified analysis by study characteristics presented in figures, the details of the "leave-one-out" analysis presented in figures, and the publication bias presented in figures. Furthermore, we excluded duplicate studies, and we included four more papers [24,26,27,47] that were not included in the previous meta-analysis but should have been as the studies were published before the search for the previous meta-analysis was done in August 2017 [29].

It is of crucial importance that authors of meta-analyses have a critical judgement of the reliability and validity of the papers they consider including in a meta-analysis, otherwise the conduct and assessment of systematic reviews may be hampered.

5. Conclusions

In conclusion, this meta-analysis of observational studies has provided new insight into the direction and magnitude of the association between dairy intake and acne overall and by dairy type, amount, and frequency. It has shed light on the knowledge gaps and the limitations of the studies included compared to previous systematic and narrative reviews with no meta-analysis, heterogeneity assessment, or bias assessment included [4,9,28].

Supplementary Materials: The following are available online at http://www.mdpi.com/2072-6643/10/8/1049/ s1, Figure S1: Meta-analysis of full-fat dairy intake vs. no dairy intake, Figure S2: Meta-analysis of any milk intake vs. no milk intake, Figure S3: Meta-analysis of whole milk intake vs. no milk intake, Figure S4: Meta-analysis of low-fat/skim milk intake vs. no milk intake, Figure S5: Meta-analysis of Cheese intake vs. no cheese intake, Figure S6: Meta-analysis of yogurt intake vs. no yogurt intake, Figure S7: Meta-analyses of frequency of milk intake and acne, Figure S8: Meta-analyses of amount of total milk intake, Figure S9: Meta-analyses of amount of whole milk intake, Figure S10: Meta-analyses of amount of low-fat/skim milk intake, Figure S11: Meta-analyses of any dairy intake vs. no dairy intake—by age group, Figure S12: Meta-analyses of any dairy intake vs. no dairy intake—by gender group, Figure S13: Meta-analyses of any dairy intake vs. no dairy intake—by number of cases, Figure S14: Meta-analyses of any dairy intake vs. no dairy intake—by continent, Figure S15: Meta-analyses of any dairy intake vs. no dairy intake—by design, Figure S16: Meta-analyses of any dairy intake vs. no dairy intake—by acne diagnosis, Figure S17: Meta-analyses of any dairy intake vs. no dairy intake—by reference group, Figure S18: Meta-analysis of any milk intake vs. no milk intake—adjusted analysis, Figure S19: Meta-analysis of whole milk intake vs. no milk intake—adjusted analysis, Figure S20: Meta-analysis of low-fat/skim milk intake vs. no milk intake—adjusted analysis, Figure S21: Meta-analysis of any dairy intake vs. no dairy intake—leave one out analysis, Figure S22: Meta-analysis of any milk intake vs. no milk intake—leave one out analysis, Figure S23: Funnel plot of standard error by log odds ratio—any dairy intake vs. no dairy intake, Figure S24: Funnel plot of standard error by log odds ratio—any milk intake vs. no milk intake, Table S1: Sensitivity analyses for the association of dairy intake and acne, Table S2: Study-specific Newcastle-Ottawa quality assessment.

Author Contributions: C.R.J. and C.E. had full access to all the data in the study and take responsibility for the integrity of the data and the accuracy of the data analysis. Study concept and design: all authors. Acquisition, analysis of data: C.R.J. and C.E. Interpretation of data: all authors. Drafting of the manuscript: C.R.J. and C.E. Critical revision of the manuscript for important intellectual content: all authors. Statistical analysis: C.R.J. and C.E. Administrative, technical, or material support: N.A. Study supervision: G.B.E.J., J.K.K., and C.E.

Funding: C.R.J. was funded by Region Zealand. The Danish General Suburban Population Study was funded by the Region Zealand Foundation, Naestved Hospital Foundation, Edith and Henrik Henriksens Memorial Scholarship, Johan and Lise Boserup Foundation, TrygFonden, Johannes Fog's Foundation, Region Zealand, Naestved Hospital, The National Board of Health, and the Local Government Denmark Foundation.

Conflicts of Interest: G.B.E.J. has received honoraria from AbbVie, MSD, Pfizer, Pierre-Fabre, and UCB for participation on advisory boards, and grants from Abbvie, Actelion, Janssen-Cilag, Leo Pharma, Novartis, and Regeneron for participation as an investigator, and received speaker honoraria from AbbVie, Galderma, Leo Pharma, and MSD. He has furthermore received unrestricted research grants from AbbVie and Leo Pharma. He has received travel grants from AbbVie, Celgene, Desitin, and Novartis. GBEJ's sponsors were not involved in any parts of this article (design, conduct, collection, management, analysis, interpretation, preparation, approval, review, decision to submit). H.K.M.B. has received a grant from the Danish Dairy Research Foundation. None of the funding agencies had any role in the design, analysis, or writing of this article.

References

1. Williams, H.C.; Dellavalle, R.P.; Garner, S. Acne vulgaris. *Lancet* **2012**, *379*, 361–372. [CrossRef]
2. Tuchayi, S.M.; Makrantonaki, E.; Ganceviciene, R.; Dessinioti, C.; Feldman, S.R.; Zouboulis, C.C. Acne vulgaris. *Nat. Rev. Dis. Primers.* **2015**, *1*, 15029. [CrossRef] [PubMed]
3. Melnik, B.C.; Schmitz, G. Role of insulin, insulin-like growth factor-1, hyperglycaemic food and milk consumption in the pathogenesis of acne vulgaris. *Exp. Dermatol.* **2009**, *18*, 833–841. [CrossRef] [PubMed]
4. Bhate, K.; Williams, H.C. Epidemiology of acne vulgaris. *Br. J. Dermatol.* **2013**, *168*, 474–485. [CrossRef] [PubMed]
5. White, G.M. Recent findings in the epidemiologic evidence, classification, and subtypes of acne vulgaris. *J. Am. Acad. Dermatol.* **1998**, *39*, S34–S47. [CrossRef]

6. Rademaker, M.; Garioch, J.J.; Simpson, N.B. Acne in schoolchildren: No longer a concern for dermatologists. *BMJ* **1989**, *298*, 1217–1229. [CrossRef] [PubMed]

7. Ghodsi, S.Z.; Orawa, H.; Zouboulis, C.C. Prevalence, severity, and severity risk factors of acne in high school pupils: A community-based study. *J. Investig. Dermatol.* **2009**, *129*, 2136–2141. [CrossRef] [PubMed]

8. Dreno, B.; Bettoli, V.; Araviiskaia, E.; Sanchez Viera, M.; Bouloc, A. The influence of exposome on acne. *J. Eur. Acad. Dermatol. Venereol.* **2018**, *32*, 812–829. [CrossRef] [PubMed]

9. Spencer, E.H.; Ferdowsian, H.R.; Barnard, N.D. Diet and acne: A review of the evidence. *Int. J. Dermatol.* **2009**, *48*, 339–347. [CrossRef] [PubMed]

10. Rich-Edwards, J.W.; Ganmaa, D.; Pollak, M.N.; Nakamoto, E.K.; Kleinman, K.; Tserendolgor, U.; Willett, W.C.; Frazier, A.L. Milk consumption and the prepubertal somatotropic axis. *Nutr. J.* **2007**, *6*, 28. [CrossRef] [PubMed]

11. Holmes, M.D.; Pollak, M.N.; Willett, W.C.; Hankinson, S.E. Dietary correlates of plasma insulin-like growth factor I and insulin-like growth factor binding protein 3 concentrations. *Cancer Epidemiol. Biomarkers Prev.* **2002**, *11*, 852–861. [PubMed]

12. Rahaman, S.M.A.; De, D.; Handa, S.; Pal, A.; Sachdeva, N.; Ghosh, T.; Kamboj, P. Association of insulin-like growth factor (IGF)-1 gene polymorphisms with plasma levels of IGF-1 and acne severity. *J. Am. Acad. Dermatol.* **2016**, *75*, 768–773. [CrossRef] [PubMed]

13. Mirdamadi, Y.; Thielitz, A.; Wiede, A.; Goihl, A.; Papakonstantinou, E.; Hartig, R.; Zouboulis, C.C.; Reinhold, D.; Simeoni, L.; Bommhardt, U.; et al. Insulin and insulin-like growth factor-1 can modulate the phosphoinositide-3-kinase/Akt/FoxO1 pathway in SZ95 sebocytes in vitro. *Mol. Cell. Endocrinol.* **2015**, *415*, 32–44. [CrossRef] [PubMed]

14. Tasli, L.; Turgut, S.; Kacar, N.; Ayada, C.; Coban, M.; Akcilar, R.; Ergin, S. Insulin-like growth factor-I gene polymorphism in acne vulgaris. *J. Eur. Acad. Dermatol. Venereol.* **2013**, *27*, 254–267. [CrossRef] [PubMed]

15. Adebamowo, C.A.; Spiegelman, D.; Danby, F.W.; Frazier, A.L.; Willett, W.C.; Holmes, M.D. High school dietary dairy intake and teenage acne. *J. Am. Acad. Dermatol.* **2005**, *52*, 207–214. [CrossRef] [PubMed]

16. Adebamowo, C.A.; Spiegelman, D.; Berkey, C.S.; Danby, F.W.; Rockett, H.H.; Colditz, G.A.; Willett, W.C.; Willett, W.C. Milk consumption and acne in teenaged boys. *J. Am. Acad. Dermatol.* **2008**, *58*, 787–793. [CrossRef] [PubMed]

17. Adebamowo, C.A.; Spiegelman, D.; Berkey, C.S.; Danby, F.W.; Rockett, H.H.; Colditz, G.A.; Willett, W.C.; Holmes, M.D. Milk consumption and acne in adolescent girls. *Dermatol. Online J.* **2006**, *12*, 1. [PubMed]

18. Ismail, N.H.; Manaf, Z.A.; Azizan, N.Z. High glycemic load diet, milk and ice cream consumption are related to acne vulgaris in Malaysian young adults: A case control study. *BMC Dermatol.* **2012**, *12*, 13. [CrossRef] [PubMed]

19. Di Landro, A.; Cazzaniga, S.; Parazzini, F.; Ingordo, V.; Cusano, F.; Atzori, L.; Cutrì, F.T.; Musumeci, M.L.; Zinetti, C.; Pezzarossa, E.; et al. Family history, body mass index, selected dietary factors, menstrual history, and risk of moderate to severe acne in adolescents and young adults. *J. Am. Acad. Dermatol.* **2012**, *67*, 1129–1135. [CrossRef] [PubMed]

20. Wolkenstein, P.; Misery, L.; Amici, J.M.; Maghia, R.; Branchoux, S.; Cazeau, C.; Voisard, J.-J.; Taïeb, C. Smoking and dietary factors associated with moderate-to-severe acne in French adolescents and young adults: Results of a survey using a representative sample. *Dermatology* **2015**, *230*, 34–49. [CrossRef] [PubMed]

21. Okoro, E.O.; Ogunbiyi, A.O.; George, A.O.; Subulade, M.O. Association of diet with acne vulgaris among adolescents in Ibadan, southwest Nigeria. *Int. J. Dermatol.* **2016**. [CrossRef] [PubMed]

22. Cerman, A.A.; Aktas, E.; Altunay, I.K.; Arici, J.E.; Tulunay, A.; Ozturk, F.Y. Dietary glycemic factors, insulin resistance, and adiponectin levels in acne vulgaris. *J. Am. Acad. Dermatol.* **2016**. [CrossRef]

23. Grossi, E.; Cazzaniga, S.; Crotti, S.; Naldi, L.; Di Landro, A.; Ingordo, V.; Cusano, F.; Atzori, L.; Cutrì, F.T.; Musumeci, M.L.; et al. The constellation of dietary factors in adolescent acne: A semantic connectivity map approach. *J. Eur. Acad. Dermatol. Venereol.* **2016**, *30*, 96–100. [CrossRef] [PubMed]

24. Jung, J.Y.; Yoon, M.Y.; Min, S.U.; Hong, J.S.; Choi, Y.S.; Suh, D.H. The influence of dietary patterns on acne vulgaris in Koreans. *Eur. J. Dermatol.* **2010**, *20*, 768–772. [CrossRef] [PubMed]

25. Ulvestad, M.; Bjertness, E.; Dalgard, F.; Halvorsen, J.A. Acne and dairy products in adolescence: Results from a Norwegian longitudinal study. *J. Eur. Acad. Dermatol. Venereol.* **2016**. [CrossRef] [PubMed]

26. Karadag, A.S.; Balta, I.; Saricaoglu, H.; Kilic, S.; Kelekci, K.H.; Yildirim, M.; Arica, D.A.; Öztürk, S.; Karaman, G.; Cerman, A.A.; et al. The effect of personal, familial, and environmental characteristics on acne vulgaris: A prospective, multicenter, case controlled study from Turkey. *G. Ital. Dermatol. Venereol.* **2017**. [CrossRef]

27. Wolkenstein, P.; Machovcova, A.; Szepietowski, J.C.; Tennstedt, D.; Veraldi, S.; Delarue, A. Acne prevalence and associations with lifestyle: A cross-sectional online survey of adolescents/young adults in 7 European countries. *J. Eur. Acad. Dermatol. Venereol.* **2017**. [CrossRef] [PubMed]

28. Veith, W.B.; Silverberg, N.B. The association of acne vulgaris with diet. *Cutis* **2011**, *88*, 84–91. [PubMed]

29. Aghasi, M.; Golzarand, M.; Shab-Bidar, S.; Aminianfar, A.; Omidian, M.; Taheri, F. Dairy intake and acne development: A meta-analysis of observational studies. *Clin. Nutr.* **2018**. [CrossRef] [PubMed]

30. Tsoy, N. The Influence of Dietary Habits on Acne. *World J. Med. Sci.* **2013**, *8*, 212. [CrossRef]

31. Tsoy, N.O. Effect of Milk and Dairy Products upon Severity of Acne for Young People. *World Appl. Sci. J.* **2013**, *24*, 403–417. [CrossRef]

32. Burris, J.; Rietkerk, W.; Woolf, K. Relationships of self-reported dietary factors and perceived acne severity in a cohort of New York young adults. *J. Acad. Nutr. Diet.* **2014**, *114*, 384–392. [CrossRef] [PubMed]

33. Poli, F.; Auffret, N.; Beylot, C.; Chivot, M.; Faure, M.; Moyse, D.; Henri, P.; Jean, R.; Brigitte, D. Acne as seen by adolescents: Results of questionnaire study in 852 French individuals. *Acta Derm. Venereol.* **2011**, *91*, 531–546. [CrossRef] [PubMed]

34. Semedo, D.; Ladeiro, F.; Ruivo, M.; D'Oliveira, C.; De Sousa, F.; Gayo, M.; Amado, J.; Lima, C.; Magalhães, F.; Brandão, R.; et al. Adult Acne: Prevalence and Portrayal in Primary Healthcare Patients, in the Greater Porto Area, Portugal. *Acta. Med. Port.* **2016**, *29*, 507–513. [CrossRef] [PubMed]

35. Law, M.P.; Chuh, A.A.; Molinari, N.; Lee, A. An investigation of the association between diet and occurrence of acne: a rational approach from a traditional Chinese medicine perspective. *Clin. Exp Dermatol.* **2010**, *35*, 31–45. [CrossRef] [PubMed]

36. Seleit, I.; Bakry, O.A.; Abdou, A.G.; Hashim, A. Body mass index, selected dietary factors, and acne severity: Are they related to in situ expression of insulin-like growth factor-1? *Anal. Quant. Cytopathol. Histpathol.* **2014**, *36*, 267–278. [PubMed]

37. Dreno, B.; Thiboutot, D.; Layton, A.M.; Berson, D.; Perez, M.; Kang, S. Large-scale international study enhances understanding of an emerging acne population: Adult females. *J. Eur. Acad. Dermatol. Venereol.* **2015**, *29*, 1096–1106. [CrossRef] [PubMed]

38. Di Landro, A.; Cazzaniga, S.; Cusano, F.; Bonci, A.; Carla, C.; Musumeci, M.L.; Patrizi, A.; Bettoli, V.; Pezzarossa, E.; Caproni, M.; et al. Adult female acne and associated risk factors: Results of a multicenter case-control study in Italy. *J. Am. Acad. Dermatol.* **2016**, *75*, 1134–1141. [CrossRef] [PubMed]

39. Skroza, N.; Tolino, E.; Semyonov, L.; Proietti, I.; Bernardini, N.; Nicolucci, F.; Viola, G.L.; Prete, G.D.; Saulle, R.; Potenza, C.; et al. Mediterranean diet and familial dysmetabolism as factors influencing the development of acne. *Scand. J. Public Health* **2012**, *40*, 466–474. [CrossRef] [PubMed]

40. LaRosa, C.L.; Quach, K.A.; Koons, K.; Kunselman, A.R.; Zhu, J.; Thiboutot, D.M.; Zaenglein, A.L. Consumption of dairy in teenagers with and without acne. *J. Am. Acad. Dermatol.* **2016**, *75*, 318–322. [CrossRef] [PubMed]

41. Agamia, N.F.; Abdallah, D.M.; Sorour, O.; Mourad, B.; Younan, D.N. Skin expression of mammalian target of rapamycin and forkhead box transcription factor O1, and serum insulin-like growth factor-1 in patients with acne vulgaris and their relationship with diet. *Br. J. Dermatol.* **2016**, *174*, 1299–1307. [CrossRef] [PubMed]

42. Stang, A. Critical evaluation of the Newcastle-Ottawa scale for the assessment of the quality of nonrandomized studies in meta-analyses. *Eur. J. Epidemiol.* **2010**, *25*, 603–615. [CrossRef] [PubMed]

43. Newcastle—Ottawa Quality Assessment Scale Case Control Studies. Available online: http://www.ohri.ca/programs/clinical_epidemiology/nosgen.pdf (accessed on 12 December 2017).

44. Huedo-Medina, T.B.; Sanchez-Meca, J.; Marin-Martinez, F.; Botella, J. Assessing heterogeneity in meta-analysis: Q statistic or I2 index? *Psychol. Methods* **2006**, *11*, 193–206. [CrossRef] [PubMed]

45. Egger, M.; Smith, G.D.; Schneider, M.; Minder, C. Bias in meta-analysis detected by a simple, graphical test. *BMJ* **1997**, *315*, 629–634. [CrossRef] [PubMed]

46. Pereira Duquia, R.; da Silva Dos Santos, I.; de Almeida, H., Jr.; Martins Souza, P.R.; de Avelar Breunig, J.; Zouboulis, C.C. Epidemiology of Acne Vulgaris in 18-Year-Old Male Army Conscripts in a South Brazilian City. *Dermatology* **2017**, *233*, 145–154. [CrossRef] [PubMed]

47. Park, S.Y.; Kwon, H.H.; Min, S.; Yoon, J.Y.; Suh, D.H. Epidemiology and risk factors of childhood acne in Korea: A cross-sectional community based study. *Clin. Exp. Dermatol.* **2015**, *40*, 844–850. [CrossRef] [PubMed]

48. Itan, Y.; Jones, B.L.; Ingram, C.J.; Swallow, D.M.; Thomas, M.G. A worldwide correlation of lactase persistence phenotype and genotypes. *BMC Evol. Biol.* **2010**, *10*, 36. [CrossRef] [PubMed]

49. Higgins, J.P.T.; Green, S. Cochrane Handbook for Systematic Reviews of Interventions. Available online: http://handbook-5-1.cochrane.org/ (accessed on 12 December 2017).

50. Menon, C.; Gipson, K.; Bowe, W.P.; Hoffstad, O.J.; Margolis, D.J. Validity of subject self-report for acne. *Dermatology* **2008**, *217*, 164–178. [CrossRef] [PubMed]

51. Anderson, P.C. Foods as the cause of acne. *Am. Fam. Physician* **1971**, *3*, 102–113. [PubMed]

52. Bergholdt, H.K.M.; Nordestgaard, B.G.; Varbo, A.; Ellervik, C. Milk intake is not associated with ischaemic heart disease in observational or Mendelian randomization analyses in 98,529 Danish adults. *Int. J. Epidemiol.* **2015**, *44*, 587–603. [CrossRef] [PubMed]

53. Juhl, C.R.; Bergholdt, H.K.M.; Miller, I.M.; Jemec, G.B.; Kanters, J.K.; Ellervik, C. Lactase persistence, milk intake and adult acne: A Mendelian randomization study of 20,416 Danish adults. *Nutrients* **2018**, *10*, 1041. [CrossRef]

54. Fardet, A.; Rock, E. Toward a new philosophy of preventive nutrition: From a reductionist to a holistic paradigm to improve nutritional recommendations. *Adv. Nutr.* **2014**, *5*, 430–446. [CrossRef] [PubMed]

55. Thorning, T.K.; Bertram, H.C.; Bonjour, J.P.; de Groot, L.; Dupont, D.; Feeney, E.; Ipsen, R.; Lecerf, J.M.; Mackie, A.; McKinley, M.C.; et al. Whole dairy matrix or single nutrients in assessment of health effects: Current evidence and knowledge gaps. *Am. J. Clin. Nutr.* **2017**, *105*, 1033–1045. [CrossRef] [PubMed]

56. Melnik, B.C. Milk—A Nutrient System of Mammalian Evolution Promoting mTORC1-Dependent Translation. *Int. J. Mol. Sci.* **2015**, *16*, 17048–17087. [CrossRef] [PubMed]

57. Melnik, B.C. Acne vulgaris: The metabolic syndrome of the pilosebaceous follicle. *Clin. Dermatol.* **2018**, *36*, 29–40. [CrossRef] [PubMed]

58. Smith, R.N.; Mann, N.J.; Braue, A.; Makelainen, H.; Varigos, G.A. A low-glycemic-load diet improves symptoms in acne vulgaris patients: A randomized controlled trial. *Am. J. Clin. Nutr.* **2007**, *86*, 107–115. [CrossRef] [PubMed]

59. Cordain, L.; Lindeberg, S.; Hurtado, M.; Hill, K.; Eaton, S.B.; Brand-Miller, J. Acne vulgaris: A disease of Western civilization. *Arch. Dermatol.* **2002**, *138*, 1584–1590. [CrossRef] [PubMed]

60. Elmstahl, H.L.; Bjorck, I. Milk as a supplement to mixed meals may elevate postprandial insulinaemia. *Eur. J. Clin. Nutr.* **2001**, *55*, 994–1009. [CrossRef] [PubMed]

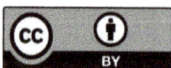

nutrients

MDPI

Article

Association between Fasting Glucose Concentration, Lipid Profile and 25(OH)D Status in Children Aged 9–11

Lukasz Szternel [1,*], Magdalena Krintus [1], Katarzyna Bergmann [1], Tadeusz Derezinski [2] and Grazyna Sypniewska [1]

[1] Department of Laboratory Medicine, Nicolaus Copernicus University, Collegium Medicum, 85094 Bydgoszcz, Poland; krintus@wp.pl (M.K.); bergmann@vp.pl (K.B.); grazynaodes@interia.pl (G.S.)
[2] Outpatient Clinic, "Esculap", 88140 Gniewkowo, Poland; tadziude@wp.pl
[*] Correspondence: lukaszszternel@wp.pl; Tel.: +48-525-854-023; Fax: +48-525-854-024

Received: 18 August 2018; Accepted: 19 September 2018; Published: 22 September 2018

Abstract: Background: The aim of this study was to assess the relationship between vitamin D status and the prevalence of dyslipidemia and impaired fasting glucose (IFG) in children. Methods and Summary: 284 children (150 boys and 134 girls) aged 9–11 were included in the study. Children with deficient 25(OH)D (25-hydroxycholecalciferol) levels $\leq$20 ng/mL (50 nmol/L) were characterized by a more frequent occurrence of impaired fasting glucose (IFG) (Odd ratios (OR) = 1.966, 95% confidence interval (CI): 1.055–3.663; p = 0.033) when compared to children with 25(OH)D >20 ng/mL. Serum 25(OH)D with concentration lower by 1 ng/mL (2.5 nmol/L) was linked to higher fasting glucose (by 0.25 mg/dL, 0.013 mmol/L; p = 0.017), higher total cholesterol (TC) by almost 1 mg/dL (0.96 mg/dL, 0.25 mmol/L; p = 0.006) and higher high-density lipoprotein cholesterol (HDL-C) (by 0.57 mg/dL, 0.015 mmol/L; p < 0.001). Conclusion: 25(OH)D deficiency may negatively affect fasting glucose and total cholesterol concentration in children aged 9–11. Vitamin D-deficient children are twice as likely to develop prediabetes as reflected by impaired fasting glucose when compared to those with a 25(OH)D level above 20 ng/mL (50 nmol/L).

Keywords: 25(OH)D deficiency; children; impaired fasting glucose; hypercholesterolemia

1. Introduction

The prevalence of obesity and vitamin D deficiency among children makes this population demographic especially vulnerable to the development of these two pervasive epidemics [1]. Research suggests an unhealthy diet coupled with a sedentary lifestyle has become the main causal factor affecting the development of obesity, which in turn is frequently accompanied by dyslipidemia. A significant amount of data supports the hypothesis that optimal vitamin D concentration is linked to a favorable lipid profile and has a positive impact on glucose homeostasis [2]. Numerous observational, epidemiological, and cross-sectional studies indicate an inverse correlation between the concentration of 25(OH)D (25-hydroxycholecalciferol) and the rate of conversion from a prediabetes state to fully symptomatic diabetes mellitus [3]. In the USA, the prevalence of prediabetes (or according to the World Health Organization (WHO) definition, "intermediate hyperglycemia") among adolescents aged 12–19 reached 13.1% between 2005 and 2006 [4]. It is estimated that annually 5%–10% of adults convert from a prediabetes state to overt diabetes, despite the fact that reversion to normoglycemia is much more common in children and adolescents. There are hypotheses indicating potentially beneficial effects of vitamin D in preventing transformation to fully symptomatic diabetes mellitus [3]. There is no consistent agreement as to whether vitamin D deficiency causes lipid abnormalities, or if these are just a consequence of excess adipose tissue mass storing 25(OH)D molecules. The inflammatory process links obesity and insulin resistance to the consequences of improper glucose homeostasis [5]. Vitamin D, being a negative marker of inflammation, seems to be a trigger molecule in the development of fully symptomatic metabolic syndrome [6]. The effects of vitamin D on lipid and carbohydrate metabolism may only be fully exploited with strong evidence from clinical trials of vitamin D supplementation.

The aim of this study is to assess the cross-sectional relationship between the status of vitamin D and the indices of metabolic pathways of lipids and glucose in a pediatric population.

2. Methods

2.1. Characteristics of the Study Participants and the Panel of Laboratory Tests

This cross-sectional study involved 284 presumably healthy children aged 9–11. The recruitment and blood collection process took place between October and November 2015. The children were selected on the basis of age (9–11 years old) from four primary schools in the Kujawsko-Pomorskie region of Poland. The second inclusion criterion was a fasting state (a minimum of 8 h since last meal) before blood drawing. Whilst school nurses and specialists in internal medicine participated in the recruitment process, the general health of the child on the day of study was subjectively evaluated by their parents. Children with any underlying liver, kidney, or endocrine diseases, or who were receiving drugs that affected vitamin D levels were excluded from the study. Immediately following blood collection, the blood samples were transported to the laboratory and centrifuged. Serum was used for further laboratory analysis. Whole blood samples were collected for HbA1c evaluation. Vitamin D status (total 25(OH)D concentration), lipid panel (total cholesterol (TC), triglycerides (TG), high-density lipoprotein cholesterol (HDL-C), low-density lipoprotein cholesterol (LDL-C)), C-reactive protein (CRP), and glucose status (fasting glucose concentration and glycated hemoglobin) were evaluated for all participants.

2.2. Laboratory and Anthropometric Measurements

Concentrations of total 25(OH)D were analyzed on an IDS-iSYS automated analyzer (Immunodiagnostic Systems Holdings PLC (Didcot Way, Boldon, UK)) using IDS-iSYS 25(OH)D^S chemiluminescence assay for the quantitative determination of 25-hydroxyvitamin D and other hydroxylated metabolites (24,25(OH)$_2$D$_3$) [7]. The percentage of 25(OH)D$_3$ and 25(OH)D$_2$ cross-reactivity was 97% and 120%, respectively. Cross-reactivity with epimers (3-epi-25(OH)D$_3$, 3-epi-25(OH)D$_2$) did not exceed 1% [8]. The reportable range for IDS-iSYS 25(OH)D^S assay ranged between 7 and 125 ng/mL (18–313 nmol/L). The assay used for the determination of 25(OH)D was traceable to isotope dilution-liquid chromatography/tandem mass spectrometry. Within-run precision of the IDS-iSYS 25(OH)D^S assay was evaluated by modified protocol CLSI EP-5A2 (Clinical and Laboratory Standard Institute, Evaluation of Precision Performance of Quantitative Measurement Methods) and ranged between 4.3% and 6.4% [8].

Lipid parameters including TC, TG, LDL-C, and HDL-C, high-sensitivity C-reactive protein (hs-CRP) and glucose concentration were measured with the use of an ABX Pentra 400 analyzer (Horiba Medical, Montpellier, France). Glycated hemoglobin was analyzed on a D-10™ Hemoglobin analyzer (BIO-RAD Diagnostics, Dublin, Ireland). All measurements were performed on fasting blood samples. The children's height and weight was measured before blood collection and body mass index (BMI) percentiles determined using an online BMI calculator based on the "OLAF" project [9].

2.3. Definitions of Decision Criteria for Study Participants

The participants were divided according to the ADA (American Diabetes Association) recommendations, where a prediabetes condition is recognized when fasting glucose concentration is between 100 mg/dL and 125 mg/dL (5.6–6.9 mmol/L). On this basis, 234 (82.4%) children had fasting glucose concentrations <100 mg/dL (<5.6 mmol/L) and 50 (17.6%) children were recognized as having impaired fasting glucose (IFG), with fasting glucose concentrations ≥100 mg/dL (≥5.6 mmol/L) [10].

Risk of dyslipidemia was assessed in accord with the currently accepted cut-off values for fasting lipids in children [11]. Vitamin D status represented by 25(OH)D concentration was also evaluated according to currently accepted recommendations [12].

2.4. Statistical Analysis

Statistical analyses were carried out using SPSS (Statistical Package for the Social Sciences version 20, Armonk, NY, USA) software. The significance level was established at $p < 0.05$. The significance of the differences were determined using the χ^2 (chi squared) test, or the Fisher exact probability test for small groups. All quantitative variables, except for TG and CRP, showed near-normal distributions. TG and CRP variables were logarithmically normalized to allow for further regression analysis.

The Fisher exact probability test was used to present significant differences in the percentage of normal glucose concentration and hyperglycemia in three subgroups of vitamin D status. Considering that only a small group had optimal 25(OH)D concentration ($n = 10$), the analysis of variables was undertaken incorporating a dichotomous division into those with deficiency states of 25(OH)D $\leq$ 20 ng/dL (<50 nmol/L) and those with 25(OH)D > 20 ng/dL (>50 nmol/L), respectively. The linear regression analysis was tested to estimate the impact of 25(OH)D and selected variables on glucose and lipid parameters. The incorporation of hs-CRP in logistic and linear regression analysis was essential to exclude any potential bias arising from possible inflammation status. In the linear regression analysis, we presented only statistically important models. Moreover, the variables included in regression analysis were chosen based on results from Pearson correlation coefficients. Multivariate logistic regression was performed for two-category variables. Because all statistical analyses were carried out in traditional units, SI units are placed in brackets.

2.5. Compliance with Ethical Standards

The study was approved by the local ethics committee (Nicolaus Copernicus University Collegium Medicum in Bydgoszcz, Poland) in accord with the Helsinki declaration and proper ethical standards (REB 338/2015). Informed consent was obtained from the parents.

3. Results

Our study consisted of 284 children: 150 girls (52.8%) and 134 boys (47.2%) aged 9–11. Characteristics of the study population are shown in Table 1.

Table 1. Characteristics of the study population ($n = 284$).

	Parameters	*n*	(%)	Mean ($\pm$SD) or Median (27–75th Percentile)	*p (<0.05)
Age	9 years	112	(39.4)	-	
	10 years	97	(34.2)	-	
	11 years	75	(26.4)	-	
Sex	Boys	150	(52.8)	-	
	Girls	134	(47.2)	-	
BMI percentiles	<5 (underweight)	16	(5.6)	26.8 ($\pm$ 6.9)	
	$\geq$5 and <85 (optimal weight)	200	(70.4)	34.4 ($\pm$ 6.0)	
	$\geq$85 and <95 (overweight)	33	(11.6)	46 ($\pm$ 6.8)	<0.001 **
	$\geq$95 (obese)	35	(12.3)	56.1 ($\pm$ 12.1)	
Glycemic status	Glucose (<100 mg/dL; 5.6 mmol/L)	234	(82.4)	90 ($\pm$ 6.5); 5.0 ($\pm$ 0.36)	
	Glucose ($\geq$100 mg/dL; 5.6 mmol/L)	50	(17.6)	105 ($\pm$ 6.5); 5.8 ($\pm$ 0.36)	<0.001
	HbA1c (<5.7 %; 38 mmol/mol)	249	(88.9)	5.3 ($\pm$ 0.2); 34.5 ($\pm$2.2)	
	HbA1c ($\geq$5.7 %; 38 mmol/mol)	31	(11.1)	5.8 ($\pm$ 0.16); 40.0 ($\pm$1.7)	

Table 1. *Cont.*

	Parameters	*n*	(%)	Mean (±SD) or Median (27–75th Percentile)	* *p* (<0.05)
	TC (<170 mg/dL; 4.4 mmol/L)	143	(50.3)	148 (± 14.1); 3.85 (± 0.37)	0.919
	TC (≥170 mg/dL; 4.4 mmol/L)	141	(49.7)	194 (± 22.0); 5.02 (± 0.57)	
	TG: 0–9 years (<75 mg/dL; 0.85 mmol/L)	67	(23.6)	53 (± 12.8); 0.60 (± 0.14)	
	TG: 10–19 years (<90 mg/dL; 1.02 mmol/L)	123	(43.3)	62 (± 15.8); 0.70 (± 0.18)	
	TG: 0–9 years (≥75 mg/dL; 0.85 mmol/L)	46	(16.2)	112 (± 39.0); 1.27 (± 0.44)	<0.001
Lipids	TG: 10–19 years (≥90 mg/dL; 1.02 mmol/L)	48	(16.9)	136 (± 42.6); 1.54 (± 0.48)	
	LDL-C (<110 mg/dL; 2.85 mmol/L)	183	(64.4)	86 (± 14.6); 2.23 (± 0.38)	<0.001
	LDL-C (≥110 mg/dL; 2.85 mmol/L)	101	(35.6)	129 (± 20.8); 3.34 (± 0.54)	
	HDL-C (>45 mg/dL; 1.17 mmol/L)	252	(88.7)	62 (± 11.2); 1.60 (± 0.29)	<0.001
	HDL-C (≤45 mg/dL; 1.17 mmol/L)	32	(11.3)	40 (± 4.4); 1.04 (± 0.11)	
	non-HDL-C (<120 mg/dL; mmol/L)	178	(62.7)	96 (± 15.3); 2.47 (± 0.40)	<0.001
	non-HDL-C (≥120 mg/dL; mmol/L)	106	(37.3)	139 (± 21.6); 3.59 (± 0.56)	
hs-CRP	(<1 mg/L)	196	(69.0)	0.2 (0.12–0.40)	<0.001
	(≥1 mg/L)	88	(31.0)	2.1 (1.5–3.8)	
25(OH)D status	Optimal (≥30 ng/mL; 75 nmol/L)	10	(3.5)	31.8 (± 1.5); 79.37 (± 3.74)	
	Insufficiency (21–29 ng/mL; 52–72 nmol/L)	167	(58.8)	23.7 (± 2.6); 59.16 (± 6.49)	0.007
	Deficiency (≤20 ng/mL; 50 nmol/L)	107	(37.7)	17.0 (± 2.3); 42.43 (± 5.74)	

* Difference between two structure indicators determined by Chi Square test. ** Optimal vs. overweight and obese. NA: not applicable. BMI: body mass index; HbA1$_c$: glycated hemoglobin; TC: total cholesterol; TG: triglycerides; LDL-C: low-density lipoprotein cholesterol (direct method); HDL-C: high-density lipoprotein cholesterol; non-HDL-C: non-high-density lipoprotein cholesterol (TC-(HDL-C)); hs-CRP: high-sensitivity C-reactive protein; 25(OH)D: 25-hydroxycholecalciferol (calcifediol); *p*: statistical significance (<0.05). Unit conversion factors: glucose ((mg/dL) × 0.05551 = mmol/L); HbA1$_c$ (10.93 × (HbA1$_c$%) − 23.5 = mmol/mol); TC, HDL-C, LDL-C ((mg/dL) × 0.0259 = mmol/L); TG ((mg/dL) × 0.0113 = mmol/L); 25(OH)D ((ng/mL) × 2.496 = nmol/L).

Overweight and obesity levels were based on BMI percentiles according to age and sex, being 11.6% and 12.3% respectively. Vitamin D deficiency, estimated by total 25(OH)D concentration, was identified in 37.7% of the children, whereas its insufficiency was identified in 58.8%. Children with impaired fasting glucose (≥100 mg/dL; 5.6 mmol/L) constituted 17.6%, and an elevated HbA1$_c$ value was seen in 11.1% (Table 1). The most commonly identified lipid abnormality was hypercholesterolemia, which was 49.7% for TC and 35.6% for LDL-C, respectively.

Our analysis revealed that 25(OH)D concentration affected glucose metabolism as reflected by changes in fasting glucose concentrations. As can be seen in Table 2, the risk of hyperglycemia (IFG) was significantly higher (*p* = 0.033) in children with 25(OH)D deficiency (≤20 ng/mL; 50 nmol/L) (OR = 1.966, 95% CI: 1.055–3.663).

Table 2. Association of 25(OH)D deficiency with other variables.

Variables	* *p* Value	OR	95% CI	
			Lower	Upper
Age	0.791	0.958	0.699	1.314
Sex	0.636	0.885	0.534	1.467
BMI percentiles	0.053	0.665	0.440	1.005
TC	0.169	1.688	0.800	3.562
TG	0.973	1.010	0.565	1.804
HDL-C	0.245	0.611	0.267	1.402
Non-HDL-C	0.624	1.267	0.493	3.257

Table 2. *Cont.*

Variables	* p Value	OR	95% CI	
			Lower	Upper
LDL-C	0.257	0.599	0.247	1.454
hs-CRP	0.935	0.975	0.531	1.791
HBA1$_C$	0.290	1.529	0.696	3.357
Glucose	0.069	1.828	0.955	3.499
Glucose **	0.033	1.966	1.055	3.663

Logistic regression (multivariate): χ^2 = 13.5; df = 11 (degrees of freedom); p = 0.258; r2 Cox and Snell = 0.047 (Cox and Snell's R squares complex samples logistic regression algorithms); r2 Nagelkerke = 0.064 (Nagelkerke R squares complex samples logistic regression algorithms) * Statistical significance was determined in logistic regression analysis. ** Logistic regression (univariate): χ^2 = 4.513; df = 1; p = 0.034; r2 Cox and Snell=0.016; r2 Nagelkerke = 0.022. 25(OH)D: 25-hydroxycholecalciferol (calcifediol); BMI: body mass index; TC: total cholesterol; TG: triglycerides; HDL-C: high-density lipoprotein cholesterol; non-HDL-C: non-high-density lipoprotein cholesterol (TC-(HDL-C)); LDL-C: low-density lipoprotein cholesterol (direct method); hs-CRP: high-sensitivity C-reactive protein; HbA1$_c$: glycated hemoglobin.

As can be seen in Figure 1, the prevalence of hyperglycemia and hypercholesterolemia was greater in the vitamin D deficiency subgroup (24.0% and 57.3%, respectively), when compared to children with concentrations of 25(OH)D over 50 nmol/L (20 ng/mL) (16.4% and 46.2%, respectively).

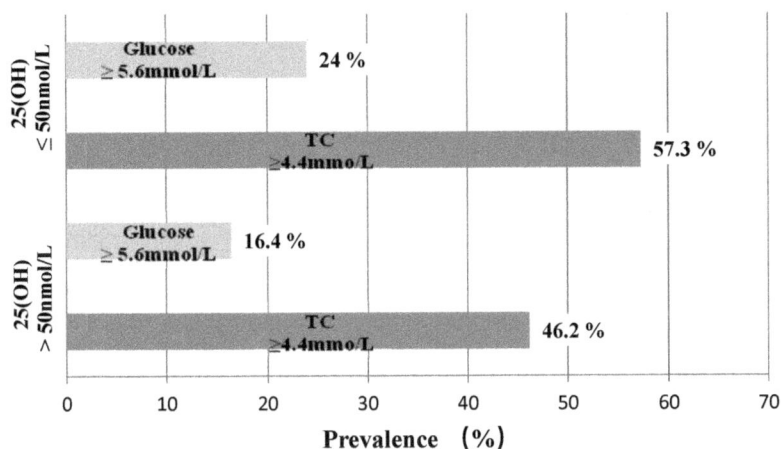

Figure 1. Occurrence of hyperglycemia/hypercholesterolemia in vitamin D-deficient children. TC: total cholesterol.

Pearson's correlation coefficients across the whole study group revealed a statistically significant weak negative correlation between 25(OH)D level and lipid variables (TG: $r = -0.160$; $p = 0.037$; HDL-C: $r = -0.209$; $p < 0.001$), and also with glucose concentrations ($r = -0.140$; $p = 0.018$). A statistically significant correlation between 25(OH)D and glucose was identified in the hypercholesterolemia subgroup ($r = -0.253$; $p = 0.002$). A weak negative correlation ($r = -0.215$; $p = 0.010$) between 25(OH)D and TC was found in the normocholesterolemic subgroup (Table 3). A significant negative correlation of 25(OH)D with HDL-C was observed in children with hyperglycemia ($r = -0.359$; $p = 0.010$).

Table 3. Pearson's correlation coefficients in normo-/hyperglycemic and normo-/hypercholesterolemic state.

Vitamin D/R-Pearson Correlation		TC	TG	HDL-C	Non-HDL-C	LDL-C	Glucose	HbA1c	hs-CRP
		Glucose: <100 mg/dL (<5.6 mmol/L) ((n = 234)—normoglycemia)							
25(OH)D	(R)[1]	−0.136	0.001	−0.163	−0.066	−0.064	−0.122	0.131	−0.001
	(p)[2]	0.037	0.990	0.012	0.314	0.330	0.063	0.046	0.989
		Glucose: ≥100 mg/dL (≥5.6 mmol/L) ((n = 50)—hyperglycemia)							
25(OH)D	(R)[1]	−0.251	−0.025	−0.359	−0.066	−0.135	−0.087	−0.008	−0.041
	(p)[2]	0.079	0.862	0.010	0.647	0.351	0.547	0.956	0.779
		Total cholesterol ≤170 mg/dL (≤4.4 mmol/L) ((n = 143)—normocholesterolemia)							
25(OH)D	(R)[1]	−0.215	−0.019	−0.187	−0.066	−0.035	−0.019	0.050	−0.053
	(p)[2]	0.010	0.820	0.026	0.436	0.677	0.821	0.554	0.531
		Total cholesterol ≥170 mg/dL (≥ 4.4 mmol/L) ((n =141)—hypercholesterolemia)							
25(OH)D	(R)[1]	−0.030	0.039	−0.181	0.091	0.030	−0.253	0.154	0.051
	(p)[2]	0.724	0.644	0.032	0.282	0.722	0.002	0.070	0.546
		All (n = 284)							
25(OH)D	(R)[1]	−0.005	−0.160	−0.209	−0.067	−0.078	−0.140	0.091	0.001
	(p)[2]	0.932	0.007	<0.001	0.262	0.193	0.018	0.129	0.991

[1] R: Pearson correlation. [2] Statistical significance ($p < 0.05$), established using Pearson's correlation analysis. 25(OH)D: 25-hydroxycholecalciferol (calcifediol); TC: total cholesterol; HDL-C: high-density lipoprotein cholesterol; non-HDL-C: non-high-density lipoprotein cholesterol (TC-(HDL-C)); LDL-C: low-density lipoprotein cholesterol (direct method); HbA1c: glycated hemoglobin; TG: triglycerides (logarithmic transformation); hs-CRP: high-sensitivity C-reactive protein (logarithmic transformation).

The linear regression model (Table 4) emphasized a significant correlation between 25(OH)D and glucose, and remained unchanged following adjustment for sex, age, and BMI percentiles.

Table 4. Impact of 25(OH)D concentration on glucose and lipids.

Model	Independent Variables	Adjusted r^2	β (beta)(Standardized coefficients)	B (Unstandardized Coefficients)	* p Value
Model 1					0.021
Glucose	25(OH)D	0.020		−0.238	0.021
	CRP log		−0.087	−1.058	0.139
Model 1 adj.					0.027
Glucose	25(OH)D	0.027	−0.142	−0.247	0.017
	CRP log		−0.107	−1.303	0.106
Model 2					<0.001
TC	25(OH)D	0.052	−0.159	−0.955	0.006
	TG log		0.183	0.124	0.002
Model 2 adj.					**0.002**
TC	25(OH)D	0.048	−0.160	−0.958	0.006
	TG log		0.192	0.130	0.003
Model 3					<0.001
HDL-C	25(OH)D	0.097	−0.202	−0.565	<0.001
	CRP log		−0.244	−4.769	<0.001
Model 3 adj.					<0.001
HDL-C	25(OH)D	0.093	−0.203	−0.568	<0.001
	CRP log		−0.249	−4.860	<0.001

* Statistical significance established using multiple linear regression analysis unadjusted and adjusted by sex, age, and BMI percentiles. Model adj.: model adjusted by sex, age, and BMI percentiles. 25(OH)D: 25-hydroxycholecalciferol (calcifediol); hs-CRP: high-sensitivity C-reactive protein (logarithmic transformation); TG: triglycerides (logarithmic transformation); TC: total cholesterol; HDL-C: high-density lipoprotein cholesterol.

Based on the first model presented, one can estimate that 25(OH)D reduced by 1 ng/mL (2.5 nmol/L) was related to slight, although significant, elevation of blood glucose concentration by

0.238 mg/dL (0.013 mmol/L). After adjustment for sex, age, and BMI, glucose concentration elevation was equal to 0.247 mg/dL (0.014 nmol/L) as a result of a unit decrease of 25 (OH)D concentration.

Our second model (Table 4) revealed a significant negative correlation between 25 (OH)D ($\beta = -0.159$; $p = 0.006$) and TC. The model presented showed a significant elevation in TC by 0.958 mg/dL (0.025 mmol/L) linked to a 25(OH)D reduction by 1 ng/mL (2.5 nmol/L). In the adjusted model, the TC elevation was identical.

The third linear regression model revealed an increase of HDL-C by 0.565 mg/dL (0.015 mmol/L), as a result of the 1 ng/mL (2.5 nmol/L) decrease in 25(OH)D concentration ($\beta = -0.203$; $p < 0.001$). Following adjustment, elevation of HDL-C reached 0.568 mg/dL (0.015 mmol/L) (Table 4).

4. Discussion

In the present study, the occurrence of IFG among children with vitamin D deficiency was almost two-fold higher (OR = 1.966) when compared to children with 25(OH)D higher than 20 ng/mL (50 nmol/L). We also observed a weak negative correlation between 25(OH)D and glucose concentration both in the whole group and in children with hypercholesterolemia.

We observed weak negative correlations between 25(OH)D and lipid components: TG and HDL-C in the whole group, HDL-C in the subgroup with hyperglycemia or TC and HDL-C in the subgroups with normo/hypercholesterolemia. Despite this weak correlation with lipid exponents, our study revealed a significant association between serum 25(OH)D and TC concentration. We found that serum 25(OH)D lower by 1 ng/mL (2.5 nmol/L) was linked to elevation in TC concentration by 0.96 mg /dL (0.025 mmol/L) and elevation of HDL-C by 0.57 mg/dL (0.015 mmol/L). The frequent occurrence of hypercholesterolemia in our study (57.3%), being a notable trend particularly in vitamin D-deficient children, is also worth noting. Evidence for the occurrence of dyslipidemia in relation to vitamin D status was inconsistent. It was observed that the concentration of TC was significantly higher in relation to vitamin D deficiency [13]. Our earlier study showed that HDL-C concentration was higher among 25(OH)D-deficient children with newly diagnosed asthma [14]. Other cross-sectional studies conducted independently by Reis et al. and Ashraf et al. did not find any significant association between low concentrations of vitamin D and abnormalities in lipid parameters [15,16]. A study by Jorde et al. revealed a cross-sectional relationship between 25(OH)D and serum lipids [17]. Meta-analysis conducted by Hao Wang et al. showed increased concentration of TC and LDL-C with simultaneously decreased concentrations of HDL-C and TG as influenced by vitamin D supplementation [18].

In this study we evaluated fasting glucose concentration, where abnormalities in this exponent of carbohydrate metabolism is considered as a first stage in prediabetes development. This condition may last several years without any additional symptoms, and depending on genetic or environmental background, may either revert to a normoglycemic state or develop into overt diabetes [19]. The prevalence of IFG among overweight and obese Hispanic children reported by Goran et al. ranged between 13% and 47% [20]. Our data indicated an inverse correlation between glucose and vitamin D concentrations, consistent with an earlier NHANES III (National Health and Nutrition Examination Survey) study where a negative relation between 25(OH)D and glycemia or diabetes occurrence was demonstrated [21]. In another study conducted on children and teenagers aged 12–19, it was seen that adjusted OR of fasting hyperglycemia among children with the lowest 25(OH)D (<15 ng/mL; 37 nmol/L) was two-and-a-half fold higher (2.54, 95% CI: 1.01–6.40) when compared to children in the highest 25(OH)D quartile (>26 ng/mL; 65 nmol/L) [15]. Our study showed that along with the decrease of 1 ng/mL (2.5 nmol/L) of 25(OH)D, serum concentration of fasting glucose increased by 0.25 mg/dL (0.014 mmol/L). The study conducted by Liu et al. indicated an association between 25(OH)D and diabetes, in contrast to that presented by Pittas et al., where it was suggested that there was insufficient data supporting hypotheses on the relation between vitamin D deficiency and its contribution to the risk of diabetes [22,23].

The most significant limitation of this study was sample size, which comprised over 100 dyslipidemic and only 50 hyperglycemic subjects. A further limitation of this study was its single-center and cross-sectional design which made it difficult to assess the influence of vitamin D on carbohydrate and lipid metabolism, with only the relationship between variables being tested. Therefore, our findings warrant confirmation in further studies. On the other hand, the strength of the present study was the simultaneous evaluation of two closely related metabolic pathways of glucose and lipids, in terms of the prevalence of vitamin D deficiency among children aged 9–11.

5. Conclusions

25(OH)D deficiency may negatively affect fasting glucose and total cholesterol concentration in children aged 9–11. Vitamin D-deficient children are twice as likely to develop prediabetes represented by IFG, when compared to those with 25(OH)D concentration above 20 ng/mL (50 nmol/L).

Author Contributions: Conceptualization, L.S. and G.S. Methodology, L.S., G.S. and M.K. Software, L.S. and K.B. Validation, G.S. Visualization, L.S. Funding Acquisition, G.S. Data Curation, L.S., M.K. and K.B. Formal Analysis, L.S. and K.B. Investigation, L.S. Project Administration, G.S. and T.D. Resources, L.S. and M.K. Supervision, T.D. and G.S. Writing—Original Draft Preparation, L.S. Writing—Review & Editing, M.K. and G.S.

Funding: This research received no external funding.

Acknowledgments: We would like to thank all of the children and their parents for participating in our study.

Conflicts of Interest: The authors declare no conflict of interest.

Abbreviations

25(OH)D	25-Hydroxycholecalciferol
ADA	American Diabetes Association
BMI	Body Mass Index
CLSI	Clinical and Laboratory Standards Institute
FG	Fasting Glucose
HbA1$_c$	Glycated Hemoglobin
HDL-C	High Density Lipoprotein Cholesterol by direct method
HS-CRP	High Sensitivity C-Reactive Protein
IFG	Impaired Fasting Glucose
LDL-C	Low Density Lipoprotein Cholesterol by direct method
NHANES	National Health and Nutrition Examination Survey
TC	Total Cholesterol
TG	Triglycerides
WHO	World Health Organization

References

1. Peterson, C. Vitamin D deficiency and childhood obesity: Interactions, implications, and recommendations. *Nutr. Diet. Suppl.* **2015**, *7*, 29–39. [CrossRef]
2. Rosen, C.J.; Adams, J.S.; Bikle, D.D.; Black, D.M.; Demay, M.B.; Manson, J.E.; Murad, M.H.; Kovacs, C.S. The nonskeletal effects of vitamin D: An Endocrine Society scientific statement. *Endocr. Rev.* **2012**, *33*, 456–492. [CrossRef] [PubMed]
3. Wimalawansa, S.J. Associations of vitamin D with insulin resistance, obesity, type 2 diabetes, and metabolic syndrome. *J. Steroid Biochem. Mol. Biol.* **2018**, *175*, 177–189. [CrossRef] [PubMed]
4. Li, C.; Ford, E.S.; Zhao, G.; Mokdad, A.H. Prevalence of pre-diabetes and its association with clustering of cardiometabolic risk factors and hyperinsulinemia among U.S. adolescents: National Health and Nutrition Examination Survey 2005–2006. *Diabetes Care* **2009**, *32*, 342–347. [CrossRef] [PubMed]
5. Mutt, S.J.; Hyppönen, E.; Saarnio, J.; Järvelin, M.R.; Herzig, K.H. Vitamin D and adipose tissue-more than storage. *Front. Physiol.* **2014**, *5*, 228. [CrossRef] [PubMed]
6. Autier, P.; Boniol, M.; Pizot, C.; Mullie, P. Vitamin D status and ill health: A systematic review. *Lancet Diabetes Endocrinol.* **2014**, *2*, 76–89. [CrossRef]

7. Enko, D.; Kriegshäuser, G.; Stolba, R.; Worf, E.; Halwachs-Baumann, G. Method evaluation study of a new generation of vitamin D assays. *Biochem. Med.* **2015**, *25*, 203–212. [CrossRef] [PubMed]

8. *Manufacturers Information Product (IDS-iSYS 25-Hydroxy Vitamin Ds IS-2700S v04)*; Immunodiagnostic Systems: The Boldons, UK, 2015.

9. Kułaga, Z.; Różdżyńska, A.; Palczewska, I.; Grajda, A.; Gurzkowska, B.; Napieralska, E.; Litwin, M. Percentile charts of height, body mass and body mass index in children and adolescents in Poland—Results of the OLAF study. *Stand. Med.* **2010**, *7*, 690–700.

10. Odrowąż-Sypniewska, G. Laboratory diagnosis of prediabetes. *Diagn. Lab.* **2016**, *52*, 57–62.

11. Myśliwiec, M.; Walczak, M.; Małecka-Tendera, E.; Dobrzańska, A.; Cybulska, B.; Filipiak, K.J.; Mazur, A.; Jarosz-Chobot, P.; Szadkowska, A.; Rynkiewicz, A.; et al. Management in familial hypercholesterolaemia in children and adolescents. Position of the Lipid Expert Forum. *Kardiol. Pol.* **2013**, *71*, 1099–1105. [CrossRef] [PubMed]

12. Sypniewska, G.; Krintus, M.; Fulgheri, G.; Siodmiak, J.; Kuligowska-Prusinska, M.; Stepien-Jaszowska, B.; Staszak-Kowalska, R.; Zawadzka-Krajewska, A.; Kierat, S.; Bergmann, K.; et al. 25-Hydroxyvitamin, D, biomarkers of eosinophilic inflammation and airway remodeling in children with newly diagnosed untreated asthma. *Allergy Asthma Proc.* **2017**, *38*, 29–36. [CrossRef] [PubMed]

13. Kumar, J.; Muntner, P.; Kaskel, F.J.; Hailpern, S.M.; Melamed, M.L. Prevalence and Associations of 25-Hydroxyvitamin D Deficiency in US Children: NHANES 2001–2004. *Pediatrics* **2009**, *124*, 362–370. [CrossRef] [PubMed]

14. Odrowąż-Sypniewska, G.; Krintus, M.; Siódmiak, J.; Jaszowska, I.; Staszak-Kowalska, R.; Zawadzka-Krajewska, A.; Kierat, S.Z.; Demkow, U. Serum 25(OH)D status and lipid profile in children with newly diagnosed asthma. *Med. Res. J.* **2015**, *3*, 113–116. [CrossRef]

15. Reis, J.P.; von Mühlen, D.; Miller, E.R.; Michos, E.D.; Appel, L.J. Vitamin D Status and Cardiometabolic Risk Factors in the United States Adolescent Population. *Pediatrics* **2009**, *124*, 371–379. [CrossRef] [PubMed]

16. Ashraf, A.; Alvarez, J.; Saenz, K.; Gower, B.; McCormick, K.; Franklin, F. Threshold for Effects of Vitamin D Deficiency on Glucose Metabolism in Obese Female African-American Adolescents. *J. Clin. Endocrinol. Metab.* **2009**, *94*, 3200–3206. [CrossRef] [PubMed]

17. Jorde, R.; Figenschau, Y.; Hutchinson, M.; Emaus, N.; Grimnes, G. High serum 25-hydroxyvitamin D concentrations are associated with a favorable serum lipid profile. *Eur. J. Clin. Nutr.* **2010**, *64*, 1457–1464. [CrossRef] [PubMed]

18. Wang, H.; Xia, N.; Yang, Y.; Peng, D.Q. Influence of vitamin D supplementation on plasma lipid profiles: A meta-analysis of randomized controlled trials. *Lipids Health Dis.* **2010**, *11*, 42. [CrossRef] [PubMed]

19. Kleber, M.; deSousa, G.; Papcke, S.; Wabitsch, M.; Reinehr, T. Impaired glucose tolerance in obese white children and adolescents: Three to five year follow-up in untreated patients. *Exp. Clin. Endocrinol. Diabetes* **2011**, *119*, 172–176. [CrossRef] [PubMed]

20. Michael, I.G.; Lane, C.; Toledo-Corral, C.; Weigensberg, M.J. Persistence of prediabetes in overweight and obese Hispanic children: Association with progressive insulin resistance, poor beta-cell function, and increasing visceral fat. *Diabetes* **2008**, *57*, 3007–3012. [CrossRef]

21. Misiorowski, W. Vitamin D in type 1 and 2 diabetes in adulthood. *Stand. Med. Pediatr.* **2015**, *9*, 639–644.

22. Liu, E.; Meigs, J.B.; Pittas, A.G.; Economos, C.D.; McKeown, N.M.; Booth, S.L.; Jacques, P.F. Predicted 25-hydroxyvitamin D score and incident type 2 diabetes in the Framingham Offspring Study. *Am. J. Clin. Nutr.* **2010**, *91*, 1627–1633. [CrossRef] [PubMed]

23. Pittas, A.G.; Chung, M.; Trikalinos, T.; Mitri, J.; Brendel, M.; Patel, K.; Lichtenstein, A.H.; Lau, J.; Balk, E.M. Systematic review: Vitamin D and cardiometabolic outcomes. *Ann. Intern. Med.* **2010**, *152*, 307–314. [CrossRef] [PubMed]

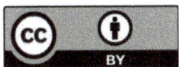

nutrients

MDPI

Review

What is the Validity of Questionnaires Assessing Fruit and Vegetable Consumption in Children When Compared with Blood Biomarkers? A Meta-Analysis

Tatiana S. Collese *, Gabriela Vatavuk-Serrati, Marcus Vinicius Nascimento-Ferreira, Augusto César Ferreira De Moraes and Heráclito Barbosa Carvalho

YCARE (Youth/Child cArdiovascular Risk and Environmental) Research Group, Department of Preventive Medicine, Faculdade de Medicina, Universidade de Sao Paulo, Sao Paulo, SP 01246-903, Brazil; gabrielavserrati@gmail.com (G.V.-S.); marcus1986@usp.br (M.V.N.-F.); augustocesar.demoraes@usp.br (A.C.F.D.M.); heracc@usp.br (H.B.C.)

* Correspondence:tcollese@usp.br; Tel.: +55-11-3061-7091; Fax: +55-11-3061-8466

Received: 27 July 2018; Accepted: 20 September 2018; Published: 1 October 2018

Abstract: Fruit and vegetable consumption has been associated with improved health outcomes in children. As an extensive number of questionnaires are currently used to assess fruit and vegetable consumption, we performed a systematic review of the criterion validity of questionnaires used to estimate fruit and vegetable consumption in children, considering blood biomarkers as the reference method. Five electronic databases (MEDLINE, CINAHL, Scopus, PsycINFO, Web of Science) were searched from database inception to 23 July 2018. The search strategy used the following sets of descriptors: children; fruits and vegetables; dietary questionnaires; blood biomarkers; and validation coefficient. The search terms were adapted for use with other databases in combination with database-specific filters. Potentially eligible articles were selected independently by two reviewers, separately, following the Preferred Reporting Items for Systematic Reviews and Meta-Analyses (PRISMA) guidelines. Two articles meeting the inclusion criteria were included. The main reason for study exclusion was the sample age range, which included adolescents. The pooled correlation coefficient was 0.32 (95% confidence interval: 0.24–0.40).This review provided insights into assessment methods of fruit and vegetable consumption in children. Although further studies are required, questionnaires for assessing fruit and vegetable consumption have fair criterion validity in children.

Keywords: systematic review; meta-analysis; children; fruits and vegetables; biomarkers; vitamins; validity

---

1. Introduction

International health associations recommend that children have a diet rich in vegetables, fruits, whole grains, low-fat dairy products, legumes, fish, and lean meat, and low in saturated fat, trans fat, and cholesterol, to help maintain a healthy weight and promote cardiovascular health [1]. Given the role that the diet plays in children's health, it is crucial to accurately determine their dietary intake and to estimate the relationship between the foods consumed and nutrients.

Regular fruit and vegetable consumption is routinely suggested as a key component of promoting health because they are an important source of nutrients, such as water, fiber, potassium, folic acid, vitamins, and phytochemicals [1,2]. Several systematic reviews and meta-analyses have found consistent associations between fruit and vegetable consumption and lower risk of cardiovascular disease, diabetes, cancer, and other chronic diseases [3–5]. Despite the well-known benefits of consuming fruits and vegetables, children are not meeting the recommended level of five servings per day [6]. Consequently, increasing fruit and vegetable consumption in children is one of the major goals of dietary interventions, worldwide [6]. Thus, valid questionnaires to assess fruit and vegetable consumption are essential to identify eating habit changes in response to interventions, and to analyze the impact of fruit consumption on health [7].

In nutritional epidemiology, the most used methods to estimate fruit and vegetable intake are subjective instruments, such as food frequency questionnaires (FFQs) and dietary recalls, because they are simple, cost-effective methods to assess long-term eating habits for large samples [8,9]. However, these subjective instruments are susceptible to both random and systematic errors [10,11], especially when applied to children, due to their limited skills to report their own dietary intake, depending on parental (or whoever is responsible for their food) literacy and motivation to complete these questionnaires [12].

As all dietary assessment methods (e.g., 24 h recalls, FFQs, smart-phone apps) have their own strengths and limitations, dietary questionnaires are usually validated against an objective measurement, such as blood biomarkers or doubly-labeled water [8,13]. Previous studies proposed that plasma vitamins, such as vitamin A, E, and C, are a reliable concentration biomarker of usual fruit and vegetable intake. Hence they are commonly used in validity studies of dietary assessment methods as independent proxy measures of fruit and vegetable consumption [14], and to evaluate whether sources of random error are independent of errors associated with measurement by questionnaire and/or inaccuracies within nutrient databases [15].

However, these plasma vitamins are still relatively recent, and a significant amount of studies are warranted in nutritional epidemiology [16]. It concerns deciphering whether these biomarkers are markers of dietary consumption or markers of altered metabolism, as a result of the food intake [16], or regarding the individual variability in absorption or availability [17]. Validation studies with blood biomarkers have been carried out in adults [10,11], but relatively few studies were conducted in children, lacking literature on key issues such as the impact of the period between fruit and vegetable consumption and the blood biomarker analysis, or the stability of blood biomarkers in children aged 3 years to less than 10 years.

Therefore, the research question of this review was "What is the criteria validity of questionnaires used to estimate fruit and vegetable consumption in children when compared with blood biomarkers?"

2. Methods

This systematic review was designed and conducted according to the guidelines of the Preferred Reporting Items for Systematic Reviews and Meta-Analyses (PRISMA) checklist (Supplementary Material 1), as described in Reference [18]. At study initiation, no similar systematic reviews were available in PROSPERO (International Prospective Register of Systematic Reviews) or the following databases: Biomed Central, Medical Literature Analysis and Retrieval System Online (MEDLINE), Web of Science, Cumulative Index to Nursing and Allied Health Literature (CINAHL), Scopus, and PsycINFO. Thus, this protocol was registered in PROSPERO (CRD42017072531).

2.1. Study Selection

Five electronic databases—MEDLINE, CINAHL, Scopus, PsycINFO, and Web of Science—were searched from inception to 20 December 2017. The searches were registered in the National Center for Biotechnology Information (US National Library of Medicine, Bethesda, MD, USA), so that continual updates on new publications would be received until 23 July 2018, and the searches were updated until this same date. References of selected articles were analyzed, and the corresponding authors were contacted to identify other relevant studies. The descriptors and medical terms used for the database search were as follows: *(Child OR Children OR school OR boy OR son OR girl OR daughter) AND (Fruit OR Vegetable) AND (Questionnaire OR 24h Dietary Recall OR 24 h-Dietary-Recall OR 24 h Dietary Recall OR Recall OR Food Frequency Questionnaire OR FFQ) AND (Biomarker OR Blood OR concentration biomarker OR serum OR serum marker OR carotenoids OR vitamins) AND (Validation OR Validity OR coefficient OR reliability).*

Two investigators examined the articles and performed the data screening, the data extraction, and the quality assessment independently. Inter-reviewer discrepancies were resolved by consensus, and a third reviewer was consulted for unresolved discrepancies. Relevant articles were obtained in full and were assessed for eligibility and exclusion criteria.

2.2. Eligibility Criteria

As the goal of this systematic review was to assess evidence, specifically for validation studies of questionnaires used to estimate fruit and vegetable consumption in children when compared with blood biomarkers, this type of review must clearly delineate the population in question. Consequently, the results may apply only to school-aged children.

The literature suggests that children are already able to help their parents to report their food intake with relative accuracy [19]. However, after 10 years of age, the World Health Organization [20] classifies the population as adolescent, with more independence and skills, which strongly influence decision making, peer affiliation, and behavior [21], allowing them to decide on and self-report their own dietary intake. In this sense, we considered only the children between three years of age until nine years and 11 months, as presented in Table 1.

Table 1. Eligibility criteria included in the systematic review.

	Eligibility Criteria
Population	Children (3 years to less than 10 years of age) in a free-living environment, without any specific condition (e.g., eating disorder, obesity, diabetes) or children under medical care.
Exposure	Fruit and/or vegetable consumption estimated by questionnaire.
Comparator	Blood biomarkers for fruit and/or vegetable consumption.
Outcome	Validation coefficients of fruit and/or vegetable consumption.
Study	Original articles.

Exclusion Criteria

Studies where the participants had different diseases (or disturbances) that could interfere with fruit and vegetable consumption were excluded. These criteria were set to increase inter-study comparability. In addition, review articles, conference papers, or books were excluded.

2.3. Data Screening and Extraction

Potentially eligible articles were selected for inclusion according to the following sequence:

1. Articles published in English, Spanish, and Portuguese were identified;
2. Titles of the articles were screened;
3. Abstracts were screened; and
4. The full texts of the articles were reviewed to determine whether they met the inclusion criteria.

Articles were saved in the EndNote Web reference manager software version 3.1 (Thomson Research Software, Carlsbad, CA, USA), and duplicates were removed. The data extracted included the author, title of the study, citation and contact details, and study eligibility (Table 1). When studies did not meet the eligibility criteria, the main reason for exclusion was documented in ink. Thereafter, a table (Supplementary Material 2) was created by each reviewer with additional details about the study, such as the sample size, settings, exposure/outcome definition and unit of measurement, statistical analysis, bias (funding sources, adjustments), key conclusions, authors, miscellaneous comments from the study authors, references to other relevant studies, limitations, correspondence required, and miscellaneous comments by the authors reviewing the included studies.

2.4. Quality Assessment

All retrieved articles were independently assessed and critically appraised using the standardized checklist of the STROBE-nut (adapted to our review) to identify sources of bias, performance, attrition, and detection. Data relevant to this review included the study design, characteristics of the research subjects, dietary assessment methods used, results, discussion, bias assessment, and ethics information.

2.5. Strategy for Data Synthesis

The reporting status of fruit and vegetable consumption in each of the included studies were determined from that listed within the results section of the included articles. The reporting status of each study was determined using three predefined categories. The categories were dependent on the level of accuracy of reported fruit and vegetable consumption, compared to measured blood biomarkers. When available from included studies, agreement estimates were extracted if the reporting status of research subjects correlated to various characteristics of the group. These characteristics included demographic statistics (age and sex), anthropometric characteristics (height, weight, and body mass index), and the study design. Limitations of each study and the evidence level were recorded as well. The agreement estimates from study questionnaires were synthesized.

2.6. Statistics

We used the Stata 14 (Stata Corp., College Station, TX, USA) program for all statistical analyses. Our outcomes were the correlation coefficients between the questionnaire and blood biomarkers, which we calculated with their corresponding 95% confidence intervals (considering $p < 0.05$ as significance level). In addition, we calculated the sample-weighted pooled correlation coefficient for the meta-analysis with the random-effects model, due to the moderate heterogeneity found in each study. We estimated the strength of the agreement of the Spearman rank correlation coefficient cutoff points using the classification for dietary assessment methods: weak < 0.20, fair = 0.21 to 0.40, moderate = 0.41 to 0.60, good = 0.61 to 0.80, and >0.80, very good [22]. Additionally, we verified the heterogeneity of the studies using the *I-squared* test (percentages and p values under 0.05 were considered significant). Heterogeneity levels of 25%, 50%, and 75% were considered low, moderate, and high, respectively [23]. We performed the Egger's regression test to verify potential publication bias (positive or negative results) and small-study effects. We also generated the funnel plot (Supplementary Material 3) to examine the potential bias graphically.

3. Results

The literature search provided 680 potentially eligible records: 4 from PsycINFO, 42 from Embase, 71 from Web of Science, 430 from Scopus, and 133 from Medline (see Appendix 1 in the Supporting Information online). After duplicates ($n = 51$) were excluded, 629 studies remained and were screened by title and, posteriorly, by abstract, according to the established inclusion criteria, resulting in 19 records for which the full-text was assessed for eligibility. Of those, the main reasons for exclusion were the population (studies included participants over 10 years of age) and biomarker (such as skin carotenoids), as shown in Figure 1. More details about these 19 study articles are stated in Supplementary Material 4. Consequently, two studies were eligible and were included in this systematic review.

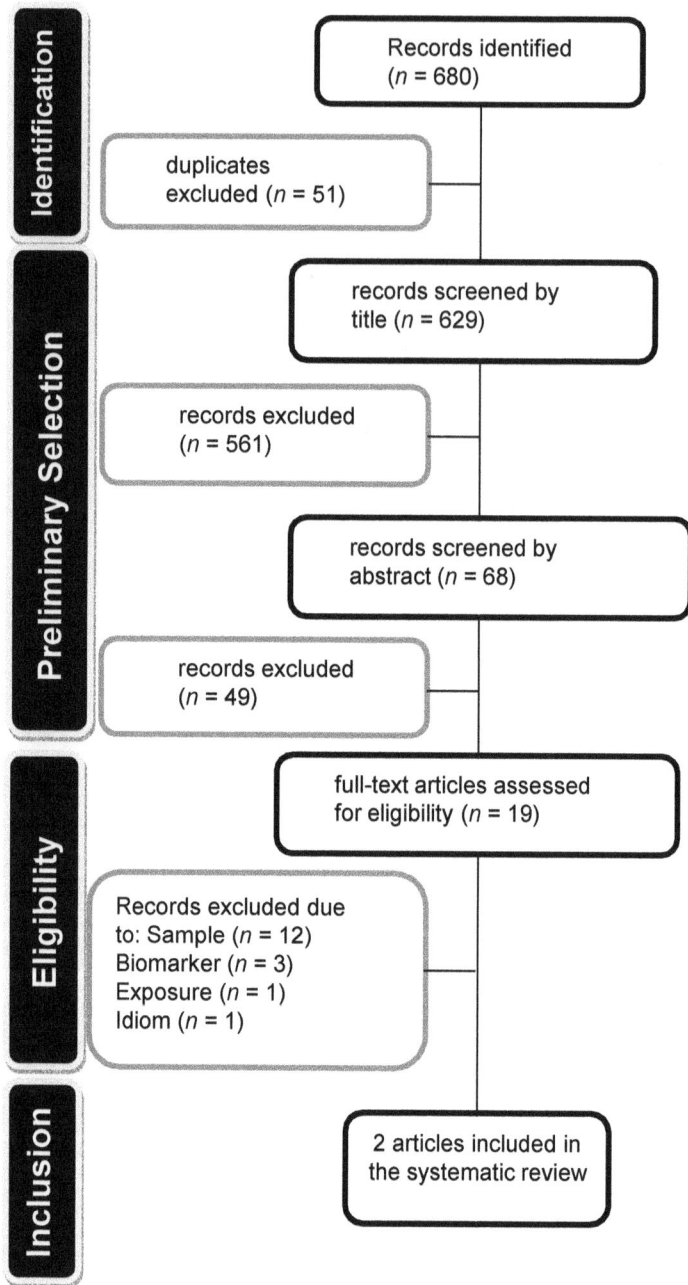

Figure 1. Flow chart of article identification, retrieval, and inclusion, for the systematic review.

The two final eligible articles included in this systematic review were published in English, but they are from different countries, one from Europe and the other from North America (Table 2). We found one study published in 1993 [24], but Medin et al. [25] was more recent, published in 2016.

Table 2. Description of the included studies.

Reference	Survey Year	Country	Study/Article Title	Sample Age (Years)	Sample Size		Study Type
					Total (*n*)	Girls (%)	
Byers et al. (1993) [24]	1990	USA	The accuracy of parental reports of their children's intake of fruits and vegetables: Validation of a food frequency questionnaire with serum levels of carotenoids and vitamins C, A, and E.	06 to 10	97	55.7	Validity
Medin et al. (2016) [25]	2013	Norway	Associations between reported intakes of carotenoid-rich foods and concentrations of carotenoids in plasma: A validation study of a web-based food recall for children and adolescents.	08 to 09 12 to 14	121	55.6	Validity

Table 3 shows that both studies asked for the parental report; however, Byers et al. [24] used the FFQ regarding the previous three months and considered fruit juice together with fruit and vegetable consumption. Medin et al. [25] used a web-based food recall, for four consecutive nights, but they assessed only vegetable intake for 4th grade children (8–9 years of age).

Nine different types of biomarkers were used to validate fruit and vegetable consumption. Both studies analyzed carotenoids (α-carotene, β-carotene, and cryptoxanthin), but Medin et al. [25] also included lycopene, lutein, and zeaxanthin in the sum of total carotenoids. On the other hand, Byers et al. [24] analyzed vitamin A (retinol), vitamin E (α-tocopherol), and vitamin C (ascorbic acid). High-performance liquid chromatography (HPLC), which is considered the gold standard analytical technique for characterization and analysis of carotenoids in biological and food samples [26], was used to assess plasma carotenoids in all studies (and for vitamin E in Byers et al. [24]), and spectrophotometry was used to assess plasma vitamin C (Table 3).

The correlation coefficients between fruit and vegetable consumption and blood biomarkers are presented in Table 4. The validity coefficients were fair to moderate, varying from 0.24 (for vitamin E) to 0.47 (carotenoids). Both studies calculated the Spearman rank correlation coefficients and adjusted the analyses for age, sex, ethnicity, and body mass index.

Table 3. Validity studies on questionnaires to assess fruit and vegetable consumption with blood biomarkers in children.

Reference	Exposure Assessment Method	Period of Report	Report	Consumption	Supplements Assessed	Nutritional Database	Blood Biomarkers	Biochemical Method	Fasting Time
Byers et al. (1993) [24]	FFQ (111 food items)	Previous 3 months	Parental	Median fruits, fruit juice, and vegetables Girls: 3.7 Boys: 2.9 (serving/day)	Not declared	Willet	α-Carotene β-Carotene Cryptoxanthin α-tocopherol Ascorbic Acid	HLPC (carotenoids, vitamin A and E), Spectrophotometry (vitamin C)	Not required
Medin et al. (2016) [25]	Web-based food recall	4 consecutive nights	Parental	Median fruits, fruit juice, and vegetables: 225.1 (g/day)	Yes + supplements containing carotenoids	USDA National Nutrient Database	α-Carotene β-Carotene β-Cryptoxanthin Lycopene Lutein Zeaxanthin	HPLC	Non-fasting

Abbreviations: FFQ: food frequency questionnaire; HPLC: high-performance liquid chromatography.

Table 4. Outcome of the included studies.

Reference	Correlations between diet and Blood				Criterion Validity	Covariates in Fully Adjusted Model	Conflict of Interest
	Vitamin A		Vitamin E	Vitamin C			
	Carotenoids	Retinol					
Byers et al. (1993) [24]	0.30	0.25	0.24	0.34	Spearman	Age, sex, ethnicity, family history of coronary artery disease, BMI, TG, serum total cholesterol, total caloric intake	Not declared
Medin et al. (2016) [25]	Vegetable intake: 0.47	-	-	-	Spearman	Age, sex, ethnicity, family structure, BMI, parental education level	None

Abbreviations: BMI: body mass index; TG: serum triglycerides.

154

The heterogeneity between studies was moderate (I-squared = 62.9%, p = 0.029), and the sample-weighted pooled correlation coefficient for biomarkers was fair (r = 0.32, 95% CI: 0.24–0.40), as shown in the Figure 2. We were not able to stratify the analysis into subgroup categories due to the small number of eligible studies included in the systematic review.

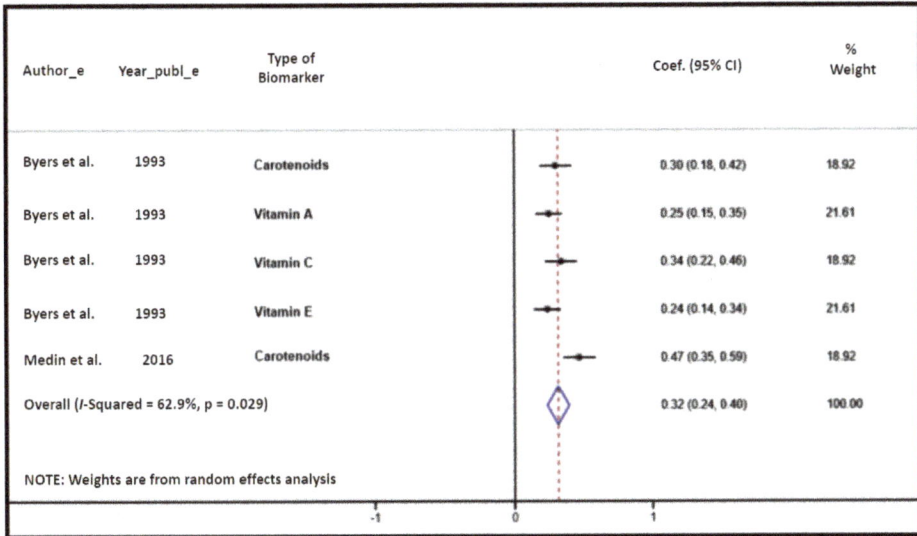

Author_e	Year_publ_e	Type of Biomarker		Coef. (95% CI)	% Weight
Byers et al.	1993	Carotenoids		0.30 (0.18, 0.42)	18.92
Byers et al.	1993	Vitamin A		0.25 (0.15, 0.35)	21.61
Byers et al.	1993	Vitamin C		0.34 (0.22, 0.46)	18.92
Byers et al.	1993	Vitamin E		0.24 (0.14, 0.34)	21.61
Medin et al.	2016	Carotenoids		0.47 (0.35, 0.59)	18.92
Overall (*I*-Squared = 62.9%, p = 0.029)				0.32 (0.24, 0.40)	100.00

NOTE: Weights are from random effects analysis

Figure 2. Forest-plot for correlation coefficients of fruit and vegetable consumption assessed by questionnaires and blood biomarkers.

4. Discussion

At present, there is no strong evidence regarding the validity of questionnaires for assessing fruit and vegetable consumption in children with blood biomarkers. Thus, we conducted a comprehensive systematic review of validity studies of questionnaires to assess fruit and vegetable consumption in children in comparison with blood biomarkers. Our findings indicated that this criteria validity was fair. This validity stems from the challenges inherent to dietary assessment through questionnaires, in addition to the fact that in children, we should consider the parent report, which is the subjective perception of the parents about their children's feeding habits [13,27].

The limited number studies (n = 2) meeting the inclusion criteria was likely due to the lack of validated dietary questionnaires, maybe because conducting blood collection in school children is less feasible, for practical and financial reasons [28], and due to the sample age range, since different age group definitions were used for children (e.g., together with infants or adolescents). For example, the study of Biltoft-Jensen et al. [29], which fulfilled our eligibility criteria, except for the population age range, which was between 8 and 11 years of age. It is correct that 11-year-old individuals are still children; however, the timing of biological maturation clearly signals entry into adolescence [21], and with more cognitive abilities that enable the researchers to apply the self-report of fruit and vegetable consumption. Therefore, it was excluded from our review.

It is important to emphasize that the credibility of our findings does not rely on the number of studies included in the meta-analysis (n = 2), as we conducted an exhaustive and reproducible literature search to produce results with the highest level of quality of evidence available. Murad et al. [30] state that a systematic review or meta-analysis should evaluate the credibility of the methods applied on the systematic review, and that this credibility depends on whether the review addressed a specific and objective question; included an exhaustive literature search; clearly indicated the reproducibility of the selection and assessment of studies; and declared the results in a convenient way that enables future research development. Furthermore, even though only two studies were eligible in our systematic review, each biomarker was considered separately in the analysis; in other words, we evaluated five different items ($n = 5$).

The sample-weighted pooled correlation coefficient found in our study ($r = 0.32$, 95% CI: 0.24–0.40) was fair, and comparisons with other validity studies carried out in children and adolescents (9–12 years) showed similar Pearson correlation coefficients for vegetable (0.26, $p = 0.13$) and fruit intake (0.49; $p = 0.003$) with total plasma carotenoids [31]. Studies carried out in adults showed a slight increase in the Spearman correlation coefficients for alpha-carotene (0.42; CI: 0.09–0.96), beta-carotene (0.40; CI: 0.09–0.99), and total plasma carotenoids (0.51; CI: 0.12–1.00) [32]. However, these correlations are not so distant from our results, and it is relevant to note that their confidence intervals were broad.

4.1. Dietary Assessment Methods

Measuring fruit and vegetable consumption is complex, with interactions of different food compounds, cultural, and socioeconomic conditions, in variable proportions [10,33]. Until this moment, an ideal questionnaire to assess fruit and vegetable consumption is unknown [28]. There is an extensive number of methods to perform this evaluation; however, all of them have both random and systematic limitations and errors [10].

It is difficult to determine from the studies included in this review who is the most accurate reporter of a child's fruit and vegetable intake, and which method is most accurate and reliable. It is important to note that mere participation in a research study may have biased the data reported for each child, because parents may have selectively reported higher consumption of fruit and vegetable of their child due to their involvement in the study. Reporting methods also depend on the difficulties associated with the method of reporting, and with the parental educational level.

4.2. Food Frequency Questionnaires

Byers et al. [24] used an FFQ to estimate fruit and vegetable consumption in children. Some advantages of the use of the FFQ are as follows: it can be given to the children's parents with limited explanation; it is a good method to obtain data regarding food eaten less than twice a week; questions can be included to allow different portion sizes (adjusted); and the food/nutrient database only needs to cover commonly eaten foods [34].

Disadvantages: it is time consuming; parents may find it difficult to decide how often their child eats fruit or vegetables; the FFQ often underestimates foods eaten regularly or in large quantities if the portion sizes used in the questionnaire are based on average intake; if a portion size is specified in the FFQ, parents may find it difficult to interpret and answer the question meaningfully; and furthermore, it depends on the level of literacy of the parents [34].

4.3. Web-Based Food Recall

Medin et al. [25] showed a higher correlation coefficient (0.47) for vegetable consumption, using a web-based food recall for four consecutive nights. The development of technology-based research tools for the assessment of intake, such as the web-based food recalls, has the potential to reach large populations and reduce language barriers through the use of images rather than verbal descriptions [19]. Technology allows for greater scale and efficiencies for researchers to rely on regular dietary intake data, for surveillance and monitoring [19]. The conversion of paper-based methods into web-based methods may have benefits, including faster completion, greater reach, and the ability to maximize the collection of complete data [19], which might explain part of the higher correlation coefficient found by Medin et al. [25], when compared to other studies that used the FFQ. Furthermore, two small details might have made a great difference in the Medin et al. [25] results: participants were given a personal gift card as an incentive for participating in the study, which may have changed their engagement in it; a voice-assisted cartoon character helped the children and parents to complete the questionnaires, with pop-up reminders to reduce the problem of food omissions, and in a more friendly way for kids—this was shown to be a promising tool for application in pediatric populations.

In addition, Medin et al. [25] included four nightly 24-h recalls. This period is more than the literature recommendation (three recalls per person) [34], and since parents answered the questionnaire at night (the end of the day), it was easier for them to remember their child's fruit and vegetable consumption on the same day, minimizing the memory bias as well [34].

However, web-based food recalls reduce the limitations in terms of misreporting. Thus, there is a need for continued development of methods, as well as to continue to evolve statistical methods to mitigate error. Training researchers, clinical staff, and research subjects on the use of the technology and the method is still highly warranted and might improve results and compliance with the dietary method [19].

To be confident about the fruit and vegetable data collected, one should combine the FFQ with food recall methods, trying to ascertain both frequent and infrequent fruit and vegetable consumption [35]. Additionally, if possible, combining technology with both dietary assessment methods is a good alternative to reduce the burden of data handling and to make this process more friendly and joyful.

4.4. Creativity

The integration of technology, pictures, drawings, cartoons, and puppets into traditional dietary questionnaires, considering the main factors inherent (Figure 3) to this approach, might provide additional insights to mitigate errors in the fruit and vegetable assessment.

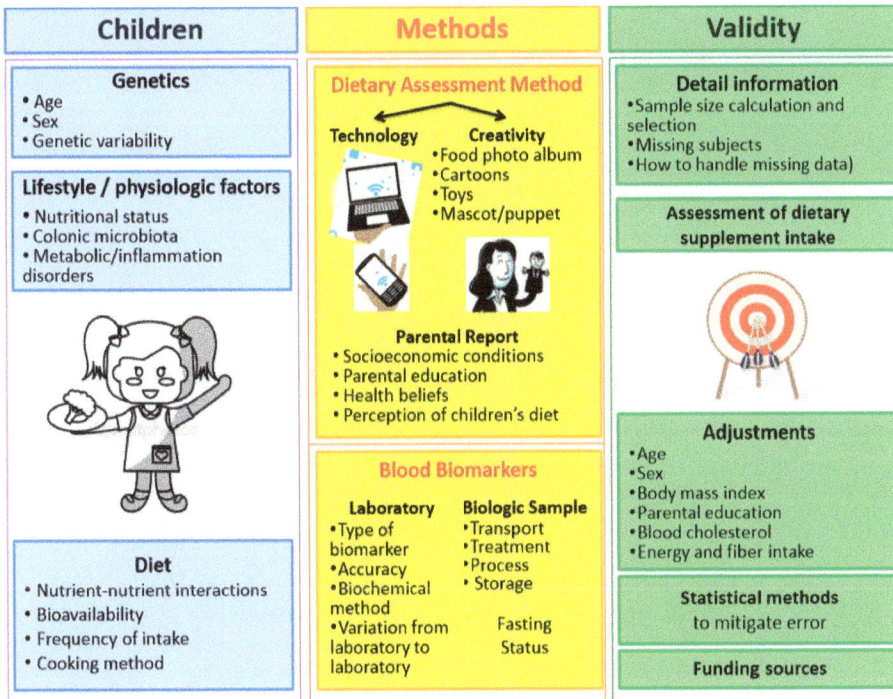

Figure 3. Main factors regarding the validity of dietary assessment methods in children.

When financial resources are scarce, like in studies conducted in low and middle-income countries, using a bit of creativity might be a good solution. For example, if it is not possible to combine the technology in the process of dietary assessment, a simple art-based method like a "mascot" (drawn on paper, as a cartoon, as a toy or a hand puppet) can make a great difference in the motivation and involvement to answer the questionnaire, turning this process into a fun moment for kids [36,37]. Additionally, pictorial assessment, such as the assessment with the help of food photography albums, food drawings or food replicas (three-dimensional models), might also be a cheaper and smart alternative to enhance motivation and give visual support to estimate fruit and vegetable portion sizes [38,39].

4.5. Administration Mode

A recent systematic review of the validity of dietary assessment methods in children when compared with doubly labeled water suggests that using a parental reporter is the most accurate method for reporting dietary intake in children aged 4–11 years [13]. However, it should be noted that parents were the proxy reporters for the children; thus, some bias can be involved in this report. For example, the parental weight status may influence the accuracy of their report, as observed in a study with obese parents, who may underestimate the food intake of their obese children [40].

4.6. Blood Biomarkers

It is important to bear in mind that there are issues pertaining to bio accessibility and bioavailability of vitamin A, E, and C in fruits and vegetables, depending on several factors, such as genotype, ripening time, cultivation method, and climatic conditions, processing, food source, food particle size and location, cooking method, and the content of fiber of the fruit or vegetable [41,42]. Moreover, different parts of the same plant may also contain different types and amounts of vitamins [41].

In addition, knowing that most vitamins have a half-life of one or 2 months [43], it is difficult to assess their blood availability and to compare it over long previous periods, such as Byers et al. [24] did with their FFQ. Blood vitamins cannot be translated into absolute levels of fruit and vegetable consumption, but these biomarkers do correlate with fruit and vegetable consumption in certain strengths, and they are commonly applied in dietary assessment studies [28].

There are other factors relating to the children that may also affect the measurement and utility of these biomarkers to properly reflect their fruit and vegetable consumption. For example, genetic variability, lifestyle or physiologic factors (e.g., colonic microbiota, body mass index, and metabolic or inflammation disorders) [44], dietary factors (e.g., frequency of intake and nutrient–nutrient interactions), blood sample (e.g., whole blood, plasma, serum, conditions of sample collection, transport, treatment, process, and storage), fasting status before examination (which neither of the studies required), and laboratory analytical methodology (e.g., accuracy, detection of limits, variation from laboratory to laboratory) [28].

Even with all these factors influencing vitamins blood levels, this method is still considered by the scientific community as a reference method for fruit and vegetable consumption in epidemiological and clinical studies.

4.7. Adjustment for Confounders

In addition, appropriate adjustments for confounding variables are critical for understanding how factors of interest are interrelated within a population, as there may be a range of plausible measurement errors that have a slight influence on these associations [45]. The two eligible studies reported adjusting for confounders; however, the variables in the adjusted model differed according to the study. Hence, we suggest that future studies should consider, at least, the sex, age, body mass index, parental education, blood cholesterol, and energy and fiber intake to be included in the fully-adjusted model.

4.8. Methodological Quality

To the best of our knowledge, there is no evidence regarding the validity of questionnaires for assessing fruit and vegetable consumption in children with blood biomarkers. However, other systematic reviews addressing the validity of dietary assessment questionnaires and objective methods, such as double label water [13] or skin biomarkers [19], have consistently reported low methodological quality of the studies as well. Other studies in the field of physical activity in children, validating questionnaires with objective methods (e.g., accelerometers), also reported low methodological quality, especially regarding the absence of information about missing subjects and how the missing data were handled [46].

In this review, only two studies were included. Based on the STROBE checklist, the major bias identified was related to the information bias, particularly due to the heterogeneity between studies in the applied methodologies. The absence of information about how the study size was calculated, or how missing data were handled was a flaw in both studies. Byers et al. [24] did not declare any adjustment for parental education level, nor information on whether fruit and vegetable intake was reported with or without the inclusion of dietary supplement intake, nor about funding sources that could influence their results.

4.9. Bias

The findings of our review indicated that more validity studies of fruit and vegetable consumption need to be carried out in school-aged children. The two eligible studies were published in English and in high-income countries. Therefore, it indicates a potential risk of publication bias, which can practically be explained by the expensive cost of conducting a validity study with blood biomarkers [28].

Moreover, most of the 19 remaining full-text articles assessed for eligibility used the plasma carotenes as a reference method, but only two articles assessed vitamin E [24,47], and one article assessed vitamin C [24]. This bias is also probably related to the costs of vitamin C, to its very sensitive biochemical methodology, and to the many difficulties and bureaucratic barriers for achieving the reactants necessary for this methodology.

As dietary assessment cannot be estimated without error, it is paramount to attempt to understand their effect on the data collected to minimize the confounding effect [17].

Byers et al. studied a sample of parents from a selective group of volunteers who reported their children's food intake once a year. Thus, the validity of their reports was probably higher than other parents, because their motivation, involvement, and knowledge in the next step of the study could be different to other parents who have never been involved in a nutritional research [24].

Another relevant issue of concern is the social approval of fruits and vegetables. As they are widely known as healthy foods [48], parents may have reported their children's fruit and vegetable consumption, either consciously or subconsciously, in ways that make them appear favorable to the researchers [17].

4.10. Heterogeneity between Studies in the Meta-Analysis

A moderate degree of heterogeneity was found in our meta-analyses ($I^2 = 62.9\%$, $p < 0.029$). At first, we found a higher degree of heterogeneity in our meta-analyses ($I^2 = 94.1\%$, $p < 0.001$), and it was more consistent with other systematic reviews regarding dietary assessment [9,19]. However, after critical point-by-point reanalysisin each article, we decided that some characteristics were not very specific to our eligibility criteria. For example, the study of Biltoft-Jensen et al. [29] that included the 11-year-old adolescents in the analysis and applied a self-report administration of the questionnaire; or the study of Royo-Bordonada et al. [47] that analyzed fruit and vegetable consumption as part of the dietary variety index (together with sausage and other foods that contributed to the dietary variety). Consequently, we had to exclude these two studies from the meta-analysis, since they had important sources of heterogeneity and did not fulfill our eligibility criteria [49]. After this exclusion, the remaining heterogeneity could be partially explained by the characteristics inherent to the different types of questionnaires used (e.g., recall period, number of items, recording bias, web-based system) and the biomarker (e.g., type of biomarker analyzed, duration of measure, different cutoff points).

4.11. Strengths and Limitations

The strengths of the current review included the use of a comprehensive search strategy and data collected from children aged 3 years to less than 10 years. To the best of our knowledge, this is the first attempt to provide estimates of the true effect sizes for assessing fruit and vegetable consumption, and to conduct a meta-analysis. Additionally, screening was performed by two independent authors; searches were updated and included papers written not only in English, but also in Spanish and Portuguese. The PRISMA statement was adopted, and a methodological quality rating was performed separately, to assist in interpreting the findings. The strength of this review was that two independent authors conducted the data extraction and the methodological quality assessment.

Despite these strengths, limitations should be noted. Although a comprehensive search was conducted, the agreement analyses were restricted to information from electronically published data, to ensure the reproducibility of the results.

Even though we considered Spanish and Portuguese for the literature search and screening, the two eligible articles were published in English. Both dietary habits and parental awareness can change considerably as children age; therefore, these findings may not be generalized to children of other ages. Moreover, although the dietary methods applied in each study were different, both methods are largely used in nutritional epidemiology [50] and in studies regarding fruit and vegetable consumption by children [51], enabling the meta-analysis, once we defined the correlation coefficients of these methods as our outcome [30].

5. Conclusions

Our findings suggest that the criterion validity of questionnaires and blood biomarkers for assessing fruit and vegetable consumption in children is fair. The assessment of food consumption—especially fruit and vegetable—in children still faces many challenges. However, having a thorough understanding of the main factors that may influence this assessment can be a promising path to enhance the validity of dietary assessment methods. Since measurement error is a key remaining difficulty, validity studies of questionnaires to assess fruit and vegetable consumption should be conducted with caution and interpreted within the broad context of the field. For example, careful study design and meticulous development of the dietary assessment tools can be validated with blood biomarkers, as long as the whole process of blood collection and analysis is adequate and rigorously controlled. Moreover, informed statistical analysis, with appropriate adjustments, can reduce the impact of these errors.

Finally, the incorporation of creativity and the development of technology, despite the challenges, can lead to advancements in the field of dietary assessment methods, and therefore, have an important role in the promising future of nutritional epidemiology.

Supplementary Materials: The following are available online at http://www.mdpi.com/2072-6643/10/10/1396/s1, Supplementary Material 1: PRISMA checklist; Supplementary Material 2: Extraction form of full-text articles assessed for eligibility; Supplementary Material 3: Funnel-plot for correlation coefficients of fruit and vegetable consumption assessed by questionnaires and blood biomarkers; Supplementary Material 4: Main reasons for exclusion of the full-text articles assessed for eligibility.

Author Contributions: T.S.C., G.V.-S., M.V.N.-F., A.C.F.D.M. and H.B.C. were responsible for the study concept and study design. T.S.C. and G.V.-S. examined the articles and performed the data screening, the data extraction, and the quality assessment. T.S.C., M.V.N.-F., and A.C.F.D.M. performed statistical analyses and interpreted the data. T.S.C. and G.V.-S. drafted the manuscript. T.S.C., G.V.-S., M.V.N.-F., A.C.F.D.M. and H.B.C. supervised the study. All authors participated in the writing of the paper, provided comments on the drafts, and approved the final version of the manuscript. All authors agree to be personally accountable for the author's own contributions and ensure that questions related to the accuracy or integrity of any part of the work, even ones in which the author was not personally involved, are appropriately investigated, resolved, and documented in the literature.

Nutrients **2018**, *10*, 1396

Funding: This research was funded by the State of São Paulo Research Foundation (FAPESP), which granted Tatiana Sadalla Collese a doctoral scholarship (proc. 2016/13922-1), Gabriela Vatavuk-Serrati a Scientific Initiation scholarship (proc. 2018/02452-0), Marcus Vinícius Nascimento-Ferreira a doctoral scholarship (proc. 2016/18436-8 and 2017/11732-3). Augusto César Ferreira De Moraes was awarded a post-doctoral scholarship from FAPESP (proc. 2014/13367-2). Heráclito Barbosa Carvalho received an advanced scientist scholarship from the National Council of Technological and Scientific Development (CNPq; proc. 300951/2015-9).

Acknowledgments: We gratefully acknowledge all of the researchers from the YCARE Research Group for their essential contributions and suggestions for improving this work.

Conflicts of Interest: The authors declare no conflict of interest.

References

1. Van Horn, L.; Carson, J.A.; Appel, L.J.; Burke, L.E.; Economos, C.; Karmally, W.; Lancaster, K.; Lichtenstein, A.H.; Johnson, R.K.; Thomas, R.J.; et al. Recommended dietary pattern to achieve adherence to the American heart association/American college of cardiology (AHA/ACC) guidelines: A scientific statement from the American heart association. *Circulation* **2016**, *134*, 505–529. [CrossRef] [PubMed]

2. Pem, D.; Jeewon, R. Fruit and vegetable intake: Benefits and progress of nutrition education interventions-Narrative review article. *Iran. J. Public Health* **2015**, *44*, 1309–1321. [PubMed]

3. Wang, X.; Ouyang, Y.; Liu, J.; Zhu, M.; Zhao, G.; Bao, W.; Hu, F.B. Fruit and vegetable consumption and mortality from all causes, cardiovascular disease, and cancer: Systematic review and dose-response meta-analysis of prospective cohort studies. *BMJ* **2014**, *349*, g4490. [CrossRef] [PubMed]

4. Zhan, J.; Liu, Y.J.; Cai, L.B.; Xu, F.R.; Xie, T.; He, Q.Q. Fruit and vegetable consumption and risk of cardiovascular disease: A meta-analysis of prospective cohort studies. *Crit. Rev. Food Sci. Nutr.* **2017**, *57*, 1650–1663. [CrossRef] [PubMed]

5. Wu, Y.; Zhang, D.; Jiang, X.; Jiang, W. Fruit and vegetable consumption and risk of type 2 diabetes mellitus: A dose-response meta-analysis of prospective cohort studies. *Nutr. Metab. Cardiovasc. Dis.* **2015**, *25*, 140–147. [CrossRef] [PubMed]

6. Myers, G.; Wright, S.; Blane, S.; Pratt, I.S.; Pettigrew, S. A process and outcome evaluation of an in-class vegetable promotion program. *Appetite* **2018**, *125*, 182–189. [CrossRef] [PubMed]

7. Biltoft-Jensen, A.; Trolle, E.; Christensen, T.; Islam, N.; Andersen, L.F.; Egenfeldt-Nielsen, S.; Tetens, I. Webdasc: A web-based dietary assessment software for 8-11-year-old Danish children. *J. Hum. Nutr. Diet.* **2014**, *27*, 43–53. [CrossRef] [PubMed]

8. Fatihah, F.; Ng, B.K.; Hazwanie, H.; Norimah, A.K.; Shanita, S.N.; Ruzita, A.T.; Poh, B.K. Development and validation of a food frequency questionnaire for dietary intake assessment among multi-ethnic primary school-aged children. *Singap. Med. J.* **2015**, *56*, 687–694. [CrossRef] [PubMed]

9. Molag, M.L.; de Vries, J.H.; Ocke, M.C.; Dagnelie, P.C.; van den Brandt, P.A.; Jansen, M.C.; van Staveren, W.A.; van't Veer, P. Design characteristics of food frequency questionnaires in relation to their validity. *Am. J. Epidemiol.* **2007**, *166*, 1468–1478. [CrossRef] [PubMed]

10. Corella, D.; Ordovas, J.M. Biomarkers: Background, classification and guidelines for applications in nutritional epidemiology. *Nutr. Hosp.* **2015**, *31*, 177–188. [PubMed]

11. Livingstone, M.B.; Robson, P.J.; Wallace, J.M. Issues in dietary intake assessment of children and adolescents. *Br. J. Nutr.* **2004**, *92*, 213–222. [CrossRef]

12. Lu, A.S.; Baranowski, J.; Islam, N.; Baranowski, T. How to engage children in self-administered dietary assessment programmes. *J. Hum. Nutr. Diet.* **2014**, *27*, 5–9. [CrossRef] [PubMed]

13. Burrows, T.L.; Martin, R.J.; Collins, C.E. A systematic review of the validity of dietary assessment methods in children when compared with the method of doubly labeled water. *J. Am. Diet. Assoc.* **2010**, *110*, 1501–1510. [CrossRef] [PubMed]

14. Burrows, T.L.; Hutchesson, M.J.; Rollo, M.E.; Boggess, M.M.; Guest, M.; Collins, C.E. Fruit and vegetable intake assessed by food frequency questionnaire and plasma carotenoids: A validation study in adults. *Nutrients* **2015**, *7*, 3240–3251. [CrossRef] [PubMed]

15. Dodd, K.W.; Midthune, D.; Kipnis, V. Re: "Application of a repeat-measure biomarker measurement error model to 2 validation studies: Examination of the effect of within-person variation in biomarker measurements". *Am. J. Epidemiol.* **2012**, *175*, 84–85. [CrossRef] [PubMed]

16. Brennan, L. Moving toward objective biomarkers of dietary intake. *J. Nutr.* **2018**, *148*, 821–822. [CrossRef] [PubMed]

17. Collins, C.E.; Watson, J.; Burrows, T. Measuring dietary intake in children and adolescents in the context of overweight and obesity. *Int. J. Obes.* **2010**, *34*, 1103–1115. [CrossRef] [PubMed]

18. Shamseer, L.; Moher, D.; Clarke, M.; Ghersi, D.; Liberati, A.; Petticrew, M.; Shekelle, P.; Stewart, L.A. Preferred reporting items for systematic review and meta-analysis protocols (PRISMA-P) 2015: Elaboration and explanation. *BMJ* **2015**, *350*, g7647. [CrossRef] [PubMed]

19. Burrows, T.L.; Rollo, M.E.; Williams, R.; Wood, L.G.; Garg, M.L.; Jensen, M.; Collins, C.E. A systematic review of technology-based dietary intake assessment validation studies that include carotenoid biomarkers. *Nutrients* **2017**, *9*, 140. [CrossRef] [PubMed]

20. World Health Organization. *Health Problems of Adolescents*; Technical Report Series 308; World Health Organization: Geneva, Switzerland, 1965.

21. Sawyer, S.M.; Azzopardi, P.S.; Wickremarathne, D.; Patton, G.C. The age of adolescence. *Lancet Child Adolesc. Health* **2018**, *2*, 223–228. [CrossRef]

22. Masson, L.F.; McNeill, G.; Tomany, J.O.; Simpson, J.A.; Peace, H.S.; Wei, L.; Grubb, D.A.; Bolton-Smith, C. Statistical approaches for assessing the relative validity of a food-frequency questionnaire: Use of correlation coefficients and the kappa statistic. *Public Health Nutr.* **2003**, *6*, 313–321. [CrossRef] [PubMed]

23. Higgins, J.P.; Thompson, S.G.; Deeks, J.J.; Altman, D.G. Measuring inconsistency in meta-analyses. *BMJ* **2003**, *327*, 557–560. [CrossRef] [PubMed]

24. Byers, T.; Trieber, F.; Gunter, E.; Coates, R.; Sowell, A.; Leonard, S.; Mokdad, A.; Jewell, S.; Miller, D.; Serdula, M.; et al. The accuracy of parental reports of their children's intake of fruits and vegetables: Validation of a food frequency questionnaire with serum levels of carotenoids and vitamins C, A, and E. *Epidemiology* **1993**, *4*, 350–355. [CrossRef] [PubMed]

25. Medin, A.C.; Carlsen, M.H.; Andersen, L.F. Associations between reported intakes of carotenoid-rich foods and concentrations of carotenoids in plasma: A validation study of a web-based food recall for children and adolescents. *Public Health Nutr.* **2016**, *19*, 3265–3275. [CrossRef] [PubMed]

26. Gupta, P.; Sreelakshmi, Y.; Sharma, R. A rapid and sensitive method for determination of carotenoids in plant tissues by high performance liquid chromatography. *Plant Methods* **2015**, *11*, 5. [CrossRef] [PubMed]

27. Rangan, A.; Allman-Farinelli, M.; Donohoe, E.; Gill, T. Misreporting of energy intake in the 2007 Australian children's survey: Differences in the reporting of food types between plausible, under- and over-reporters of energy intake. *J. Hum. Nutr. Diet.* **2014**, *27*, 450–458. [CrossRef] [PubMed]

28. Jenab, M.; Slimani, N.; Bictash, M.; Ferrari, P.; Bingham, S.A. Biomarkers in nutritional epidemiology: Applications, needs and new horizons. *Hum. Genet.* **2009**, *125*, 507–525. [CrossRef] [PubMed]

29. Biltoft-Jensen, A.; Bysted, A.; Trolle, E.; Christensen, T.; Knuthsen, P.; Damsgaard, C.T.; Andersen, L.F.; Brockhoff, P.; Tetens, I. Evaluation of web-based dietary assessment software for children: Comparing reported fruit, juice and vegetable intakes with plasma carotenoid concentration and school lunch observations. *Br. J. Nutr.* **2013**, *110*, 186–195. [CrossRef] [PubMed]

30. Murad, M.H.; Montori, V.M.; Ioannidis, J.P.; Jaeschke, R.; Devereaux, P.J.; Prasad, K.; Neumann, I.; Carrasco-Labra, A.; Agoritsas, T.; Hatala, R.; et al. How to read a systematic review and meta-analysis and apply the results to patient care: Users' guides to the medical literature. *JAMA* **2014**, *312*, 171–179. [CrossRef] [PubMed]

31. Nguyen, L.M.; Scherr, R.E.; Ermakov, I.V.; Gellermann, W.; Jahns, L.; Keen, C.L.; Miyamoto, S.; Steinberg, F.M.; Young, H.M.; Zidenberg-Cherr, S. Evaluating the relationship between plasma and skin carotenoids and reported dietary intake in elementary school children to assess fruit and vegetable intake. *Arch. Biochem. Biophys.* **2015**, *572*, 73–80. [CrossRef] [PubMed]

32. McNaughton, S.A.; Marks, G.C.; Gaffney, P.; Williams, G.; Green, A. Validation of a food-frequency questionnaire assessment of carotenoid and vitamin e intake using weighed food records and plasma biomarkers: The method of triads model. *Eur. J. Clin. Nutr.* **2005**, *59*, 211–218. [CrossRef] [PubMed]

33. Vandevijvere, S.; Geelen, A.; Gonzalez-Gross, M.; van't Veer, P.; Dallongeville, J.; Mouratidou, T.; Dekkers, A.; Bornhorst, C.; Breidenassel, C.; Crispim, S.P.; et al. Evaluation of food and nutrient intake assessment using concentration biomarkers in European adolescents from the healthy lifestyle in Europe by nutrition in adolescence study. *Br. J. Nutr.* **2013**, *109*, 736–747. [CrossRef] [PubMed]

34. Emmett, P. Assessing diet in longitudinal birth cohort studies. *Paediatr. Perinat. Epidemiol.* **2009**, *23*, 154–173. [CrossRef] [PubMed]

35. Crispim, S.P.; Geelen, A.; Souverein, O.W.; Hulshof, P.J.; Ruprich, J.; Dofkova, M.; Huybrechts, I.; De Keyzer, W.; Lillegaard, I.T.; Andersen, L.F.; et al. Biomarker-based evaluation of two 24-h recalls for comparing usual fish, fruit and vegetable intakes across European centers in the Efcoval study. *Eur. J. Clin. Nutr.* **2011**, *65*, 38–47. [CrossRef] [PubMed]

36. Androutsos, O.; Apostolidou, E.; Iotova, V.; Socha, P.; Birnbaum, J.; Moreno, L.; De Bourdeaudhuij, I.; Koletzko, B.; Manios, Y. Process evaluation design and tools used in a kindergarten-based, family-involved intervention to prevent obesity in early childhood. The toybox-study. *Obes. Rev.* **2014**, *15*, 74–80. [CrossRef] [PubMed]

37. Birkin, S. Monkey mascot used to gather children's opinions. *Nurs. Child Young People* **2017**, *29*, 7.

38. Townsend, M.S.; Shifts, M.K.; Styne, D.M.; Drake, C.; Lanoue, L.; Woodhouse, L.; Allen, L.H. Vegetable behavioral tool demonstrates validity with my plate vegetable cups and carotenoid and inflammatory biomarkers. *Appetite* **2016**, *107*, 628–638. [CrossRef] [PubMed]

39. Bernal-Orozco, M.F.; Vizmanos-Lamotte, B.; Rodriguez-Rocha, N.P.; Macedo-Ojeda, G.; Orozco-Valerio, M.; Roville-Sausse, F.; Leon-Estrada, S.; Marquez-Sandoval, F.; Fernandez-Ballart, J.D. Validation of a Mexican food photograph album as a tool to visually estimate food amounts in adolescents. *Br. J. Nutr.* **2013**, *109*, 944–952. [CrossRef] [PubMed]

40. McGloin, A.F.; Livingstone, M.B.; Greene, L.C.; Webb, S.E.; Gibson, J.M.; Jebb, S.A.; Cole, T.J.; Coward, W.A.; Wright, A.; Prentice, A.M. Energy and fat intake in obese and lean children at varying risk of obesity. *Int. J. Obes. Relat. Metab. Disord.* **2002**, *26*, 200–207. [CrossRef] [PubMed]

41. Saini, R.K.; Nile, S.H.; Park, S.W. Carotenoids from fruits and vegetables: Chemistry, analysis, occurrence, bioavailability and biological activities. *Food Res. Int.* **2015**, *76*, 735–750. [CrossRef] [PubMed]

42. Paiva, S.A.; Russell, R.M. Beta-carotene and other carotenoids as antioxidants. *J. Am. Coll. Nutr.* **1999**, *18*, 426–433. [CrossRef] [PubMed]

43. Burri, B.J.; Neidlinger, T.R.; Clifford, A.J. Serum carotenoid depletion follows first-order kinetics in healthy adult women fed naturally low carotenoid diets. *J. Nutr.* **2001**, *131*, 2096–2100. [CrossRef] [PubMed]

44. Collins, C.E.; Boggess, M.M.; Watson, J.F.; Guest, M.; Duncanson, K.; Pezdirc, K.; Rollo, M.; Hutchesson, M.J.; Burrows, T.L. Reproducibility and comparative validity of a food frequency questionnaire for Australian adults. *Clin. Nutr.* **2014**, *33*, 906–914. [CrossRef] [PubMed]

45. Lee, P.H.; Burstyn, I. Identification of confounder in epidemiologic data contaminated by measurement error in covariates. *BMC Med. Res. Methodol.* **2016**, *16*, 54. [CrossRef] [PubMed]

46. Nascimento-Ferreira, M.V.; De Moraes, A.C.F.; Toazza Oliveira, P.V.; Rendo-Urteaga, T.; Gracia-Marco, L.; Forjaz, C.L.M.; Moreno, L.A.; Carvalho, H.B. Assessment of physical activity intensity and duration in the paediatric population: Evidence to support an a priori hypothesis and sample size in the agreement between subjective and objective methods. *Obes. Rev.* **2018**, *19*, 810–824. [CrossRef] [PubMed]

47. Royo-Bordonada, M.A.; Gorgojo, L.; Ortega, H.; Martin-Moreno, J.M.; Lasuncion, M.A.; Garces, C.; Gil, A.; Rodriguez-Artalejo, F.; de Oya, M. Investigators of the Four Provinces Study. Greater dietary variety is associated with better biochemical nutritional status in Spanish children: The four provinces study. *Nutr. Metab. Cardiovasc. Dis.* **2003**, *13*, 357–364. [CrossRef]

48. Lichtenstein, A.H. Fruits and vegetables get a golden halo once again: Is there more to the story? *Circulation* **2015**, *132*, 1946–1948. [CrossRef] [PubMed]

49. Pereira, M. Heterogeneidade e viés de publicação em revisões sistemáticas. *Epidemiol. Serv. Saúde* **2014**, *23*, 775–778. [CrossRef]

50. Freedman, L.S.; Commins, J.M.; Moler, J.E.; Arab, L.; Baer, D.J.; Kipnis, V.; Midthune, D.; Moshfegh, A.J.; Neuhouser, M.L.; Prentice, R.L.; et al. Pooled results from 5 validation studies of dietary self-report instruments using recovery biomarkers for energy and protein intake. *Am. J. Epidemiol.* **2014**, *180*, 172–188. [CrossRef] [PubMed]

51. Riordan, F.; Ryan, K.; Perry, I.J.; Schulze, M.B.; Andersen, L.F.; Geelen, A.; Van't Veer, P.; Eussen, S.; Dagnelie, P.; Wijckmans-Duysens, N.; et al. A systematic review of methods to assess intake of fruits and vegetables among healthy European adults and children: A DEDIPAC (DEterminants of DIet and Physical Activity) study. *Public Health Nutr.* **2017**, *20*, 417–448. [CrossRef] [PubMed]

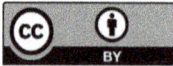

nutrients

Article

Cardiovascular Biomarkers in Association with Dietary Intake in a Longitudinal Study of Youth with Type 1 Diabetes

Namrata Sanjeevi *, Leah M. Lipsky and Tonja R. Nansel

Social and Behavioral Sciences Branch, Division of Intramural Population Health Research, Eunice Kennedy Shriver National Institute of Child Health and Human Development, Bethesda, MD 20817, USA; leah.lipsky@nih.gov (L.M.L.); nanselt@mail.nih.gov (T.R.N.)
* Correspondence: namrata.sanjeevi@nih.gov; Tel.: +1-301-827-0831

Received: 14 September 2018; Accepted: 17 October 2018; Published: 19 October 2018

Abstract: Despite cardioprotective effects of a healthy diet in the general population, few studies have investigated this relationship in individuals with type 1 diabetes, who are at elevated risks of cardiovascular disease (CVD) due to hyperglycemia. The objective of this study was to examine the association of CVD biomarkers with overall diet quality, as measured by the Healthy Eating Index-2015 (HEI-2015), and its dietary components in youth with type 1 diabetes. Youth with type 1 diabetes ($n = 136$, 8–16.9 years) were enrolled in an 18-month behavioral nutrition intervention trial. Dietary intake from three-day diet records, CVD biomarkers (total cholesterol (TC), high-density lipoprotein cholesterol (HDL-C), low-density lipoprotein cholesterol (LDL-C); triglycerides (TG), C-reactive protein (CRP), 8-iso-prostaglandin-F2alpha ($8\text{-iso-PGF}_{2\alpha}$), systolic and diastolic blood pressure (SBP and DBP, respectively), and glycated hemoglobin (HbA1c) were assessed at baseline, 6, 12 and 18 months. Linear mixed-effects models estimated associations of dietary intake with CVD biomarkers, adjusting for HbA1c and other covariates. Separate models estimated associations of time-varying change in dietary intake with time-varying change in CVD biomarkers. HEI-2015 was not associated with CVD biomarkers, but whole grain intake was inversely associated with TC, HDL-C and DBP, and a greater increase in whole fruit intake was associated with lower DBP. Added sugar, saturated fat and polyunsaturated fat were positively related to serum TG, HDL-C, and DBP, respectively. Findings suggest that the intake of specific dietary components, including whole grains, whole fruits, added sugar and PUFA, may influence cardiometabolic health in youth with type 1 diabetes, independent of glycemic control.

Keywords: type 1 diabetes; cardiovascular disease; whole grains; glycemic control; serum lipids

---

1. Introduction

Cardiovascular disease (CVD) is the major cause of mortality and morbidity in patients with type 1 diabetes, whose risk is several-fold higher than the general population [1,2]. This increased risk starts early in life; 15–45% of youth with type 1 diabetes have at least two CVD risk factors, and subclinical CVD abnormalities are observed within the first decade of diagnosis [3]. While glycemic control is central to CVD prevention in type 1 diabetes [4], identifying additional risk modifiers would inform timely interventions.

Several studies in the general population have indicated associations of dietary intake with CVD indicators; however, few studies have examined these relationships in individuals with type 1 diabetes. Better cardiometabolic health in the general population is consistently associated with better overall diet quality [5,6], greater intake of whole plant foods [7–17], and lower intakes of added sugar [18,19], saturated fat [20,21] and sodium [22,23]. Associations of dietary intake with CVD risk in individuals with type 1 diabetes may differ from that of the general population due to the characteristic glucose fluctuations and hyperglycemia that trigger inflammatory responses, thereby increasing CVD risk [24,25]. However, only two studies have examined associations of overall diet quality with CVD risk factors in individuals with type 1 diabetes, finding an inverse association of overall diet quality with blood pressure in adults [26] and dyslipidemia in youth [27,28]. Furthermore, associations of CVD biomarkers with the intake of individual food groups and nutrients other than fiber [29–31], saturated and total fat [31] in adults, and sugar-sweetened beverages [32] in youth have not been examined. Although diet quality indices reflect overall dietary patterns, a composite score based on several dietary components may mask associations of individual food groups or nutrients with cardiovascular health. Understanding associations with individual dietary components also is critical for developing behavioral targets for reducing CVD risk in patients with type 1 diabetes. Additionally, although oxidative stress and inflammation are known CVD risk factors [24], only one study has investigated dietary associations with inflammation in patients with type 1 diabetes, suggesting an inverse relationship of fiber intake with inflammation. No study has examined associations of diet with oxidative stress. Thus, the objective of this research was to investigate relationships of CVD biomarkers (serum lipids, blood pressure, inflammation and oxidative stress) with overall diet quality, as measured by Healthy Eating Index-2015 (HEI-2015), and its dietary components in youth with type 1 diabetes followed prospectively for 18 months.

2. Materials and Methods

This is a secondary analysis of a randomized controlled trial of a family-based behavioral nutrition intervention conducted from 2010–2013 at a tertiary diabetes center in Boston, Massachusetts. Youth eligibility criteria included: Age 8.0 to 16.9 years, diagnosed diabetes duration of $\geq$1 year, daily insulin dose of $\geq$0.5 units per kilogram, HbA1c of 6.5% (48 mmol/mol)–10.0% (86 mmol/mol) at the most recent clinic visit, insulin pump use or $\geq$3 injections per day, $\geq$1 clinic visit in the past year, and able to communicate in English. Youth were excluded due to the daily use of premixed insulin, the transition to insulin pump therapy three months prior to study, the use of real-time continuous glucose monitoring three months prior to study, participation in another intervention study six months prior to study, the use of medications that significantly interfere with glucose metabolism, the presence of gastrointestinal disease, multiple food allergies, or significant mental illness. Of 622 eligible youth, 24% (*n* = 148) provided consent and 22% (*n* = 139) completed baseline measures. Data from one sibling each of 3 sibling pairs was excluded resulting in 136 youth, and 125 participants were retained through the study duration of 18 months.

Intervention details have been described previously [33]. The intervention aimed to increase the intake of whole plant foods (whole fruits, vegetables, whole grains, legumes, nuts, and seeds). The control group had an equal frequency of contact with the research staff, but did not receive any nutrition advice besides that included as part of regular type 1 diabetes care.

Youth and parents provided assent and written informed consent, respectively, at the time of enrollment. Written informed consent was obtained from youth turning 18 during the study. Study procedures were approved by institutional review boards of the participating institutions. Sample size was ascertained to detect meaningful differences in dietary intake and HbA1c between the treatment and control groups [33].

2.1. Measures

2.1.1. CVD Biomarkers

Youth blood and urine samples obtained at baseline, 6, 12 and 18 months were stored at room temperature for 20–30 min after withdrawal, centrifuged for 15 min at ~3000 RPM at 4 °C, then aliquoted and frozen at −80 °C for later analysis. Serum concentrations of triglycerides (TG), total cholesterol (TC), high-density lipoprotein cholesterol (HDL-C) and low-density lipoprotein cholesterol (LDL-C) were assessed using enzyme linked immunosorbent assay (ELISA). Systolic and diastolic blood pressure (SBP and DBP) were abstracted from medical records at each visit. A high sensitivity enzyme-linked immunosorbent assay (Architect c8000, Abbott) with a lower detection limit of 0.2 mg/L was used to quantify CRP in the serum samples, and 8-iso-prostaglandin $F_{2\alpha}$ (8-iso-PGF$_{2\alpha}$), an indicator of oxidative stress, was determined from urine frozen at $-80\ ^\circ$C using enzyme linked immunosorbent assay (ELISA).

2.1.2. Diet Assessment

Families completed 3-day youth diet records at baseline and 3, 6, 9, 12, and 18 months based on instructions from research assistants on accurate measurement and reporting of food and beverage intake. Potion size estimation was facilitated by scales and measuring utensils. Families were asked to include detailed description of each food item, such as brand names and item labeling (e.g., low fat or 1% milk). The completed records were reviewed by research staff, and clarified for any missing information, as needed. A registered dietitian obtained two nonconsecutive 24-h dietary recalls for visits in which a family did not complete the diet record (1.7% of assessments).

Three-day diet records were analyzed using Nutrition Data System for Research 2012 (NDSR 2012; Nutrition Coordinating Center, University of Minnesota) software to obtain intake estimates of key dietary components of the Dietary Guidelines of Americans 2015 (DGA 2015), including total and whole fruits, total vegetables, greens and beans, whole and refined grains, dairy, total protein foods, seafood, nuts and seeds, sodium, percentage of energy from added sugars and saturated fat, and fatty acids. Intake of food groups and sodium per 1000 kcal were determined. The dietary subgroup, fatty acids, is represented as the ratio of the sum of poly- and mono-unsaturated fat (PUFA and MUFA, respectively) to saturated fat ((PUFA + MUFA): SFA). Overall diet quality was measured using the Healthy Eating Index-2015 (HEI-2015), an a priori index that measures in adherence to DGA 2015 recommendations. The score is comprised of twelve component scores, which are summed to obtain the total score that ranges from 0 to 100; a greater score indicates greater conformance to the DGA 2015.

2.1.3. Clinical and Demographic Data

HbA1c was assessed at baseline, 3, 6, 9, 12 and 18 months using a laboratory assay standardized to the Diabetes Control and Complications Trial (reference range, 4–6%, (20–42 mmol/mol)). Tosoh (Tosoh Medics, South San Francisco, CA, USA) was used for initial HbA1c assays ensued by Roche Cobas Integra (Indianapolis, IN, USA). No clinically significant bias was detected between the Tosoh and Roche methods based on results from the two instruments on identical samples.

Date of diabetes diagnosis, insulin regimen, age, sex, height, weight, Tanner stage and use of cardiac medications (anticoagulants, ace inhibitors and statins) were abstracted from the medical records at each study visit. Tanner stage from the previous visit was used for missing visit data. Body mass index (BMI, kg/m^2) was computed from height and weight measurements, and baseline diabetes duration was calculated based on date of diagnosis. Parents reported youth race/ethnicity at baseline. Items from the Behavioral Risk Factor Surveillance System assessed total moderate and vigorous physical activity at baseline, 6, 12 and 18 months [34].

2.2. Statistical Analysis

Differences in characteristics between treatment groups were analyzed using independent samples *t*-tests for continuous variables and Pearson's chi-square tests for categorical variables. Serum TG and CRP were log-transformed to improve normality. Linear mixed-effects models estimated associations of time-varying continuous independent variables (HEI-2015, and intake per 1000 kcal of total fruits, whole fruits, total vegetables, dark green vegetables, beans, whole grains, dairy, total protein foods, seafood, nuts and seeds, refined grains and sodium, percentage of energy from added sugars and saturated fat, and fatty acids), with time-varying continuous dependent variables (TG, TC, LDL-C, HDL-C, CRP, 8-iso-PGF$_{2\alpha}$, SBP and DBP). Models included a random intercept representing the subject-specific baseline variation in the outcome. Covariates included baseline sex, treatment assignment, and diabetes duration, and time-varying age, body mass index, Tanner stage, insulin regimen, physical activity, use of cardiac medications, and HbA1c. Adjustments for multiple comparisons were not performed due to the exploratory nature of the secondary data analysis [35,36]. Since 42.6%, 85.5%, 76.7% and 54.7% of participants reported zero intake of dark green vegetables, beans, seafood, and nuts and seeds, respectively, these variables were dichotomized as having either zero or greater than zero intake. Additional models estimated associations of each of the dichotomized food group variable with CVD risk factors. Further, to enable within-subject analysis of the association of change in diet with change in CVD biomarkers, the change from baseline in each dietary intake variable and CVD biomarkers was calculated for each assessment period. Separate models estimated associations of time-varying change in dietary intake with time-varying change in CVD biomarkers. Models were controlled for baseline age, sex, treatment assignment, diabetes duration, Tanner stage, insulin regimen, HbA1c, physical activity, body mass index and use of cardiac medication for the respective assessment period. SPSS version 21 were used for all analyses.

3. Results

Baseline demographic and diet characteristics for study participants are shown in Tables 1 and 2, respectively. At baseline, 19.4%, 11.2%, 28.4%, and 3.7% of participants were not within the recommended concentrations [37,38] for TG (<150 mg/dL), TC (<200 mg/dL), LDL-C (<100 mg/dL) and HDL-C (≥35 mg/dL), respectively.

Table 1. Baseline demographic characteristics of youth with type 1 diabetes overall and by treatment assignment.

	Overall (N = 136)	Treatment (N = 66)	Control (N = 70)	p-Value
Age, years	12.7 ± 2.6	12.5 ± 2.7	13.0 ± 2.5	0.27
Body mass index, kg/m^2	21.3 ± 4.2	21.0 ± 4.1	21.6 ± 4.3	0.37
Weight status [1]				
Underweight	1 (0.7)	1 (1.5)	0 (0)	0.55
Normal weight	91 (66.9)	42 (63.6)	49 (70.0)	
Overweight	28 (20.6)	17 (25.8)	11 (15.7)	
Obese	16 (11.8)	6 (9.1)	10 (14.3)	
HbA1c, (%, (mmol/mol))	8.1 ± 1.0 (65 ± 11)	8.1 ± 1.1 (65 ± 12)	8.1 ± 1.0 (65 ± 12)	0.95
Duration of diabetes, years	6.0 ± 3.1	5.6 ± 2.5	6.4 ± 3.6	0.15
Insulin dose, Units/day	49.8 ± 26.8	46.9 ± 23.9	52.7 ± 29.3	0.24
Tanner stage	2.5 ± 1.4	2.4 ± 1.4	2.6 ± 1.5	0.38
Youth race/ethnicity				
Non-Hispanic white	123 (90.4)	58 (87.9)	65 (92.9)	0.17
Non-Hispanic black	5 (3.7)	2 (3.0)	3 (4.3)	
Hispanic	7 (5.2)	6 (9.1)	1 (1.4)	
American Indian/Alaska Native	1 (0.7)	0 (0)	1 (1.4)	
TG (mg/dL)	111.1 ± 56.9	101.3 ± 42.4	120.2 ± 66.8	0.05
TC (mg/dL)	165.2 ± 27.9	162.7 ± 24.3	167.6 ± 30.8	0.32
HDL-C (mg/dL)	56.6 ± 13.6	56.5 ± 14.0	56.6 ± 13.3	0.98
LDL-C (mg/dL)	86.4 ± 24.0	85.7 ± 19.7	87.0 ± 27.5	0.75
CRP (mg/L)	1.1 ± 1.9	0.9 ± 1.4	1.4 ± 2.3	0.09
8-iso-PGF$_{2\alpha}$ (ng/mL)	1.6 ± 1.3	1.7 ± 1.5	1.4 ± 1.1	0.33
SBP (mm Hg)	108.7 ± 7.1	108.6 ± 7.8	108.8 ± 6.5	0.90
DBP (mm Hg)	66.4 ± 5.5	66.7 ± 5.9	66.2 ± 5.2	0.60

TG, triglycerides; TC, total cholesterol; HDL-C, high-density lipoprotein cholesterol; LDL-C, low-density lipoprotein cholesterol; CRP, C-reactive protein; 8-iso-PGF2, 8-iso-prostaglandin-F2-alpha; SBP, systolic blood pressure; DBP, diastolic blood pressure. Data are presented as mean ± SD or *n* (%). [1] Underweight = BMI%ile < 5; Normal weight = 5 ≤ BMI%ile < 85; Overweight = 85 ≤ BMI%ile < 95; Obese = 95 ≤ BMI%ile.

Table 2. Baseline dietary characteristics of youth with type 1 diabetes overall and by treatment assignment.

Dietary Components	Overall (N = 136)	Treatment (N = 66)	Control (N = 70)	p-Value
HEI-2015	46.05 ± 11.70	45.33 ± 12.44	46.73 ± 11.01	0.49
Total fruits [1]	0.44 ± 0.40	0.45 ± 0.38	0.42 ± 0.43	0.70
Whole fruits [1]	0.32 ± 0.37	0.32 ± 0.32	0.33 ± 0.41	0.90
Total vegetables [1]	0.49 ± 0.35	0.49 ± 0.38	0.49 ± 0.31	0.99
Dark green vegetables [1]	0.09 ± 0.12	0.07 ± 0.11	0.10 ± 0.12	0.09
Beans [1]	0.03 ± 0.09	0.04 ± 0.12	0.02 ± 0.05	0.19
Whole grains [1]	0.52 ± 0.53	0.47 ± 0.38	0.57 ± 0.64	0.26
Dairy [1]	0.68 ± 0.33	0.68 ± 0.34	0.67 ± 0.33	0.85
Protein foods [1]	2.54 ± 1.24	2.53 ± 1.27	2.55 ± 1.21	0.94
Seafood [1]	0.16 ± 0.40	0.11 ± 0.29	0.20 ± 0.48	0.07
Nuts and seeds [1]	0.34 ± 0.73	0.33 ± 0.89	0.34 ± 0.54	0.93
Refined grains [1]	3.44 ± 1.09	3.58 ± 1.04	3.30 ± 1.13	0.13
Sodium [2]	1.69 ± 0.33	1.69 ± 0.31	1.68 ± 0.34	0.85
Added sugars, % kcal	11.97 ± 5.16	11.39 ± 4.47	12.53 ± 5.71	0.20
Saturated fat, % kcal	12.39 ± 2.75	12.37 ± 2.68	12.41 ± 2.83	0.93
Fatty acid [3]	1.69 ± 0.49	1.72 ± 0.52	1.65 ± 0.46	0.42

[1] Expressed as total number of cup- or ounce-equivalents per 1000 kcal; [2] expressed as grams per 1000 kcal; [3] calculated as (polyunsaturated fat + monounsaturated fat)/saturated fat.

Associations between dietary intake and serum lipids after adjustments of HbA1c and other covariates are indicated in Table 3. In the adjusted model, serum lipids were not associated with overall diet quality. However, whole grain intake was inversely associated with TC and HDL-C. Added sugar and saturated fat intakes were positively associated with TG and HDL-C, respectively. Other dietary components (including dark green vegetables, beans, seafood, and nuts and seeds) were not associated with serum lipids. Findings were unchanged when the food groups, dark green vegetables, beans, seafood, and nuts and seeds, were treated as categorical variables (Table S1).

Associations of dietary intake with inflammation, oxidative stress and blood pressure are shown in Table 4. These CVD biomarkers were not associated with overall diet quality; however, 8-iso-PGF$_{2\alpha}$ was inversely associated with refined grain intake, and lower DBP was related to greater whole grain intake and greater (PUFA + MUFA): SFA. To determine the specific fatty acids associated with DBP, we further examined the association of the intake of individual fatty acid with DBP. Although MUFA intake (% kcal) was not associated with DBP ($\beta = 0.08$, SE = 0.10, $p = 0.38$), PUFA intake (% kcal) was positively related to DBP ($\beta = 0.23$, SE = 0.09, $p = 0.008$). Dark green vegetables, beans, seafood and nuts and seeds were not associated with inflammation, oxidative stress and blood pressure (Table 4), and findings were unchanged when these food groups were treated as categorical variables (Table S2).

Associations between time-varying changes in dietary intake with time-varying changes in CVD biomarkers are indicated in Tables S3 and S4 Greater increase in whole grain intake was associated with a decrease in LDL-C and HDL-C. Increase in whole fruit intake was inversely associated with DBP, whereas increase in fatty acid ratio was positively associated with DBP. Increase in time-varying total vegetable, whole grain and added sugar intake was positively associated with TG, but increase in time-varying refined grain intake was inversely associated with TG and 8-iso-PGF$_{2\alpha}$. Further, increase in time-varying dairy intake was positively associated with SBP.

Table 3. Association of diet quality and food group and nutrient intake with serum lipids in youth with type 1 diabetes [1].

Dietary Components	TG [2] (mg/dL)		TC (mg/dL)		HDL-C (mg/dL)		LDL-C (mg/dL)	
	β ± SE	p	β ± SE	p	β ± SE	p	β ± SE	p
HEI-2015	0.0003 ± 0.001	0.77	−0.16 ± 0.10	0.11	−0.07 ± 0.05	0.16	−0.12 ± 0.09	0.19
Total fruits [3]	0.01 ± 0.03	0.78	1.31 ± 3.21	0.68	0.06 ± 1.49	0.97	1.07 ± 3.00	0.72
Whole fruits [3]	0.01 ± 0.04	0.70	3.22 ± 3.96	0.42	0.67 ± 1.86	0.72	1.59 ± 3.68	0.67
Total vegetables [3]	0.03 ± 0.03	0.28	2.44 ± 2.83	0.39	0.05 ± 1.36	0.97	−2.74 ± 2.66	0.30
Dark green vegetables [3]	−0.02 ± 0.06	0.75	−9.18 ± 6.31	0.15	−2.63 ± 2.85	0.36	−8.50 ± 5.89	0.15
Beans [3]	−0.14 ± 0.10	0.18	−17.17 ± 10.77	0.11	−2.81 ± 5.06	0.58	−5.16 ± 10.22	0.61
Whole grains [3]	0.01 ± 0.02	0.61	−4.60 ± 2.05	0.03	−1.98 ± 0.99	0.046	−3.42 ± 1.92	0.08
Dairy [3]	0.01 ± 0.03	0.79	−1.97 ± 3.78	0.60	−0.64 ± 1.81	0.72	−1.61 ± 3.44	0.64
Protein foods [3]	−0.01 ± 0.01	0.30	0.05 ± 0.88	0.95	0.25 ± 0.41	0.55	0.39 ± 0.83	0.63
Seafood [3]	0.01 ± 0.03	0.61	0.09 ± 2.66	0.97	−0.90 ± 1.27	0.48	1.77 ± 2.47	0.47
Nuts and seeds [3]	0.004 ± 0.02	0.84	0.15 ± 1.74	0.93	0.12 ± 0.85	0.89	0.06 ± 1.64	0.97
Refined grains [3]	−0.02 ± 0.01	0.08	0.54 ± 1.05	0.61	0.31 ± 0.51	0.54	1.72 ± 0.98	0.08
Sodium [4]	−0.05 ± 0.03	0.10	2.13 ± 3.33	0.52	0.21 ± 1.52	0.89	5.38 ± 3.10	0.08
Added sugars, % kcal	0.004 ± 0.002	0.04	0.22 ± 0.21	0.30	−0.10 ± 0.10	0.32	0.09 ± 0.20	0.64
Saturated fat, % kcal	−0.002 ± 0.003	0.61	0.35 ± 0.37	0.35	0.34 ± 0.17	0.04	0.19 ± 0.35	0.58
Fatty acid [5]	−0.002 ± 0.02	0.90	−0.50 ± 2.10	0.81	−0.74 ± 0.96	0.45	−1.12 ± 1.93	0.56

TG, triglycerides; TC, total cholesterol; HDL-C, high-density lipoprotein cholesterol; LDL-C, low-density lipoprotein cholesterol; HEI-2015, healthy eating index-2015. [1] Models were controlled for baseline treatment assignment, sex, diabetes duration, and time-varying age, body mass index, Tanner stage, insulin regimen, physical activity, use of cardiac medication, and glycemic control (HbA1c); [2] log-transformed to meet the normality assumption; [3] expressed as total number of cup- or ounce-equivalents per 1000 kcal; [4] expressed as grams per 1000 kcal; [5] calculated as (polyunsaturated fat + monounsaturated fat)/saturated fat.

Table 4. Association of diet quality and food group and nutrient intake with inflammation, oxidative stress and blood pressure in youth with type 1 diabetes [1].

Dietary Components	CRP [2] (mg/L) β ± SE	p	8-iso-PGF$_{2\alpha}$ (ng/mL) β ± SE	p	SBP (mmHg) β ± SE	p	DBP (mmHg) β ± SE	p
HEI-2015	0.0002 ± 0.002	0.90	0.002 ± 0.007	0.77	0.01 ± 0.02	0.59	0.01 ± 0.02	0.53
Total fruits [3]	0.04 ± 0.06	0.46	−0.23 ± 0.22	0.31	−0.25 ± 0.71	0.73	0.10 ± 0.66	0.88
Whole fruits [3]	0.07 ± 0.08	0.39	−0.17 ± 0.28	0.54	−0.73 ± 0.86	0.40	−0.11 ± 0.88	0.90
Total vegetables [3]	−0.02 ± 0.05	0.67	0.06 ± 0.21	0.77	−0.02 ± 0.69	0.97	0.69 ± 0.63	0.28
Dark green vegetables [3]	−0.04 ± 0.12	0.72	−0.42 ± 0.50	0.40	−0.52 ± 1.46	0.72	−1.10 ± 1.38	0.42
Beans [3]	−0.30 ± 0.21	0.15	0.85 ± 1.05	0.42	−0.64 ± 2.67	0.81	−0.93 ± 2.43	0.70
Whole grains [3]	0.04 ± 0.04	0.26	−0.09 ± 0.16	0.60	0.03 ± 0.47	0.96	−0.98 ± 0.46	0.04
Dairy [3]	−0.004 ± 0.07	0.95	−0.47 ± 0.27	0.08	0.89 ± 0.81	0.27	−0.99 ± 0.73	0.18
Protein foods [3]	−0.01 ± 0.02	0.55	0.09 ± 0.07	0.22	−0.11 ± 0.20	0.59	0.20 ± 0.17	0.23
Seafood [3]	0.02 ± 0.05	0.65	−0.09 ± 0.21	0.69	−0.18 ± 0.63	0.78	0.78 ± 0.61	0.20
Nuts and seeds [3]	0.02 ± 0.04	0.61	0.25 ± 0.14	0.08	0.29 ± 0.45	0.53	0.21 ± 0.43	0.62
Refined grains [3]	−0.02 ± 0.02	0.42	−0.18 ± 0.08	0.04	0.05 ± 0.25	0.85	0.04 ± 0.23	0.86
Sodium [4]	0.02 ± 0.06	0.79	−0.42 ± 0.27	0.12	−0.53 ± 0.78	0.50	0.19 ± 0.78	0.80
Added sugars, % kcal	−0.00003 ± 0.004	0.99	0.01 ± 0.02	0.58	−0.04 ± 0.05	0.34	−0.01 ± 0.04	0.89
Saturated fat, % kcal	0.01 ± 0.007	0.43	0.02 ± 0.03	0.57	0.01 ± 0.08	0.87	−0.12 ± 0.08	0.13
Fatty acid [5]	0.02 ± 0.04	0.59	0.19 ± 0.15	0.20	0.19 ± 0.45	0.67	0.98 ± 0.42	0.02

CRP, C-reactive protein; 8-iso-PGF$_{2\alpha}$, 8-iso-prostaglandin F$_{2\alpha}$; SBP, systolic blood pressure; DBP, diastolic blood pressure; HEI-2015, healthy eating index-2015. [1] Models were controlled for baseline treatment assignment, sex, diabetes duration, time-varying age, Tanner stage, body mass index, insulin regimen, physical activity, use of cardiac medication and glycemic control (HbA1c); [2] log-transformed to meet the normality assumption; [3] expressed as total number of cup- or ounce-equivalents per 1000 kcal; [4] expressed as grams per 1000 kcal; [5] calculated as (polyunsaturated fat + monounsaturated fat)/saturated fat.

4. Discussion

In contrast to the general population [5,39], CVD biomarkers were not associated with greater adherence to DGA 2015, as measured by HEI, in this sample of youth with type 1 diabetes. However, greater intake of whole grains and whole fruits, and lower added sugar and PUFA were associated with more favorable CVD biomarkers. Much of the current study findings regarding the association of intake of specific dietary components with CVD biomarkers are comparable to the general population. However, CVD etiology in type 1 diabetes differs from that of the general population, as hyperglycemia is known to increase CVD risk. Findings suggest that these dietary components may be associated with CVD risk in persons with type 1 diabetes independent of glycemic control.

Several studies in the general population have indicated the protective role of whole grains in reducing CVD risk factors, including blood pressure [40] and TC [7,8,10]. In contrast, no study has examined this relationship in individuals with type 1 diabetes. Improved endothelial function due to whole grain consumption [41] could explain the association of greater intake with lower blood pressure in this sample. The inverse association of whole grain intake with TC, independent of HbA1c could be attributed to increased clearance or decreased biosynthesis of cholesterol [42]. This pathway also is consistent with the inverse relationship between whole grain consumption and HDL-C found in this study. Although this result is in contrast to previous research in the general population [8,10], it is comparable to another study finding that a whole grain diet significantly lowered HDL-C in overweight and obese adults [43]. The inverse association of whole grain intake with HDL-C is not considered atherogenic in this sample, given the negligible number of participants (3.7%) with low HDL-C (<35 mg/dL) at baseline. However, it is important to consider the impact of whole grain consumption on HDL-C in future CVD-related research in patients with type 1 diabetes. Associations of whole grain intake with cholesterol are further supported by within-subject analyses, where increase in whole grain intake was inversely related to LDL-C and HDL-C. Further, improved endothelial function could explain the inverse association of whole fruits with DBP, which is consistent to previous research in the general population [44]. However, other relationships of time-varying changes in whole grain, refined grain and dairy intake with that of CVD biomarkers are not supported by known biological mechanisms. Findings for within-subject analyses should be interpreted with caution, given the modest degree of individual change over time, resulting in increased chances of spurious findings.

The positive association of added sugar intake with serum TG is consistent with previous literature in the general population [18,19]. This result could be attributed to hepatic de novo lipogenesis induction by common sugars [45], resulting in increased serum TG, independent of glycemic control. This finding is also somewhat comparable to another study in youth with type 1 diabetes, whereby increased sugar-sweetened beverage intake was related to greater serum lipids [46]. The positive association of saturated fat intake with HDL-C is comparable to previous research [47], and may be explained by increased transport rates of HDL-C ester by dietary fat [47]. While additional studies are needed, these findings indicate some consistency in the relationship of food group and nutrient intake with serum lipids in individuals with type 1 diabetes as compared with the general population.

The inverse relationship of refined grain intake with oxidative stress contrasts previous research indicating the detrimental effects of refined grain intake on CVD biomarkers [9]. This may be attributed to the use of urinary 8-iso-PGF$_{2\alpha}$ as an oxidative stress marker, which is a less sensitive measure than its metabolite, 2,3-dinor-5,6-dihydro-15-F2t-isoprostane [48]. Future research using more sensitive markers of oxidative stress could better elucidate the association of refined grain intake with oxidative stress. Finally, greater DBP was associated with increased PUFA intake. Given PUFA includes omega-6 and omega-3 PUFA, a high intake could be obtained for an individual consuming excess omega-6 and minimal omega-3 PUFA. Although total omega-6 PUFA intake could not be obtained for the current study, stimulation of vasoconstriction by omega-6 PUFA-derived eicosanoids [49] could explain the relationship of PUFA intake with DBP reported in this study.

The study findings are subject to certain limitations. These findings are observational, precluding inferences on causality. The eligibility criteria for the primary study, recruitment from a single clinic,

22% recruitment rate and predominantly white sample limit generalizability of the results to all youth with type 1 diabetes. Since youth with poor glycemic control (most recent HbA1c prior to recruitment >10.0%) were not recruited, the study may have excluded patients most affected by adverse CVD biomarkers. The lack of adjustment for multiple comparisons could have increased the family-wise error rate. Nevertheless, the detected associations of diet with CVD biomarkers are supported by biological mechanisms. Although food records are among the most valid method of assessing dietary intake, they are susceptible to reporting and response biases [50]. However, this study is strengthened by the prospective design utilizing repeated measures of exposures and outcomes, assessment of several CVD risk factors, and adjustment of potentially important covariates in the analyses.

5. Conclusions

Nutrition recommendations for youth with type 1 diabetes include general healthful eating for reducing risk of complications, and there are limited disease-specific nutrition guidelines. However, characteristic hyperglycemia in individuals with type 1 diabetes may attenuate dietary influences on CVD biomarkers. The current study suggests that overall diet quality was not associated with CVD biomarkers in youth with type 1 diabetes. However, specific dietary components were associated with CVD biomarkers, independent of glycemic control. Additional studies are needed to corroborate if intake of greater whole grains, lower added sugar and PUFA may favorably influence CVD biomarkers in this population. Examining whether these dietary associations differ by glycemic control could inform efforts that promote cardiovascular health in patients with type 1 diabetes.

Supplementary Materials: The following are available online at http://www.mdpi.com/2072-6643/10/10/1552/s1.

Author Contributions: T.R.N. and L.M.L. designed the research and obtained funding. N.S. conceptualized the research question and wrote the manuscript, and all authors contributed to the manuscript editing, and read and approved the final manuscript.

Funding: This research was supported by the intramural research program of the National Institutes of Health, Eunice Kennedy Shriver National Institute of Child Health and Human Development, contract #'s HHSN267200703434C and HHSN2752008000031/HHSN275002.

Conflicts of Interest: The authors declare no conflicts of interest.

References

1. Margeirsdottir, H.D.; Larsen, J.R.; Brunborg, C.; Overby, N.C.; Dahl-Jorgensen, K.; Norwegian Study Group for Childhood, D. High prevalence of cardiovascular risk factors in children and adolescents with type 1 diabetes: A population-based study. *Diabetologia* **2008**, *51*, 554–561. [CrossRef] [PubMed]
2. Rawshani, A.; Sattar, N.; Franzén, S.; Rawshani, A.; Hattersley, A.T.; Svensson, A.M.; Eliasson, B.; Gudbjörnsdottir, S. Excess mortality and cardiovascular disease in young adults with type 1 diabetes in relation to age at onset: A nationwide, register-based cohort study. *Lancet* **2018**, *392*, 477–486. [CrossRef]
3. de Ferranti, S.D.; de Boer, I.H.; Fonseca, V.; Fox, C.S.; Golden, S.H.; Lavie, C.J.; Magge, S.N.; Marx, N.; McGuire, D.K.; Orchard, T.J.; et al. Type 1 diabetes mellitus and cardiovascular disease: A scientific statement from the American Heart Association and American Diabetes Association. *Circulation* **2014**, *130*, 1110–1130. [CrossRef] [PubMed]
4. Mannucci, E.; Dicembrini, I.; Lauria, A.; Pozzilli, P. Is glucose control important for prevention of cardiovascular disease in diabetes? *Diabetes Care* **2013**, *36* (Suppl. 2), S259–S263. [CrossRef]
5. Nicklas, T.A.; O'Neil, C.E.; Fulgoni, V.L., 3rd. Diet quality is inversely related to cardiovascular risk factors in adults. *J. Nutr.* **2012**, *142*, 2112–2118. [CrossRef] [PubMed]
6. Kuczmarski, M.F.; Mason, M.A.; Allegro, D.; Zonderman, A.B.; Evans, M.K. Diet quality is inversely associated with C-reactive protein levels in urban, low-income African-American and white adults. *J. Acad. Nutr. Diet.* **2013**, *113*, 1620–1631. [CrossRef] [PubMed]
7. Newby, P.K.; Maras, J.; Bakun, P.; Muller, D.; Ferrucci, L.; Tucker, K.L. Intake of whole grains, refined grains, and cereal fiber measured with 7-d diet records and associations with risk factors for chronic disease. *Am. J. Clin. Nutr.* **2007**, *86*, 1745–1753. [CrossRef] [PubMed]

8. McKeown, N.M.; Meigs, J.B.; Liu, S.; Wilson, P.W.; Jacques, P.F. Whole-grain intake is favorably associated with metabolic risk factors for type 2 diabetes and cardiovascular disease in the Framingham Offspring Study. *Am. J. Clin. Nutr.* **2002**, *76*, 390–398. [CrossRef] [PubMed]

9. Masters, R.C.; Liese, A.D.; Haffner, S.M.; Wagenknecht, L.E.; Hanley, A.J. Whole and refined grain intakes are related to inflammatory protein concentrations in human plasma. *J. Nutr.* **2010**, *140*, 587–594. [CrossRef] [PubMed]

10. Damsgaard, C.T.; Biltoft-Jensen, A.; Tetens, I.; Michaelsen, K.F.; Lind, M.V.; Astrup, A.; Landberg, R. Whole-Grain Intake, Reflected by Dietary Records and Biomarkers, Is Inversely Associated with Circulating Insulin and Other Cardiometabolic Markers in 8- to 11-Year-Old Children. *J. Nutr.* **2017**, *147*, 816–824. [CrossRef] [PubMed]

11. Mellendick, K.; Shanahan, L.; Wideman, L.; Calkins, S.; Keane, S.; Lovelady, C. Diets Rich in Fruits and Vegetables Are Associated with Lower Cardiovascular Disease Risk in Adolescents. *Nutrients* **2018**, *10*, 136. [CrossRef] [PubMed]

12. Djousse, L.; Arnett, D.K.; Coon, H.; Province, M.A.; Moore, L.L.; Ellison, R.C. Fruit and vegetable consumption and LDL cholesterol: The National Heart, Lung, and Blood Institute Family Heart Study. *Am. J. Clin. Nutr.* **2004**, *79*, 213–217. [CrossRef] [PubMed]

13. Holt, E.M.; Steffen, L.M.; Moran, A.; Basu, S.; Steinberger, J.; Ross, J.A.; Hong, C.P.; Sinaiko, A.R. Fruit and vegetable consumption and its relation to markers of inflammation and oxidative stress in adolescents. *J. Am. Diet. Assoc.* **2009**, *109*, 414–421. [CrossRef] [PubMed]

14. Bazzano, L.A.; Thompson, A.M.; Tees, M.T.; Nguyen, C.H.; Winham, D.M. Non-soy legume consumption lowers cholesterol levels: A meta-analysis of randomized controlled trials. *Nutr. Metab. Cardiovasc. Dis.* **2011**, *21*, 94–103. [CrossRef] [PubMed]

15. Salehi-Abargouei, A.; Saraf-Bank, S.; Bellissimo, N.; Azadbakht, L. Effects of non-soy legume consumption on C-reactive protein: A systematic review and meta-analysis. *Nutrition* **2015**, *31*, 631–639. [CrossRef] [PubMed]

16. Sabate, J.; Oda, K.; Ros, E. Nut consumption and blood lipid levels: A pooled analysis of 25 intervention trials. *Arch. Intern. Med.* **2010**, *170*, 821–827. [CrossRef] [PubMed]

17. Yu, Z.; Malik, V.S.; Keum, N.; Hu, F.B.; Giovannucci, E.L.; Stampfer, M.J.; Willett, W.C.; Fuchs, C.S.; Bao, Y. Associations between nut consumption and inflammatory biomarkers. *Am. J. Clin. Nutr.* **2016**, *104*, 722–728. [CrossRef] [PubMed]

18. Kell, K.P.; Cardel, M.I.; Bohan Brown, M.M.; Fernandez, J.R. Added sugars in the diet are positively associated with diastolic blood pressure and triglycerides in children. *Am. J. Clin. Nutr.* **2014**, *100*, 46–52. [CrossRef] [PubMed]

19. Welsh, J.A.; Sharma, A.; Cunningham, S.A.; Vos, M.B. Consumption of added sugars and indicators of cardiovascular disease risk among US adolescents. *Circulation* **2011**, *123*, 249–257. [CrossRef] [PubMed]

20. Te Morenga, L.; Montez, J.M. Health effects of saturated and trans-fatty acid intake in children and adolescents: Systematic review and meta-analysis. *PLoS ONE* **2017**, *12*, e0186672. [CrossRef] [PubMed]

21. King, D.E.; Egan, B.M.; Geesey, M.E. Relation of dietary fat and fiber to elevation of C-reactive protein. *Am. J. Cardiol.* **2003**, *92*, 1335–1339. [CrossRef] [PubMed]

22. Aburto, N.J.; Ziolkovska, A.; Hooper, L.; Elliott, P.; Cappuccio, F.P.; Meerpohl, J.J. Effect of lower sodium intake on health: Systematic review and meta-analyses. *BMJ* **2013**, *346*, f1326. [CrossRef] [PubMed]

23. Zhu, H.; Pollock, N.K.; Kotak, I.; Gutin, B.; Wang, X.; Bhagatwala, J.; Parikh, S.; Harshfield, G.A.; Dong, Y. Dietary sodium, adiposity, and inflammation in healthy adolescents. *Pediatrics* **2014**, *133*, e635. [CrossRef] [PubMed]

24. Pistrosch, F.; Natali, A.; Hanefeld, M. Is hyperglycemia a cardiovascular risk factor? *Diabetes Care* **2011**, *34* (Suppl. 2), S128–S131. [CrossRef]

25. Goldberg, I.J. Clinical review 124: Diabetic dyslipidemia: Causes and consequences. *J. Clin. Endocrinol. Metab.* **2001**, *86*, 965–971. [CrossRef] [PubMed]

26. Gingras, V.; Leroux, C.; Desjardins, K.; Savard, V.; Lemieux, S.; Rabasa-Lhoret, R.; Strychar, I. Association between Cardiometabolic Profile and Dietary Characteristics among Adults with Type 1 Diabetes Mellitus. *J. Acad. Nutr. Diet.* **2015**, *115*, 1965–1974. [CrossRef] [PubMed]

27. Liese, A.D.; Bortsov, A.; Gunther, A.L.; Dabelea, D.; Reynolds, K.; Standiford, D.A.; Liu, L.; Williams, D.E.; Mayer-Davis, E.J.; D'Agostino, R.B., Jr.; et al. Association of DASH diet with cardiovascular risk factors in youth with diabetes mellitus: The SEARCH for Diabetes in Youth study. *Circulation* **2011**, *123*, 1410–1417. [CrossRef] [PubMed]

28. Zhong, V.W.; Lamichhane, A.P.; Crandell, J.L.; Couch, S.C.; Liese, A.D.; The, N.S.; Tzeel, B.A.; Dabelea, D.; Lawrence, J.M.; Marcovina, S.M.; et al. Association of adherence to a Mediterranean diet with glycemic control and cardiovascular risk factors in youth with type I diabetes: The SEARCH Nutrition Ancillary Study. *Eur. J. Clin. Nutr.* **2016**, *70*, 802–807. [CrossRef] [PubMed]

29. Toeller, M.; Buyken, A.E.; Heitkamp, G.; de Pergola, G.; Giorgino, F.; Fuller, J.H. Fiber intake, serum cholesterol levels, and cardiovascular disease in European individuals with type 1 diabetes. EURODIAB IDDM Complications Study Group. *Diabetes Care* **1999**, *22* (Suppl. 2), B21.

30. Bernaud, F.S.; Beretta, M.V.; do Nascimento, C.; Escobar, F.; Gross, J.L.; Azevedo, M.J.; Rodrigues, T.C. Fiber intake and inflammation in type 1 diabetes. *Diabetol. Metab. Syndr.* **2014**, *6*, 66. [CrossRef] [PubMed]

31. Toeller, M.; Buyken, A.E.; Heitkamp, G.; Scherbaum, W.A.; Krans, H.M.; Fuller, J.H. Associations of fat and cholesterol intake with serum lipid levels and cardiovascular disease: The EURODIAB IDDM Complications Study. *Exp. Clin. Endocrinol. Diabetes* **1999**, *107*, 512–521. [CrossRef] [PubMed]

32. Liese, A.D.; Crandell, J.L.; Tooze, J.A.; Kipnis, V.; Bell, R.; Couch, S.C.; Dabelea, D.; Crume, T.L.; Mayer-Davis, E.J. Sugar-sweetened beverage intake and cardiovascular risk factor profile in youth with type 1 diabetes: Application of measurement error methodology in the SEARCH Nutrition Ancillary Study. *Br. J. Nutr.* **2015**, *114*, 430–438. [CrossRef] [PubMed]

33. Nansel, T.R.; Laffel, L.M.; Haynie, D.L.; Mehta, S.N.; Lipsky, L.M.; Volkening, L.K.; Butler, D.A.; Higgins, L.A.; Liu, A. Improving dietary quality in youth with type 1 diabetes: Randomized clinical trial of a family-based behavioral intervention. *Int. J. Behav. Nutr. Phys. Act.* **2015**, *12*, 58. [CrossRef] [PubMed]

34. Centers for Disease Control and Prevention. *Behavioral Risk Factor Surveillance System Survey Questionnaire*; Centers for Disease Control and Prevention: Atlanta, GA, USA, 2001.

35. Bender, R.; Lange, S. Multiple test procedures other than Bonferroni's deserve wider use. *BMJ* **1999**, *318*, 600. [CrossRef] [PubMed]

36. Althouse, A.D. Adjust for Multiple Comparisons? It's Not That Simple. *Ann. Thorac. Surg.* **2016**, *101*, 1644–1645. [CrossRef] [PubMed]

37. Cox, R.A.; Garcia-Palmieri, M.R. Cholesterol, Triglycerides, and Associated Lipoproteins. In *Clinical Methods: The History, Physical, and Laboratory Examinations*; Walker, H.K., Hall, W.D., Hurst, J.W., Eds.; Butterworth Publishers: Boston, MA, USA, 1990.

38. Gooding, H.C.; de Ferranti, S.D. Cardiovascular risk assessment and cholesterol management in adolescents: Getting to the heart of the matter. *Curr. Opin. Pediatr.* **2010**, *22*, 398–404. [CrossRef] [PubMed]

39. Shah, B.S.; Freeland-Graves, J.H.; Cahill, J.M.; Lu, H.; Graves, G.R. Diet quality as measured by the healthy eating index and the association with lipid profile in low-income women in early postpartum. *J. Am. Diet. Assoc.* **2010**, *110*, 274–279. [CrossRef] [PubMed]

40. Flint, A.J.; Hu, F.B.; Glynn, R.J.; Jensen, M.K.; Franz, M.; Sampson, L.; Rimm, E.B. Whole grains and incident hypertension in men. *Am. J. Clin. Nutr.* **2009**, *90*, 493–498. [CrossRef] [PubMed]

41. Katz, D.L.; Nawaz, H.; Boukhalil, J.; Chan, W.; Ahmadi, R.; Giannamore, V.; Sarrel, P.M. Effects of oat and wheat cereals on endothelial responses. *Prev. Med.* **2001**, *33*, 476–484. [CrossRef] [PubMed]

42. Develaraja, S.; Reddy, A.; Yadav, M.; Jain, S.; Yadav, H. Whole Grains in Amelioration of Metabolic Derangements. *J. Nutr. Health Food Sci.* **2016**, *4*, 1–11.

43. Kirwan, J.P.; Malin, S.K.; Scelsi, A.R.; Kullman, E.L.; Navaneethan, S.D.; Pagadala, M.R.; Haus, J.M.; Filion, J.; Godin, J.P.; Kochhar, S.; et al. A Whole-Grain Diet Reduces Cardiovascular Risk Factors in Overweight and Obese Adults: A Randomized Controlled Trial. *J. Nutr.* **2016**, *146*, 2244–2251. [CrossRef] [PubMed]

44. Borgi, L.; Muraki, I.; Satija, A.; Willett, W.C.; Rimm, E.B.; Forman, J.P. Fruit and Vegetable Consumption and the Incidence of Hypertension in Three Prospective Cohort Studies. *Hypertension* **2016**, *67*, 288–293. [CrossRef] [PubMed]

45. Schwarz, J.M.; Clearfield, M.; Mulligan, K. Conversion of Sugar to Fat: Is Hepatic de Novo Lipogenesis Leading to Metabolic Syndrome and Associated Chronic Diseases? *J. Am. Osteopath. Assoc.* **2017**, *117*, 520–527. [CrossRef] [PubMed]

46. Bortsov, A.V.; Liese, A.D.; Bell, R.A.; Dabelea, D.; D'Agostino, R.B., Jr.; Hamman, R.F.; Klingensmith, G.J.; Lawrence, J.M.; Maahs, D.M.; McKeown, R.; et al. Sugar-sweetened and diet beverage consumption is associated with cardiovascular risk factor profile in youth with type 1 diabetes. *Acta Diabetol.* **2011**, *48*, 275–282. [CrossRef] [PubMed]

47. Hayek, T.; Ito, Y.; Azrolan, N.; Verdery, R.B.; Aalto-Setala, K.; Walsh, A.; Breslow, J.L. Dietary fat increases high density lipoprotein (HDL) levels both by increasing the transport rates and decreasing the fractional catabolic rates of HDL cholesterol ester and apolipoprotein (Apo) A-I. Presentation of a new animal model and mechanistic studies in human Apo A-I transgenic and control mice. *J. Clin. Investig.* **1993**, *91*, 1665–1671. [PubMed]

48. Dorjgochoo, T.; Gao, Y.T.; Chow, W.H.; Shu, X.O.; Yang, G.; Cai, Q.; Rothman, N.; Cai, H.; Li, H.; Deng, X.; et al. Major metabolite of F2-isoprostane in urine may be a more sensitive biomarker of oxidative stress than isoprostane itself. *Am. J. Clin. Nutr.* **2012**, *96*, 405–414. [CrossRef] [PubMed]

49. Patterson, E.; Wall, R.; Fitzgerald, G.F.; Ross, R.P.; Stanton, C. Health implications of high dietary omega-6 polyunsaturated Fatty acids. *J. Nutr. Metab.* **2012**, *2012*, 539426. [CrossRef] [PubMed]

50. Ortega, R.M.; Perez-Rodrigo, C.; Lopez-Sobaler, A.M. Dietary assessment methods: Dietary records. *Nutr. Hosp.* **2015**, *31* (Suppl. 3), 38–45.

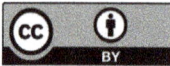

nutrients

MDPI

Article

Food Perceptions and Dietary Changes for Chronic Condition Management in Rural Peru: Insights for Health Promotion

Silvana Perez-Leon [1,*], M. Amalia Pesantes [1], Nathaly Aya Pastrana [2], Shivani Raman [3], Jaime Miranda [1] and L. Suzanne Suggs [2]

[1] CRONICAS Center of Excellence in Chronic Diseases, Universidad Peruana Cayetano Heredia, Lima 15074, Peru; maria.pesantes.v@upch.pe (M.A.P.); jaime.miranda@upch.pe (J.M.)
[2] BeCHANGE Research Group, Institute of Public Communication, Università della Svizzera italiana, 6900 Lugano, Switzerland; nathaly.aya.pastrana@usi.ch (N.A.P.); suzanne.suggs@usi.ch (L.S.S.)
[3] Department of Sociology, Rice University, Houston, TX 77005, USA; sir3@rice.edu
* Correspondence: silvanaplq@gmail.com; Tel.: +51-1-241-6978

Received: 8 September 2018; Accepted: 19 October 2018; Published: 23 October 2018

Abstract: Peru is undergoing a nutrition transition and, at the country level, it faces a double burden of disease where several different conditions require dietary changes to maintain a healthy life and prevent complications. Through semistructured interviews in rural Peru with people affected by three infectious and noninfectious chronic conditions (type 2 diabetes, hypertension, and neurocysticercosis), their relatives, and focus group discussions with community members, we analyzed their perspectives on the value of food and the challenges of dietary changes due to medical diagnosis. The findings show the various ways in which people from rural northern Peru conceptualize good (*buena alimentación*) and bad (*mala alimentación*) food, and that food choices are based on life-long learning, experience, exposure, and availability. In the context of poverty, required changes are not only related to what people recognize as healthy food, such as fruits and vegetables, but also of work, family, trust, taste, as well as affordability and accessibility of foods. In this paper we discuss the complexity of introducing dietary changes in poor rural communities whose perspectives on food are poorly understood and rarely taken into consideration by health professionals when promoting behavior change.

Keywords: dietary changes; health promotion; health behavior; Peru; chronic conditions

1. Introduction

Over the past several decades, low- and middle-income countries (LMICs) have experienced a nutrition transition. Countries that have faced hunger and malnutrition as their main concerns are now confronting an additional problem of overweight and obesity and are experiencing increasing rates of noncommunicable diseases (NCD) such as diabetes and hypertension [1]. Additionally, LMICs are still struggling to reduce the incidence of infectious diseases that are often caused by contaminated food or poor hygiene practices. One example is neurocysticercosis (NCC), a neglected tropical disease (NTD) characterized by parasitic infection of the brain that primarily affects the poor [2].

Peru is undergoing a nutrition transition. The Ministry of Health of Peru has estimated that 20% of the burden of disease in 2011 was associated with overweight and obesity [3]. NCDs are the main cause of mortality in Peru [3], while NTDs continue to affect vulnerable groups of the population such as those living in rural areas with limited access to water and sanitation facilities. In the north of Peru, the prevalence of type 2 diabetes (T2D) and hypertension (HT) is high (10% and 26%, respectively) [4,5], and NCC is considered to be endemic in this part of the country [2].

Type 2 diabetes (T2D) and hypertension (HT) require dietary changes to manage the conditions and though patients with NCC do not require specific changes in their diet, its prevention has a close relation with the consumption of uncooked pork and poor sanitary practices. The control of NCC requires breaking the life cycle of the Taenia solium [6], where the main intervention to stop transmission in LMICs is improving sanitary practices [7,8]. The prevention of both NCDs and NCC share the need to promote changes in dietary habits in the population.

Most studies in LMICs have addressed the problem of nutrition transition from the perspective of accessibility and affordability [9–12] but nutrition is a complex issue since what people eat is not only about nutritional value, as food choices and preferences are influenced by many factors [13]. The cultural and social contexts in which individuals are brought up, live, and work have a strong influence on the food choices made, as they affect their views of foods and eating behaviors [13]. Diet is also an important aspect of social life and is related with sharing, belonging to a group, and celebration [14]. Thus, promoting and supporting dietary changes requires a thorough understanding of local cultural norms, values, beliefs, and practices that underlie certain unhealthy habits [15].

In this study, we examine the perspectives on the value of food and the challenges of dietary changes among people living with T2D, HT, and/or NCC from four rural communities in Northern Peru. We contrast and compare local perspectives of what and why a particular food item is perceived as "good" or "bad". Our findings are particularly relevant for culturally appropriate design of health promotion aiming to achieve the U.N. Sustainable Development Goals for ending all forms of malnutrition and ensuring healthy lives.

2. Materials and Methods

2.1. Study Design

The study is part of a multicountry research for development project that aims to address the health challenges faced in low- and middle-income countries as a result of the double burden that NTDs and NCDs place on local health systems [16].

The data were collected as part of a qualitative study aimed at understanding local health perceptions and use of health facilities of people with chronic conditions and other community dwellers. Data were collected through semistructured interviews and focus group discussions using a predetermined set of questions (see Tables S1–S3, interview and focus group guidelines) and complemented with field notes. This analysis utilized the data related to local dietary habits and changes in the patient's life due to the disease (see Table S1 questions 10, 18, 19; Table S2 questions 13, 20; Table S3 questions A4, A5, D1).

2.2. Study Site

All data were collected in the province of Ayabaca, located in the highlands of the Piura region in northern Peru (Figure S1. Map of Ayabaca). Ayabaca is divided into 10 districts and has an approximate population of 140,000 (Information is gathered in 2015) [17], with 73% of the population living in poverty (Information is gathered in 2009) [17]. Two rural communities and their district's capital towns were selected for this study: Pingola (Ayabaca district) and Sicacate (Montero district). The main economic activity in both communities is agriculture. Men predominately work as agricultural farmers, while women work as housewives (cooking, cleaning, caring for children, etc.) and in some cases, manage small shops (*bodegas*).

2.3. Study Participants and Selection Rationale

Study participants were caregivers, head of households, people living with T2D, HT, and/or NCC, and community dwellers. The latter participated in the focus group discussions. All participants were 18 years old or older and provided verbal consent.

Interviews allowed the discovery of opinions and personal experiences on the selected chronic conditions of the caregivers, heads of households, and patients with T2D, HT, and NCC. The rationale for interviewing caregivers, heads of household, and patients was to have complementary views of the condition from each family. All caregivers and head of households were relatives of those affected by T2D, HT, or NCC. Due to the difficulties to find patients diagnosed with NCC in these communities, we included persons with epilepsy. Epilepsy is one of the main symptoms for those with NCC, which is endemic in Ayabaca [2].

Focus groups examined the common perceptions of community members on T2D, HT, and NCC as well as other health problems, and focus group participants were homogeneous in age and sex. In order to have the perspective of a vulnerable group within the selected communities, additional focus groups were conducted with women beneficiaries of JUNTOS, the national cash transfer program targeting poor women with children under five years old. Some focus groups did not take place because no participants showed up. Each "failed" focus group was replaced with four individual interviews. Additionally, when the focus groups had less than six participants, the research team conducted a "small" focus group and complimented it with additional interviews.

2.4. Recruitment

For semistructured interviews, fieldworkers used word of mouth to find people with the conditions of T2D, HT, and NCC, their caregiver and head of households, followed by a snowball sampling methodology.

For the recruitment of focus groups, fieldworkers invited people gathered in different parts of the communities to participate, e.g., church, marketplace, main square, etc., and asked them to invite friends of the same age and sex.

2.5. Data Collection

At the beginning of the focus group discussions and interviews, sociodemographic data were collected from all participants. All interviews and focus groups were audio-recorded.

2.5.1. Data Collection Teams

Data were collected by four people with degrees in social sciences, who had previous experience in qualitative research in rural areas, and who underwent a four-day training. They were divided into two teams, one per district, ensuring sex parity [18]. Evidence suggests that the gender of the interviewer influences participant's involvement and interaction [19,20] and that matching the gender of the interviewer and interviewee can facilitate discussion on sensitive topics [20]. For this reason, teams were made up of one male and one female fieldworker, which allowed the research team to conduct focus group discussions and interviews by the interviewer who was the same sex of the interviewee(s).

Data from semistructured interviews and focus groups were complemented with field notes taken by a doctoral student that accompanied the fieldwork team.

2.5.2. Collection Period

Most data were collected between 2 and 21 February 2017. However, one research team returned to the field site from 10 to 12 March 2017, to conduct a focus group discussion with young men who were unavailable during the initial data collection period. Because the data collection period coincided with the rainy season in these communities, participation in focus groups discussions was low.

2.6. Data Analysis

All interviews and focus group discussions were transcribed and the fieldworkers entered the data into matrices. The matrices were reviewed by the research assistant and the lead researcher, and were then uploaded into ATLAS.ti 8 (Scientific Software Development GmbH, Berlin, Germany), including the field notes.

A codebook was created (see Table S4: Codebook) and entered into ATLAS.ti 8. To ensure quality of coding, weekly discussions were held between the lead researcher, two research assistants, and a doctoral student, in which the codes were analyzed and concerns were addressed.

2.7. Structure of the Analysis

In the interviews and focus groups, participants were asked about the food consumed on a regular basis, to have an overview of the diet in the communities of the study. To assess community perceptions of "good" food, we asked informants "*¿Para usted cómo es una buena alimentación?*", which can be translated as "What is a good meal/food/nutrition for you?". The question translated into English does not completely preserve its meaning in Spanish. The words *"buena alimentación"* can have different uses, for example, in some cases it can be interpreted as having good nutrition and in other cases it may mean consuming large amounts of food. The intention of this question was to examine the different meanings the informants give to *"buena alimentación"*, thus understanding which elements they consider most relevant when they talk about nutrition, food, and diets.

We also asked informants "*¿Por qué es importante tener una buena alimentación?*" (Why is it important to have a good meal/food/nutrition?)" in order to understand community perceptions about the importance of buena alimentación. In some cases based on the interview, fieldworkers explored if the food was related to physical strength.

To understand what changes to diet were made by patients after their diagnoses and how family life was affected because of the diagnosis, both patients and their caregiver/head of households were interviewed. Patients were asked what changes they had made in their life since they were diagnosed with their disease (*¿Qué cambios ha hecho en su vida desde que fue diagnosticado con diabetes/ hipertensión/ neurocisticercosis ?*) and what were the most difficult aspects of living with the disease (*¿Cuáles son los aspectos más difíciles de vivir con su enfermedad?*). Caregivers and heads of households were asked about how family life had been affected as a result of living with a person with T2D/HT/NCC (*¿Cómo afecta la vida familiar el vivir con una persona con diabetes / hipertensión / cisticercosis?*) and what were the main changes that had occurred since this relative was diagnosed with T2D/HT/NCC (*¿Cuáles son los principales cambios que han ocurrido desde que él / ella se le diagnosticó diabetes / hipertensión / cisticercosis?*).

2.8. Ethics

The study was approved by the *Comité Institucional de Ética* (Institutional Review Board) at Universidad Peruana Cayetano Heredia in Lima, Peru (code 393-22-16), and by the Institutional Review Board at the University of Geneva in Geneva, Switzerland (IRB No. 2016-01242).

3. Results

A total of 138 individuals participated in the study. In total, 16 semistructured interviews were conducted with individuals living with T2D ($n = 4$), HT ($n = 7$), and NCC or epilepsy ($n = 5$), the caregivers ($n = 8$), and head of household ($n = 5$). Additionally, 12 focus group discussions were arranged where 82 community dwellers participated as well as 27 individual interviews that replaced or complimented some focus groups.

3.1. Overview of the Diet in the Communities

As stated previously, the main economic activity in both communities is agriculture. Half of the production in these communities is for sale and half for selfconsumption or to feed their animals. The main products grown are maize, bananas, sugar cane, cassava, potatoes, and cultivated pasture grasses [21].

When asked about the foods consumed on a regular basis, participants sometimes gave a list of ingredients or food preparations, while other times they described the characteristics of each meal.

Based on their answers, it appeared that most people have three meals, breakfast, lunch, and dinner, and that the quantity of food consumed at each meal was usually big in comparison to the amounts people from urban areas eat:

People are used to eat a lot, not like in the city where for example in the morning they have coffee and bread. (Female, 70 years old)

We eat a lot. Here is not like the city where they eat bread, here if there is no rice or cassava it is not a meal. (. . .) Here people eat a lot, the big dish and double portion. (Male, 18–34 years group)

For breakfast, participants said they could have rice and fried chicken or rice and fish or egg. At noon, some people have a snack and later they will have lunch which often consists of rice and another starchy local food such as potato, yucca, and plantains with legumes (*menestras*) (see Figures S2–S4). At dinner, participants stated they would have a soup with noodles, some vegetables, chicken or with egg. Red meat and pork were not commonly consumed, while chicken and fish (salted fish) were mentioned as part of the regular diet. Though pork is not consumed in their day-to-day diets, people often mentioned it as a traditional meal, something easily found in local restaurants. Vegetables do not appear to be a common ingredient. According to participants, the consumption of vegetables is related to their availability according to seasonal changes, as one participant explained: *"during the rainy seasons (January, February and March) we eat more vegetables like lettuce and carrot. In April and May we eat more tamalitos, more corn."(Man, 56 years old)*. It is hard to find vegetables in the local bodegas and if they are available, they are expensive. We observed that noodles were a staple food in the communities, as they are affordable. Though the interview and focus group participants did not frequently report this consumption, the observational notes that complemented this information showed that noodles and cookies are regularly sold products in the small shops of the communities and noodles are a common ingredient seen in the meals of local people.

Overall, participants described a high consumption of carbohydrates and legumes that they usually grow. Meat consumption (especially chicken and salted fish) was frequent but in smaller quantities. Few participants mentioned fruits except for bananas which are part of the local diet.

3.2. What Do People Consider to Be a "Good" and "Bad" Food in These Communities?

As expected, informants responded to the question *"¿Para usted cómo es una buena alimentación?* (What is good meal/food/nutrition for you?)", in different ways. In most cases, they mentioned specific types of foods they consider to be a buena alimentación (good meal/food/nutrition) or, on the contrary, foods they view as a "mala alimentacion" (bad meal/food/nutrition). In other cases, informants mentioned characteristics of their meals (whether meals are "balanced"), certain methods of food preparation, or aspects of the food production process.

Informants most often responded by mentioning specific foods that they consider to be a *buena alimentación* or *mala alimentación*. In the following tables (Tables 1 and 2) we summarize the most frequently mentioned food categories and the number of transcripts where each type of food was mentioned. These tables include responses from both interviews and focus groups, not all the informants answered this question. Out of 67 transcripts, 62 had a response.

Table 1. "Buena alimentación".

Type of Food	No. of Transcripts n = 62 n (%)
Vegetables (lettuce, cabbage, chard, cauliflower, cucumber, celery, carrot, beet, onion, etc.)	37 (59.7%)
Meat (chicken, beef, pork, lamb, fish, etc.)	28 (45.2%)
Legumes (beans, lentils, peas, etc.)	27 (43.5%)
Grains (rice, wheat/*sango*, quinoa, cereals, etc.)	24 (38.7%)
Fruits (banana, apple, orange, etc.)	16 (25.8%)
Potatoes, cassava, sweet potatoes	9 (14.5%)
Eggs and dairy (eggs, milk, cheese, yogurt, etc.)	8 (12.9%)

Table 2. "Mala alimentación".

Type of Food	No. of Transcripts $n = 62$ n (%)
Meat (pork, chicken, etc.)	18 (29.0%)
Rice	12 (19.4%)
Fried foods	5 (8.1%)
Processed foods (bread, noodles, etc.)	5 (8.1%)
Junk food	3 (4.8%)
Other (potato, sweets, flours, fats, soda, alcohol, unboiled water)	7 (11.3%)

Of those informants who identified meat as a *mala alimentación* ($n = 18$), most identified pork ($n = 9$) and/or chicken ($n = 6$) as the most harmful meats. Informants characterized pork as *mala alimentación* due to its high fat content and its link to NCC. For those diagnosed with NCC or epilepsy, almost all (4/5) mentioned pork as a *mala alimentación*.

Informants also characterized a *buena alimentación* by mentioning specific methods of food preparation. Several mentioned that *"comidas sancochadas"*, or foods that have been cooked in boiling water, are preferable to fried foods: *"(I think a good meal is) usually boiled food, because most of the people eat fried, or making steamed fish or ceviche. Because if you eat fried food it has fat. For me healthier food is steamed." (Woman, 38 years old)*.

One participant mentioned that buena alimentación consists of maintaining good hygiene in the process of preparing food: *"We need to have a proper hygiene to be able to feed us. If we don't have the cookware well cleaned, the hands washed and the nails cut, then we are not going to have a good nutrition". (Woman, 18–34 years group)*. The importance of hygienical preparation was also mentioned in a conversation with a local restaurant owner.

In addition to mentioning aspects of food preparation, informants also characterized *buena alimentación* by describing the food production process. Informants considered the foods grown in their communities or in the "olden days" to be *buena alimentación* because they are free of hormones, pesticides, herbicides, fertilizers, and other chemicals. On the other hand, they viewed foods from the city or "modern" time as *mala alimentación* because they are produced using the abovementioned chemicals:

> The food here is healthy because the food is natural. Here you can still find natural food, mainly what comes from the farms because the products do not have fertilizers, so the food is natural. (Man, 70 years old)

> They inject them too much, those chicken don't have nutrients. What is good is milk, lentil, beef, mutton, pork, which is also nutritious as they eat corn. (Woman, 35 years or older group)

> The truth is that we do not know from where they bring the vegetables that are sold in the market, we do not have trust. (. . .) When you grow vegetables in your garden you have trust. But those plants that come from other places are not recommended to eat because they irrigate them with wastewater. (Women, 35 years or older group)

> The food now is not like before. (Before) it was natural (. . .) now it has a lot of chemical, the plant absorbs the chemical. (Women, 35 years old)

Several informants' characterized rice (see Table 2) as *mala alimentación* because they consider that it requires a greater use of chemicals to grow: *"The rice is more chemical, the rice is to fill the stomach." (Man, 35 or older years group)*.

Several also described *buena alimentación* as eating "balanced" food/meals. While most did not specify what they meant by "balanced" food/meals, two informants provided the following descriptions:

> You have to eat meat, salad and when there is no meat it can be legumes and to drink it can be chicha morada (typical beverage made of purple corn). (Woman with HT, 48 years old)

I think the meals have to be balanced. Eating cereals, fruits, vegetables in large amounts, fish and eating more white than red meat. Red meat is a little more harmful. From time to time you can eat a desert, like yogurt. (Man, 24 years old)

The reasons provided to the question "*¿Por qué es importante tener una buena alimentación?* (Why is it important to have a good meal/food/nutrition?)" are summarized in Table 3. In many cases, informants mentioned more than one of the listed reasons. Therefore, the categories below are not independent of one another, rather, they are often interrelated (e.g., "to maintain good health" co-occurs with "to prevent diseases"). This table includes responses from both interviews and focus groups, not all the informants answered this question. Out of the 67 transcripts, 36 had a response.

Table 3. Reasons for "*buena alimentación*".

Reasons	No. of Transcripts $n = 36$ n (%)
To maintain good health (in general)	18 (50.0%)
To carry out day-to-day activities/tasks [1]	16 (44.4%)
To prevent diseases	12 (33.3%)
To have physical strength and endurance	11 (30.6%)
To maintain a strong immune system	2 (5.6%)
To maintain good mental health	2 (5.6%)
Other [2]	5 (13.9%)

[1] Working in agriculture, domestic work, caring for children, attending school/studying, etc. [2] To maintain good sexual health, to maintain strong bones, to maintain healthy skin, to control weight, to have good physical appearance/"*estar regias*".

Most often, informants stated that it is important to have *buena alimentación* in order to maintain good health in general. Many also expressed that it is important to have *buena alimentación* in order to prevent diseases. They often mentioned maintaining good health in conjunction with preventing diseases: "*To not get sick also, have a good health.*" (*Women with HT, 48 years old*). One female informant specifically mentioned that *buena alimentación* is important for preventing anemia; however, no one mentioned T2D, HT, or NCC.

The second most commonly mentioned reason for maintaining *buena alimentación* was important for having sufficient strength and endurance to carry out day-to-day labor and activities. Responses often corresponded to their roles within their family and in the community. Men commonly mentioned working in agriculture, while women most often mentioned performing domestic tasks and caring for children.

Because if we are weak we cannot do anything, what are we supposed to do? You cannot work, not even with your wife you can work. (Man with NCC, 36 years old)

To have strength to work, for example we are weaving and it's time to have lunch, we make some food and then again we weave with strength. (Woman with T2D, 68 years old)

In response to a question about what foods give strength to perform agricultural work, responses commonly mentioned included mote (Peruvian corn), *sango* (food prepared with corn), and sweet potato as foods that provide strength and endurance. "*The sweet potato is also good, it lasts all day, from 8:00 am when you eat, until 19:00.*" (*Man with NCC, 36 years*) Participants described *mala alimentación* as foods that do not provide sufficient strength and endurance to perform daily labors:

The bread does not make your stomach full, for example here you cannot eat bread because the work is hard. If you eat bread at breakfast it will only last until 10:00 am and you have no strength." (Man, 41 years old)

Some participants also mentioned that *buena alimentación* is important for attending school and studying.

3.3. Changes in Diet Due to a Chronic Disease

The answers provided by patients and their family members regarding dietary changes and its implications were complementary and thus the family is the unit of analysis ($n = 17$). Three themes emerged in the data regarding the types of changes patients and their caregivers/heads of household made in their diets and the difficulties they faced in accomplishing these changes.

One of the main responses had to do with dietary changes in the patient's life. Patients with T2D or HT and their relatives ($n = 12$) reported undergoing dietary changes. They spoke about reducing or eliminating certain types of foods or ingredients such as sugar (5) (sweets, certain fruits, potatoes, yucca, rice, noodles, and harinas, colloquial way of saying carbohydrates); salt (7), pork (5), and red meats (3). They also spoke about decreasing their intake of fats/oils (3) or avoiding preparing fried meals (1). The reduction/elimination of other foods like alcoholic beverages (1) and food coloring (1) was scarcely mentioned.

Several patients with T2D and HT and their families said the patient had increased their consumption of vegetables (6) and fruits (1), or they mentioned the types of food they consumed, such as chicken (1) and beans (1). Some mentioned they had reduced the amount of food they ate at each meal (3). Two families of patients with HT reported not making any changes in their diet due to their disease.

The patients with T2D or HT and their families expressed several challenges associated with making dietary changes. They expressed struggles in adhering to dietary changes (5) due to the difficulty of eliminating certain foods from their diet and not being able to eat the way they would like to: *"The most difficult (thing) is not being able to eat what I like, what I have been taught to eat"(Woman with T2D, 68 years old)*, eating food they did not enjoy like vegetables, not being able to cook their own food or not being able to buy vegetables: *"It is going to be two months or three months that I have not been able to buy vegetables, I am afraid that my blood pressure will go up, they say because of high blood pressure you can die."(Woman with HT, 64 years old)*. Another challenge was having to decline the food being served in social occasions (2), like parties or restaurants, which was uncomfortable.

Though most patients with T2D and HT reported making dietary changes, most of the interviewed families said they cooked the same meal for everyone (7). No case of separate meal preparation was reported; however, they did mention various ways of adapting the patients' diets to the recommendations they received from the health professionals. For example, in some cases the family separated the patient's portion before adding spices, and in other cases the entire family adopted a new diet as a result of the patient's chronic condition: *"Now we cannot prepare some foods, tamal (food made of corn), tortillas (food made of corn), sweets, those things we cannot prepare. We used to drink sodas, but now none of us drinks sodas because its poison (...) now (we drink) only water." (Woman caregiver of TD2, 46 years old)*. Relatives said that some members of the family would later add spices to the food or would secretly eat some "unhealthy" types of food: *"The food I prepare is tasteless; if they (family) want they can add more salt." (Woman with T2D, 52 years)* In some cases, patients would try to adapt their diet with the food already prepared by their family *"Everything is already prepared from early in the morning, so I take out a chicken breast and with a napkin I take out the fat." (Woman with T2D, 64 years)*.

Some patients with NCC and their families also mentioned some dietary changes, including the reduction/elimination of pork (3), duck (2), fish (2), turkey (1), and *"bocadillo"* (1) (typical sweets from the district). *"They gave me my treatment for epilepsy and told me to not eat pork, which I should not eat until I die." (Woman with NCC, 50 years)*. They also mentioned having difficulties to stop eating some of these foods: *"I do not eat pork now, though I really liked eating pork." (Man with NCC, 36 years)*. Two families of patients with NCC reported not making any changes in their diet.

4. Discussion

Our study shows the various ways in which people from rural northern Peru value food and the multiplicity of factors that play a role in identifying food as good/healthy or not. Understanding food- and diet-related contexts like the one in Ayabaca, and similar rural settings facing a nutritional transition, and the complexity attached to it, is fundamental to end all forms of malnutrition (encompassing both undernutrition and overnutrition) and promoting healthy lifestyles and well-being for all and throughout the life course, as proposed by the sustainable development goals 2 and 3 [22].

Our study highlights the challenges of dietary changes in patients with chronic conditions in a rural area and the relevance of understanding the local context. In the communities where we conducted this study, perceptions of *buena* and *mala alimentación* are strongly linked to the extent to which foods enable individuals to perform day-to-day tasks and activities, and this finding is consistent with other studies in Peru [23]. For this reason, individuals are accustomed to consuming high-carbohydrate foods such as rice, potato, corn, and grains, often in large portion sizes. On the other hand, there is conflict between the people recognizing vegetables and fruits as "good" food, and the insufficient consumption of these fruits and vegetables because they are not available or are not affordable. As other studies have reported [24,25], we also found that when foods are not available within the community, participants do not buy them outside due to negative perceptions about consuming food from an unknown source. Yet, there is an increasing consumption of cheap processed foods, such as noodles.

Our findings show the complexity of introducing dietary changes in rural communities where the perspectives on food are poorly understood and rarely taken into consideration when promoting food- or diet-related behavior change. T2D and HT are diseases for which much of their management can occur in the community, at the primary care level, and where the prevention of NCC needs adequate control at the community as well. So the food people intake will have consequences in the management of their disease or in the prevention of new diseases.

For patients with T2D, HT, and NCC, following dietary recommendations received by health professionals is challenging. On the one hand, people have difficulties not being able to eat food they like, the food they grew up with, the food that they perceive as nutritious or tasteful, nor eat certain foods in the quantities they are used to. On the other hand, the food recommended by the health professionals are things they do not like to eat. Furthermore, diet modifications involve negotiation or arrangements with the family, which is key to successfully adapt to the recommended diet [26]. In this sense, involving the family is a key element for dietary modifications. As Vanstone and colleagues show in their review, "support at home is universally described as an essential component of successful dietary modification" [27,28]. Patients in our study know and say they make dietary modifications, but the compliance of healthy dietary practices seems more complex to accomplish. As what is reported in other studies [27,28], making dietary changes recommended by health professionals is challenging. This study helps understand how dietary recommendations for chronic conditions in rural agrarian communities need to be reconciled with working conditions, access to food, perceptions of food, and family.

Our results align with some crosscutting themes such as food availability, introducing dietary changes, and health promotion. What people eat, especially what poor people eat, is not only about what people identify as healthy, but the availability of such foods. Food availability is one of the four pillars of food security [29]. Thus, a poor person's socioeconomic status can exert a strong influence on food choice behaviors [30–32]. It is necessary to transform food systems into sustainable and sensitive nutrition systems that will provide a variety of healthy foods, devoting special attention to the most vulnerable [9].

The availability of cheap unhealthy choices is a growing problem in many LMICs [33–35] and it is also happening in rural Peru [36]. Understanding local eating habits must take into account the role of structural factors on food choices [37]. Thus, our study supports the finding that individual choices, especially those of the poor, are influenced by broader social and environmental factors [32,38].

Our findings are consistent with studies across the globe that show that knowledge is not enough to influence behavior [39–41]. Theories of human behaviors, such as eating behavior, suggest that a combination of environmental and personal factors influence behavior [42]. Environmental factors include cultural determinants (e.g., nationality, ethnicity, identity), physical (e.g., policies, availability, accessibility), and social (e.g., parental behavior, peer influence, advertisement exposure) [43]. Personal determinants, such as liking and preference, are the strongest determinants of diet habits [44–46]. Introducing, achieving, and sustaining healthier dietary changes will require a combination of all those factors, beyond availability and affordability.

This study highlights that patients, caregivers, and community members living in rural Peru have reasonable knowledge of what a healthy diet consists of, yet making food choices is a complex issue influenced by work, family, trust, taste, as well as affordability and accessibility. It also highlights that perceptions of the value of certain foods are not necessarily consistent with the advice received about healthy diet from health educators and health workers. Health promotion efforts therefore must include not only factual information about nutrients, but also provide opportunities to taste new foods, cook in new ways that are sustainable, and learn about what foods and vendors from outside the community are prepared in ways that respect local preferences. For example, it would be beneficial for health professionals to have a good idea of what foods are produced locally in order to recommend these items in the diet, but also to provide a clear understanding of the relationship between what a person needs versus how much is needed, in accordance with their daily activities (i.e., caloric expenditure).

Some limitations are worth noting. During the recruitment process, it was not always possible to achieve the desired sample size of patient, caregiver, and head of household. The participation in focus groups was low due to the rainy season and there were difficulties recruiting young men in the focus groups. Additional interviews with community dwellers were conducted so as to reach data saturation. Additionally, our study did not include the perspective of health workers' views, which would be helpful in better understanding their challenges in promoting healthy eating. Furthermore, we did not collect information about the availability of food at local stores and their prices in a systematic way that would enable us to fully understand accessibility and affordability of food choices in our sample. Finally, objective measures of the reality in the homes of participants were not collected and so it was not possible to know with certainty if perceptions matched the reality in the home. Nonetheless, the methodology and sampling procedure utilized allow for an overview of the situation regarding food perceptions in these communities.

5. Conclusions

This study shows the important influence of culture and social conditions on food perceptions and dietary changes in rural Peru. The findings highlight that poor people in rural northern Peru, just like others across the globe, make decisions and have knowledge about food that are based on life-long learning, experience, exposure, and availability. The study also stresses that knowledge alone does not influence eating behavior and that making dietary change is difficult. Thus, promoting healthy diets without contextualizing information and recommendations is sure to produce suboptimal results. Health promotion focused on nutrition for rural, poor communities must take into account the activities of daily life, access and affordability of foods, but also food taste preferences and traditions.

Supplementary Materials: The following are available online at www.mdpi.com/2072-6643/10/11/1563/s1, Figure S1: Map of Ayabaca, reproduced from reference [47], Figure S2: Meal made of soup with potatoes, pasta, and beans, Figure S3: Traditional meal named "Sango" made with maize flour and water with a fires egg, Figure S4: Meal in a community meeting, containing potatoes, rice, carrots, and onions with one serving of meat, Table S1: Interview Guide for Patients, Table S2: Interview guide for caregivers and head of household, Table S3: Guide for focus group discussions, Table S4: Codebook.

Author Contributions: Conceptualization, N.A.P. and L.S.S.; Methodology, M.A.P., N.A.P., and L.S.S.; Formal Analysis, S.R., S.P.-L., N.A.P., and M.A.P.; Investigation, S.P.-L. and N.A.P.; Resources, J.M.; Data Curation, S.R. and S.P.-L.; Writing-Original Draft Preparation, S.P.-L.; Writing-Review & Editing, M.A.P., S.R., N.A.P., J.M., and L.S.S.; Supervision, M.A.P.; Project Administration, M.A.P.; Funding Acquisition, J.M., M.A.P., and L.S.S.

Funding: This research was funded under the r4d Public Health call of the Swiss Programme for Research on Global Issues for Development by the Swiss National Science Foundation and the Swiss Development Cooperation grant number 40P740_160366/1.

Acknowledgments: We want to thank David Beran, who provided critical feedback on earlier versions of the manuscript and whose encouragement was key to complete the manuscript.

Conflicts of Interest: The authors declare no conflict of interest. The funders had no role in the design of the study; in the collection, analyses, or interpretation of data; in the writing of the manuscript, and in the decision to publish the results.

References

1. Popkin, B.M.; Adair, L.S.; Ng, S.W. Global nutrition transition and the pandemic of obesity in developing countries. *Nutr. Rev.* **2012**, *70*, 3–21. [CrossRef] [PubMed]
2. Moyano, L.M.; O'Neal, S.E.; Ayvar, V.; Gonzalvez, G.; Gamboa, R.; Vilchez, P.; Rodriguez, S.; Reistetter, J.; Tsang, V.C.W.; Gilman, R.H.; et al. High Prevalence of Asymptomatic Neurocysticercosis in an Endemic Rural Community in Peru. *PLoS Negl. Trop. Dis.* **2016**, *10*, e0005130. [CrossRef] [PubMed]
3. Diez-Canseco, F.; Saavedra-Garcia, L. Programas sociales y reducción de la obesidad en el Perú: Reflexiones desde la investigación. *Revista Peruana De Medicina Experimental Y Salud Pública* **2017**, *34*, 105–112. [CrossRef] [PubMed]
4. Bernabé-Ortiz, A.; Carrillo-Larco, R.M.; Gilman, R.H.; Checkley, W.; Smeeth, L.; Miranda, J.J. Contribution of modifiable risk factors for hypertension and type-2 diabetes in Peruvian resource-limited settings. *J. Epidemiol. Community Health* **2016**, *70*, 49–55. [CrossRef] [PubMed]
5. Bernabe-Ortiz, A.; Perel, P.; Miranda, J.J.; Smeeth, L. Diagnostic accuracy of the Finnish Diabetes Risk Score (FINDRISC) for undiagnosed T2DM in Peruvian population. *Prim. Care Diabetes* **2018**, in press. [CrossRef] [PubMed]
6. Maurice, J. Of pigs and people—WHO prepares to battle cysticercosis. *Lancet* **2014**, *384*, 571–572. [CrossRef]
7. Summary of the Twenty-First Meeting of the International Task Force for Disease Eradication (II). Available online: http://www.cartercenter.org/resources/pdfs/news/health_publications/itfde/ITFDE-summary-071013.pdf (accessed on 7 February 2018).
8. Wielinga, P.R.; Schlundt, J. Food Safety: At the center of a One Health approach for combating zoonoses. *Curr. Top. Microbiol. Immunol.* **2013**, *366*, 3–17. [CrossRef] [PubMed]
9. Panorama de la Seguridad Alimentaria y Nutricional en América Latina y el Caribe. Available online: http://www.fao.org/3/a-i7914s.pdf2017 (accessed on 6 September 2018).
10. Ortiz-Hernández, L.; Delgado-Sánchez, G.; Hernández-Briones, A. Cambios en factores relacionados con la transición alimentaria y nutricional en México. *Gaceta Médica De México* **2006**, *142*, 181–193. [PubMed]
11. Sánchez, L.S.I.; Ibarra, L.S.V.; Bernal, V.G.; Guerrero, F.H. Transición Alimentaria en México. *Razón Y Palabra* **2016**, *58*, 568–573.
12. Peña, M.; Bacallao, J. *La Obesidad en la Pobreza: Un Nuevo Reto para la Salud Pública*; PAO: Washington, DC, USA, 2000; ISBN 978-92-75-31576-7.
13. Shepherd, R. Social determinants of food choice. *Proc. Nutr. Soc.* **1999**, *58*, 807–812. [CrossRef] [PubMed]
14. Mintz, S.W.; Bois, C.M.D. The Anthropology of Food and Eating. *Annu. Rev. Anthropol.* **2002**, *31*, 99–119. [CrossRef]
15. Dickey, M.K.; John, R.; Carabin, H.; Zhou, X.-N. Focus group discussions among the Bai in China to inform a social marketing campaign for sanitation promotion. *J. Water Sanit. Hyg. Dev.* **2016**, *6*, 121–131. [CrossRef]
16. Tackling NCDs and NTDs: The COHESION Approach to Addressing the SDGs. Health Network Shareweb of the Swiss Agency for Development and Cooperation SDC. Available online: https://www.shareweb.ch/site/Health/aboutus/Pages/Contributions-January-2018/Tackling-NCDs-and-NTDs.aspx (accessed on 4 September 2018).
17. PERÚ Instituto Nacional de Estadística e Informática 2015. Available online: https://www.inei.gob.pe/ (accessed on 4 July 2018).
18. World Health Organization. *Gender Mainstreaming for Health Managers: A Practical Approach*; WHO: Geneva, Switzerland, 2011.
19. Kamuya, D.M.; Catherine, S.M.; Theobald, S. Gendered negotiations for research participation in community-based studies: Implications for health research policy and practice. *BMJ Glob. Health* **2017**, *2*, e000320. [CrossRef] [PubMed]

20. Padfield, M.; Procter, I. The Effect of Interviewer's Gender on the Interviewing Process: A Comparative Enquiry. *Sociology* **1996**, *30*, 355–366. [CrossRef]

21. IV Censo Nacional Agropecuario 2012—Base de Datos REDATAM. Available online: http://censos.inei.gob.pe/Cenagro/redatam/ (accessed on 16 October 2018).

22. Transforming our World: The 2030 Agenda for Sustainable Development. Available online: http://undocs.org/A/RES/70/1 (accessed on 4 September 2018).

23. Pesantes, M.A.; Diez-Canseco, F.; Bernabé-Ortiz, A.; Ponce-Lucero, V.; Miranda, J.J. Taste, Salt Consumption, and Local Explanations around Hypertension in a Rural Population in Northern Peru. *Nutrients* **2017**, *9*. [CrossRef] [PubMed]

24. Lipus, A.C.; Leon, J.S.; Calle, S.C.; Andes, K.L. "It Is Not Natural Anymore": Nutrition, Urbanization, and Indigenous Identity on Bolivia's Andean Plateau. *Qual. Health Res.* **2018**. [CrossRef] [PubMed]

25. Garro, L.C. Intracultural variation in causal accounts of diabetes: A comparison of three Canadian Anishinaabe (ojibway) communities. *Cult. Med. Psych.* **1996**, *20*, 381–420. [CrossRef]

26. Pesantes, M.A.; Del Valle, A.; Diez-Canseco, F.; Bernabé-Ortiz, A.; Portocarrero, J.; Trujillo, A.; Cornejo, P.; Manrique, K.; Miranda, J.J. Family Support and Diabetes: Patient's Experiences From a Public Hospital in Peru. *Qual. Health. Res.* **2018**, *28*. [CrossRef] [PubMed]

27. Vanstone, M.; Rewegan, A.; Brundisini, F.; Giacomini, M.; Kandasamy, S.; DeJean, D. Diet modification challenges faced by marginalized and nonmarginalized adults with type 2 diabetes: A systematic review and qualitative meta-synthesis. *Chronic Illn.* **2017**, *13*, 217–235. [CrossRef] [PubMed]

28. Vanstone, M.; Giacomini, M.; Smith, A.; Brundisini, F.; DeJean, D.; Winsor, S. How diet modification challenges are magnified in vulnerable or marginalized people with diabetes and heart disease: A systematic review and qualitative meta-synthesis. *Ont. Health Technol Assess. Ser.* **2013**, *13*, 1–40. [PubMed]

29. Power, E.M. Conceptualizing Food Security for Aboriginal People in Canada. *Can. J. Public Health* **2008**, *99*, 95–97. [PubMed]

30. Drewnowski, A.; Rolls, B.J. *Obesity Treatment and Prevention: New Directions*; Karger Publishers: Basel, Switzerland, 2012.

31. O'Neill, M.; Rebane, D.; Lester, C. Barriers to healthier eating in a disadvantaged community. *Health Educ. J.* **2004**, *63*, 220–228. [CrossRef]

32. Irala-Estévez, J.D.; Groth, M.; Johansson, L.; Oltersdorf, U.; Prättälä, R.; Martínez-González, M.A. A systematic review of socio-economic differences in food habits in Europe: Consumption of fruit and vegetables. *Eur. J. Clin. Nutr.* **2000**, *54*, 706–714. [CrossRef] [PubMed]

33. Stuckler, D.; McKee, M.; Ebrahim, S.; Basu, S. Manufacturing epidemics: The role of global producers in increased consumption of unhealthy commodities including processed foods, alcohol, and tobacco. *PLoS Med.* **2012**, *9*, e1001235. [CrossRef] [PubMed]

34. Doak, C.M.; Adair, L.S.; Monteiro, C.; Popkin, B.M. Overweight and Underweight Coexist within Households in Brazil, China and Russia. *J. Nutr.* **2000**, *130*, 2965–2971. [CrossRef] [PubMed]

35. Monteiro, C.A.; Conde, W.L.; Popkin, B.M. Income-Specific Trends in Obesity in Brazil: 1975–2003. *Am. J. Public Health* **2007**, *97*, 1808–1812. [CrossRef] [PubMed]

36. Díaz, V.R. *Análisis Económico de la Ingesta de Alimentos en el Perú: Informe Final*; Instituto de Estudios Peruanos: Lima, Peru, 2010.

37. Attree, P. Low-income mothers, nutrition and health: A systematic review of qualitative evidence. *Matern. Child Nutr.* **2005**, *1*, 227–240. [CrossRef] [PubMed]

38. Committee on Preventing the Global Epidemic of Cardiovascular Disease: Meeting the Challenges in Developing Countries. *Promoting Cardiovascular Health in the Developing World: A Critical Challenge to Achieve Global Health*; National Academies Press: Washington, DC, USA, 2010; ISBN 978-0-309-14774-3.

39. Rothman, A.J.; Gollwitzer, P.M.; Grant, A.M.; Neal, D.T.; Sheeran, P.; Wood, W. Hale and Hearty Policies:How Psychological Science Can Create and Maintain Healthy Habits. *Perspect. Psychol. Sci.* **2015**, *10*, 701–705. [CrossRef] [PubMed]

40. Gupta, A.; Smithers, L.G.; Harford, J.; Merlin, T.; Braunack-Mayer, A. Determinants of knowledge and attitudes about sugar and the association of knowledge and attitudes with sugar intake among adults: A systematic review. *Appetite* **2018**, *126*, 185–194. [CrossRef] [PubMed]

41. Wardle, J.; Parmenter, K.; Waller, J. Nutrition knowledge and food intake. *Appetite* **2000**, *34*, 269–275. [CrossRef] [PubMed]

42. Rasmussen, M.; Krølner, R.; Klepp, K.-I.; Lytle, L.; Brug, J.; Bere, E.; Due, P. Determinants of fruit and vegetable consumption among children and adolescents: A review of the literature. Part I: Quantitative studies. *Int. J. Behav. Nutr. Phys. Act.* **2006**, *3*, 22. [CrossRef] [PubMed]

43. Sorokowska, A.; Pellegrino, R.; Butovskaya, M.; Marczak, M.; Niemczyk, A.; Huanca, T.; Sorokowski, P. Dietary customs and food availability shape the preferences for basic tastes: A cross-cultural study among Polish, Tsimane' and Hadza societies. *Appetite* **2017**, *116*, 291–296. [CrossRef] [PubMed]

44. Drewnowski, A. Taste Preferences and Food Intake. *Annu. Rev. Nutr.* **1997**, *17*, 237–253. [CrossRef] [PubMed]

45. Blanchette, L.; Brug, J. Determinants of fruit and vegetable consumption among 6–12-year-old children and effective interventions to increase consumption. *J. Hum. Nutr. Diet.* **2005**, *18*, 431–443. [CrossRef] [PubMed]

46. Haß, J.; Hartmann, M. What determines the fruit and vegetables intake of primary school children?—An analysis of personal and social determinants. *Appetite* **2018**, *120*, 82–91. [CrossRef] [PubMed]

47. AgainErick. Map Ayabaca Province. Available online: https://commons.wikimedia.org/w/index.php?curid=3229022 (accessed on 21 August 2018).

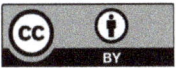

![nutrients logo] *nutrients*

MDPI

Review

The Role of Nutrients in Reducing the Risk for Noncommunicable Diseases during Aging

Maaike J. Bruins [1,*], Peter Van Dael [1] and Manfred Eggersdorfer [2]

[1] Nutrition Science & Advocacy, DSM Nutritional Products, CH-4303 Kaiseraugst, Switzerland; peter.van-dael@dsm.com

[2] University Medical Center Groningen, 9713 GZ Groningen, The Netherlands; m.l.eggersdorfer@rug.nl

* Correspondence: maaike.bruins@dsm.com; Tel.: +41-618-158-761

Received: 20 September 2018; Accepted: 27 December 2018; Published: 4 January 2019

Abstract: An increasing aging population worldwide accounts for a growing share of noncommunicable diseases (NCDs) of the overall social and economic burden. Dietary and nutritional approaches are of paramount importance in the management of NCDs. As a result, nutrition programs are increasingly integrated into public health policies. At present, programs aimed at reducing the burden of NCDs have focused mostly on the excess of unhealthy nutrient intakes whereas the importance of optimizing adequate essential and semi-essential nutrient intakes and nutrient-rich diets has received less attention. Surveys indicate that nutrient intakes of the aging population are insufficient to optimally support healthy aging. Vitamin and mineral deficiencies in older adults are related to increased risk of NCDs including fatigue, cardiovascular disease, and cognitive and neuromuscular function impairments. Reviewed literature demonstrates that improving intake for certain nutrients may be important in reducing progress of NCDs such as musculoskeletal disorders, dementia, loss of vision, and cardiometabolic diseases during aging. Current knowledge concerning improving individual nutrient intakes to reduce progression of chronic disease is still emerging with varying effect sizes and levels of evidence. Most pronounced benefits of nutrients were found in participants who had low nutrient intake or status at baseline or who had increased genetic and metabolic needs for that nutrient. Authorities should implement ways to optimize essential nutrient intake as an integral part of their strategies to address NCDs.

Keywords: chronic disease; noncommunicable disease; nutrient inadequacies and deficiencies; nutrient interventions; public health; musculoskeletal disorders; dementia; eye disorders; cardiovascular disease

---

1. Introduction

Globally, significant gains in human longevity have been made in the last couple of decades as evidenced by an average 5.5-year increase in life expectancy between 2000 and 2016 [1]. In many countries average life expectancy currently exceeds 80 years [1]. These longevity gains have come at a cost, however, with the most obvious being an increase in age-related diseases [2]. Noncommunicable diseases (NCDs) such as diabetes, musculoskeletal disorders, cardiovascular diseases, neurological disorders, and cancers increase with age, and place a burden on individuals and healthcare systems [3]. Supporting healthy aging by preventing NCDs is a major priority for agencies such as the World Health Organization (WHO) and United Nations [4,5].

The WHO estimates that NCDs contribute 1.6 billion disability-adjusted life-years (DALYs) to the global burden of disease and identified unhealthy diets and physical inactivity are among the main modifiable risk factors, together with excess alcohol and tobacco use [6]. Nutrition is an important determinant of human health by providing the essential building blocks for growth, development, and maintenance of a healthy status throughout life [7,8]. In this context, the co-existing burdens of undernutrition and overnutrition represent a paradigm shift for health authorities requiring appropriate dietary management recommendations [9]. Modern lifestyles and easy access to high-energy, low-nutrient rich foods are considered part of the problem [3,10–12]. For example, the economic costs of unhealthy diets and low physical activity in the EU were calculated to be €1.3 billion per year [13].

Currently, health authorities mainly target problems associated with obesity and cardiovascular diseases by focusing on reducing excess intake of calories, sugar, salt, and saturated fats. However, the importance of a positive message associated with promoting adequate nutrient intake as part of a balanced diet should not be overlooked [4]. There is considerable variation in the consumption of food items that need to be encouraged and food items which should be limited, both between and within different countries. This was reflected in a recent study in European countries showing suboptimal nutrient-density of diets and significant proportions of the population consuming excess amounts of salt, sugar and saturated fat, as well as significant proportions of the population not meeting the required or adequate intakes for various essential nutrients (Table 1) [12].

Table 1. Percentage of adults with nutrient intakes meeting the estimated average requirement (EAR) or adequate intake (AI) or exceeding the maximum reference value (MRV) [12].

% Meeting EAR or AI	EAR or AI	Denmark *n* = 2025 people	Czech Republic *n* = 1869 people	Italy *n* = 2831 people	France *n* = 2624 people
Protein, g/d	0.66 g/kg BW	84%	88%	99%	98%
MUFA, E%	10–20 E%	69%	92%	75%	77%
Dietary fiber, g/d	25	19%	4%	12%	9%
Calcium, mg/d	750	70%	31%	43%	62%
Iron, mg/d	M: 6; F: 7	92%	96%	98%	98%
Potassium, mg/d	3500	31%	4%	19%	18%
Magnesium, mg/d	M: 350; F: 300	46%	25%	20%	23%
Zinc, mg/d	M: 7.5; F: 6.2	90%	48%	97%	91%
Vitamin A, µg RE/d	M: 570; F490	77%	38%	66%	77%
Vitamin C, mg/d	M: 90; F: 80	50%	35%	62%	44%
Vitamin E, mg/d	M: 13; F: 11	5%	44%	47%	34%
Vitamin D, µg/d	15	3%	1%	1%	1%
Vitamin B$_1$, mg/d	0.6	97%	98%	47%	100%
Vitamin B$_2$, mg/d	M: 1.1; F: 0.9	80%	35%	84%	92%
Vitamin B$_{12}$, µg/d	4	55%	36%	52%	50%
Folate, µg DFE/d	250	59%	24%	77%	51%
% exceeding MRV	**MRV**				
SFA, E%	<10 E%	86%	80%	62%	91%
Added sugar, E%	<10 E%	32%	21%	24%	
Sodium, mg/d	<2400 mg/d	80%	98%	13%	85%

RE: retinol equivalents, DFE: dietary folate equivalents, E%: energy percentage, MUFA: mono-unsaturated fatty acids, SFA: saturated fatty acids. The red, orange, yellow, light green and dark green signals, respectively, represent ≤5%, 6–35%, 36–65%, 66–95%, and ≥96% of people meeting the EAR.

The health consequences of poor nutrition almost certainly accumulate over the lifespan of the individual. Table 2 presents information regarding some of the more frequently reported chronic clinical signs associated with certain vitamin and mineral deficiencies in older adults. Clinical signs and symptoms are mostly nonspecific and difficult to diagnose. During the aging process, a number of changes occur, such as increased medication use, reduced food intake due to lower food appeal, and compromised nutrient absorption. These complex changes prevent elderly persons from meeting their nutritional requirements. This consequently leads to increased risk of malnutrition, frailty, and reduced quality of life (QoL) [14–17].

Table 2. Critical nutrients in older adults [18].

Micronutrient	Challenges, Clinical Signs, and Symptoms in Older Adults
Vitamin B12 (cobalamin)	Deficiencies common in older adults, often underdiagnosed. Role in reducing elevated homocysteine, a cardiovascular risk factor. Absorption decreases mainly due to high prevalence of age-related atrophic gastritis. Among the common causes of anaemia in older adults, leading to weakness and fatigue. Low status increases the risk for cardiovascular disease and cognitive impairment.
Folate	Deficiencies common in older adults. Role in reducing elevated homocysteine, a cardiovascular risk factor. Closely related to vitamin B12 and B6. Among the common causes of anaemia in older adults, leading to weakness and fatigue. Deficiencies linked to depression and dementia.
Vitamin B6	Deficiencies common in older adults. Role in reducing elevated homocysteine, a cardiovascular risk factor. Closely related to vitamin B12 and folate.
Thiamine (vitamin B1)	Deficiencies common in older adults, often underdiagnosed. Risk factor for heart failure, peripheral neuropathy, and encephalopathy.
Calcium	Deficiencies common in senior women. Mean intake decreases with age, probably related to general change in diet. Associated with low bone mass, rapid bone loss, and high fracture rates.
Vitamin D	Older adults are less exposed to sun and have diminished ability of the skin to synthesize vitamin and the liver and kidney to hydrolyze vitamin D with age. Deficiency is a risk factor low bone mass, rapid bone loss, high fracture rates, and muscle weakness.
Vitamin C	Prevalence of inadequate intake is very high among adults. May help elderly maintain immune cells and function. Smoking increases need.
Iron	Women's iron requirements decrease after the menopause. Deficiencies are mainly seen among hospitalized, institutionalized, or chronically ill older adults. Among the common causes of anaemia in older adults, leading to weakness and fatigue.
Zinc	Deficiency is common in the elderly. Risk factor for immune deficiency and susceptibility to infection in the elderly.
Selenium	Deficiency deficiency may increase risk of diseases of aging such as cardiovascular disease, reduced immune response, and cognitive decline.
Magnesium	Often deficient in older adults. Maintains muscle integrity and function.

Health policies and interventions to improve dietary intake at the population level are essential to reverse the global trend towards unhealthy dietary patterns and physical inactivity. However, more individualized approaches may be needed to address persistent nutritional gaps and prevent future morbidity in high-risk groups such as the older population [19,20]. An estimated 5% to 10% of community-dwelling adults >70 years of age are undernourished; this proportion rises to 30% to 65% among institutionalized elderly patients. In the older adult population, nutrients of concern include, among others, calcium, vitamin D, and vitamin B_6 and B_{12} [15,20,21]. Vitamin D deficiency was found not only to be a problem in the elderly, but to be a global problem common across all age ranges [22]. Genetic variations play a role in dietary response and genetic variations also play a role in determining nutrient status and requirements [23]. By understanding the genome that affects the individual requirements for and response to nutrition, diseases of aging that have a nutritional component can be addressed in a targeted way.

In general, activities endorsing lifestyles that include healthy diets have usually focused on limiting the consumption of salt, sugar, and saturated fat. However, focus on the need to meet adequate dietary intake of essential nutrients through a healthy diet is considered equally important.

This review focuses on the role of nutrients in the risk reduction of NCDs in disorders prevalent in the aging population and for which the societal costs are substantial [24]. The evidence for a connection between NCDs and inadequate intake or status of specific nutrients such as vitamins, carotenoids, omega-3 fatty acids, and other bioactive substances is reviewed. Furthermore, the impact of interventions aimed at correcting these inadequacies will be discussed.

2. Musculoskeletal Health in the Older Adult

The gradual loss of bone mass and disruption of bone architecture associated with osteoporosis results in an increased risk of bone fractures, particularly of the hip, spine, and wrist. It is an age-related chronic, complex, multifactorial skeletal disorder which affects both men and women, particularly postmenopausal women [25]. Osteoporosis places a huge personal and economic burden on society. In Europe, for example, the disability caused by the disease is greater than that caused by cancers (with the exception of lung cancer) and is comparable or greater than that caused by a variety of chronic NCDs, such as rheumatoid arthritis, asthma and hypertension-related heart disease [26].

In a WHO report it was noted that the remaining lifetime risk of an osteoporotic fracture in women aged 50 years in developed countries was >40% (>20% for hip fracture) [27]. At the time of this report, osteoporotic fractures had the sixth highest disease burden in the Americas and Europe combined, as estimated by disability-adjusted life years [27,28]. In 27 countries in the European Union, based upon the overall epidemiology of 22 million women and 5.5 million men with osteoporosis, it was calculated that this would result in 3.5 million new bone fractures (hip, 610,000; vertebral, 520,000; forearm, 560,000; and others 1.8 million) [28]. The economic burden to manage these incident and prior bone fractures was calculated to be €37 billion.

In the elderly, both micronutrient and macronutrient deficiencies appear to contribute to the pathogenesis of skeletal fractures as a consequence of age-related bone loss and frailty [16]. Nutrients that play a role in bone metabolism include vitamin D and vitamin K, calcium, magnesium, phosphorus, proteins, and fatty acids.

2.1. Vitamin D in Musculoskeletal Health

Vitamin D is involved in bone homeostasis by enhancing calcium and phosphorus absorption from the intestine and maintaining adequate levels in blood. Low vitamin D levels have been mainly implicated in musculoskeletal disorders including bone and muscle health [29]. Serum levels of 25(OH)D have been associated with bone turnover markers levels [30].

Vitamin D comprises a group of secosteroids (calciferols), and in humans the two most important compounds in this group are vitamin D_3 (cholecalciferol) and vitamin D_2 (ergocalciferol) [22]. A major part of vitamin D comes from UV-B induced production in the skin and only about 20% from dietary intake. Dietary sources are limited to mainly oily fish and foods fortified with the vitamin [31]. Lack of vitamin D from the diet and increased awareness of the harmful skin effects of excessive sunlight exposure have contributed to low vitamin D status and even deficiency globally.

Serum 25-hydroxyvitamin D is the most widely used indicator for vitamin D status in clinical practice and, while 25–50 nmol/L is generally defined as insufficiency with regards to bone health, for optimal calcium absorption and control of secondary hyperparathyroidism a level closer to 75 nmol/L has been proposed [16,22,32,33]. Most researchers agree that 25-hydroxyvitamin D levels below 50 nmol/L are associated with lower bone mineral density [22]. Likewise, the effect of vitamin D deficiency on fracture risk is difficult to quantify, but large population studies found that hip fracture risk was higher in those with a 25-hydroxyvitamin D level below 50–62.5 nmol/L [34,35]. Based on a serum 25-hydroxyvitamin D level of <30 nmol/L it was reported that on average 13% of 55,844 European individuals had moderate or severe vitamin D deficiency, and this increased to 40% of individuals with mild to severe deficiency if a level of <50 nmol/L was included [36]. The authors noted that vitamin D deficiency was present across Europe and was both a clinical and public health concern requiring urgent action. Similar levels of vitamin D deficiency and concern have been reported by many research groups worldwide [22,36–38]. Figure 1 highlights the variable levels of vitamin D deficiency across Europe [39].

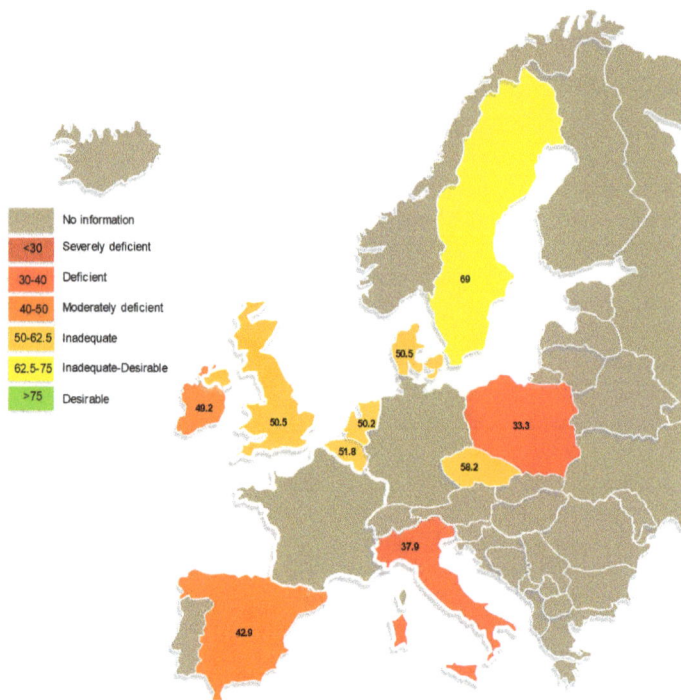

Figure 1. Europe map of vitamin D deficiency in older adults (mean 25(OH)D status (nmol/L) in adults aged ≥50 years) (based on: [39]).

The role of vitamin D and related analogues, with or without calcium, for preventing bone fractures in post-menopausal women and older men was the subject of a Cochrane review [25]. This systematic review included 53 trials and 91,791 older women or men aged over 65 years from community, hospital, and nursing-home settings, and assessed the impact of vitamin D for the prevention of hip or other types of fracture. In this analysis vitamin D alone did not appear to have a significant effect on fracture prevention, whereas vitamin D in combination with calcium significantly reduced the likelihood of hip fractures ($P = 0.01$), non-vertebral fractures and any type of fracture. Hip fracture incidence was particularly reduced in institutionalized residents with a risk reduction of 25%. In a separate systematic review (30 randomized controlled trials (RCTs) involving 5615 subjects of mean age 61 years), vitamin D supplementation was shown to produce a small but statistically significant improvement in global muscle strength. The most benefit was observed in individuals who presented with a 25-hydroxyvitamin D level below 30 nmol/L (compared with those with a level ≥30 nmol/L), and in subjects aged 65 years or older [29].

The economic value of vitamin D supplementation has been the subject of several health economic evaluations showing that increasing vitamin D status through supplementation or fortification can prevent fractures and improve QoL in older adults and associated health care costs [40–44].

2.2. Vitamin K in Musculoskeletal Health

Two forms of vitamin K exist: vitamin K_1 (phylloquinone, mainly found in green leafy vegetables) and vitamin K_2 (menaquinone, mainly found in fermented dairy and produced by lactic acid bacteria in the intestine). Vitamin K is required for promoting osteoblast differentiation, upregulating transcription of specific genes in osteoblasts, and activating bone-associated vitamin K dependent proteins, which play critical roles in extracellular bone matrix mineralization. Less is known about vitamin K and health, but there is growing evidence suggesting a synergistic effect between vitamins K and D in bone [40]. A number of studies reported that vitamin K is essential for optimization of bone health with benefits in preventing bone loss [41]. Vitamin K_2 supplementation combined with vitamin D and calcium for 2 years in a randomized placebo-controlled trial resulted in a significant increase in bone-mineral density and content in older women [42]. In another recent RCT it was found that combined vitamin K_2, vitamin D and calcium supplementation for 6 months increased the bone mineral density of lumbar 3 spine vertebra compared to vitamin D and calcium alone in postmenopausal Korean women [43].

Current research investigating the effect of vitamin D alone or in combination with other nutrients on fractures, cardiovascular disease, diabetes, cognitive function, immunity, and other benefits is ongoing in two large scale studies in older adults (DO-HEALTH in Europe, FIND in Finland). In addition, many research groups engage in basic science to study the combined action of vitamin K2, vitamin D, and calcium, and their function on the molecular level. More studies are required that target vitamin D supplementation in combination with other nutrients such as calcium and vitamin K where it is needed, in people with vitamin D deficiency or older people, who are more likely to be frail in institutionalized residents.

3. Cognitive Disorders

Dementia is a term that describes a decline in cognitive abilities including memory, and reduction in a person's ability to perform everyday activities [44]. Dementia prevalence is forecast to increase dramatically in future years [45]. At present about 50 million people have dementia worldwide, and this is projected to reach 80 million by 2030 and 150 million by 2050 [46]. Alzheimer's disease (AD) is the most common form of dementia in people aged >60 years, accounting for 60–70% of the total number of cases and is the major focus of this section [46]. Vascular dementia is the second most common cause of dementia with at least 20% of dementia cases.

Alzheimer's disease is a complex, progressive, multifactorial, neurodegenerative disease [24,45]. The presentation generally involves progressive memory loss, impaired thinking, disorientation, and changes in personality and mood. As the disease advances there is a marked reduction in cognitive and physical functioning [47,48]. Genetic factors account for about 70% of the risk contributing to AD, while modifiable factors related to general health and lifestyle may also be involved [48]. Risk factors for vascular dementia are predominantly modifiable and of vascular origin (including hypertension, diabetes mellitus, dyslipidemia, and the metabolic syndrome). Managing non-genetic risk factors effectively may provide opportunity to prevent and treat the progressive cognitive decline associated with AD [47]. The focus of this section of the review is on nutritional status and its potential role in AD.

The Role of Nutrition in Dementia

In terms of a link between nutrient status in older adults and cognition, evidence exists for B-vitamins, and vitamin C, D, and E, as well as the omega-3 long chain polyunsaturated fatty acids (LCPUFAs) docosahexaenoic acid (DHA) and eicosapentaenoic acid (EPA), as reviewed by Antal et al. [48] and summarized here (unless otherwise noted).

Folic acid and vitamin B_6 and B_{12} are important in the nervous system at all ages, but particularly in elderly people, deficiency contributes to aging brain processes [49]. Low status of folic acid and vitamins B_6 and B_{12} are among the risk factors for elevated homocysteine. With respect to dementia, there is reasonable evidence linking lower levels of folic acid, vitamin B_6, vitamin B_{12}, and higher concentrations of homocysteine with age-related cognitive decline [50]. One of the mechanisms involved may the impaired methylation processes due to folic acid and vitamin B_{12} deficiency that lead to accumulation of homocysteine affecting mood and some cognitive functions [50]. In several RCTs supplementation with folic acid, vitamin B_{12}, and vitamin B_6 for at least 2 years has been investigated [44]. However, the findings of a recent meta-analysis reported that B vitamins had

Nutrients **2019**, *11*, 85

little to no effect with respect to preventing cognitive decline [51]. Notably, individuals with high homocysteine levels had significant cognitive decline and B-vitamins were found to improve memory only in this subgroup [52]. Also, evidence exists that in elderly subjects with an increased risk of dementia, B-vitamins can slow brain shrinkage over two years by up to 30% [53]. At present, the evidence is insufficiently compelling to support B-vitamin supplementation to prevent cognitive decline and dementia.

Dehydroascorbic acid, a metabolite of vitamin C, is a potent antioxidant, an essential cofactor in many enzymatic reactions, and has a role in metabolizing cholesterol. Large dietary surveys undertaken in Germany, the Netherlands, the UK, and the US indicated inadequate vitamin C intake in up to half of respective populations [54]. As with vitamin E, however, studies of vitamin C in patients with AD have been equivocal. The overall conclusion of the Team of Alzheimer Drug Discovery Foundation is that maintaining adequate levels of vitamin C through diet may offer more benefit than supplementation.

The metabolically active form of vitamin D, 1,25-dihydroxy vitamin D, binds to vitamin D receptors that are present in brain regions involved in cognition. Proposed mechanisms for the protective effects of vitamin D against cognitive decline include clearing Aβ peptide, regulating intraneuronal calcium, anti-inflammatory activity, antioxidative activity, preventing and reducing ischemia, and regulating choline acetyltransferase neurotrophic agents. There is strong evidence that patients with AD have lower vitamin D status than healthy controls and that lower vitamin D status is associated with increased risk of developing dementia. Although vitamin D supplementation alone was insufficient to improve cognition in a study of patients with newly diagnosed AD, the Vitamin D Council recommends that middle-aged and older adults maintain vitamin D blood levels in the higher range of normal (175–200 nmol/L; 70–80 ng/mL).

Vitamin E possesses antioxidant properties which may prevent hyperphosphorylated tau protein dysfunction and has been shown to reduce the rate of Aβ protein-induced death in cultures of hippocampal and cortical cells [55]. The γ-tocopherol isomer is particularly effective in scavenging free radicals that cause inflammation [55]. By scavenging Aβ protein-associated free radicals, vitamin E may have a neuroprotective effect during oxidative stress. However, while promising in principle, studies of α-tocopherol supplementation in patients with AD have not been convincing and dietary vitamin E may provide greater protection against age-related neurodegenerative conditions.

Brain membranes are composed mainly of phospholipids, predominantly the LCPUFAs DHA and arachidonic acid (ARA). DHA has multiple actions in maintaining neurological function. Lower plasma DHA has been associated with cognitive decline in both healthy elderly people and AD patients [56]. Investigations to date of the therapeutic potential of supplementation or higher dietary intake of DHA in patients with AD have produced conflicting results, although it is possible that cognitive impairment in the study populations was already resistant to intervention. Given the essential role of DHA in the human brain, a general recommendation to maintain an adequate dietary intake of DHA throughout adulthood appears to be a reasonable approach to prevent cognitive decline.

Due to a high concentration of oxygen free radicals relative to antioxidative defenses in the brain, it may be especially vulnerable to oxidative stress and consequent damage to lipids and proteins [57]. AD is also associated with lower levels of acetylcholine in the hippocampal and cortical regions, resulting in memory impairment. Fruits, vegetables, coffee, and cereal grains contain high levels of polyphenols. In vitro and animal studies of specific dietary flavonoids and plant extracts have shown reduction of oxidative stress and inhibition of acetylcholinesterase, suggesting a dual protective role for polyphenols against cognitive decline and dementia [57]. Although no conclusions can be drawn about the relative benefits of any particular plant polyphenol over another, the findings emphasize the importance of life-long consumption of foods with high content of these antioxidants.

Trials that have reported no effect of nutrients generally included older adults who were unlikely to have a marked decline in cognitive function [52]. Trial design should consider including older individuals with deficiencies that increases their risk of cognitive decline, and who may benefit from nutrition intervention. Sensitive assessment tools and surrogate markers are needed that examine specific aspects of brain structure and function such as neuroimaging techniques to advance the understanding of nutrition interventions that could reduce the risk of dementia.

4. Eye Disorders

Impairments of the essential senses of vision and hearing are the second-leading cause of years of lived with disability [58]. The most common causes of vision loss among the elderly are age-related macular degeneration, glaucoma, cataracts, and diabetic retinopathy [59]. Aging is the greatest risk factor associated with the development of age-related macular degeneration, but also environmental and lifestyle factors such as smoking, oxidative stress, and diet may significantly affect the risk [60]. Recent studies suggest that increasing exposure to blue light emitted by electronics and energy-efficient lightbulbs over time could lead to damaged retinal cells which on the long-term can cause vision problems like age-related macular degeneration [61]. Eye health problems in the ever-increasing aging generation, and "exposure to blue light" may result in a new NCD.

Carotenoids have a range of functions in human health and, in particular, there is evidence that they have beneficial effects on eye health [62]. Two dietary carotenoids, lutein and zeaxanthin are macular pigments found in the human retina [63]. Macular pigment has local antioxidant properties and absorbs high energy, short wavelength blue light protecting the retina from photochemical damage [64]. Macular pigment can neutralize ROS, protect against UV-induced peroxidation, and reduce the formation of lipofuscin and associated oxidative-stress induced damage [63]. Thus, the carotenoids provide potential benefits for ocular function and health.

Individuals who have low macular pigment optical density levels (0.2 or lower) may benefit from supplementation with lutein/zeaxanthin which can help increase macular pigment optical density levels [65–72]. For retinal protection, macular pigment optical density values of 0.4 to 0.6 are desirable, especially in older adults [73]. Dietary intake of lutein and zeaxanthin may differ with age, sex, and ethnicity. Across all age groups the intake of lutein is higher than for zeaxanthin and this is independent of sex and ethnicity. In addition, lower zeaxanthin to lutein ratios are reported for groups at risk of age-related macular degeneration (e.g., the elderly and females) [74]. A number of studies, including some in healthy subjects, have demonstrated that lutein/zeaxanthin supplementation can improve visual performance, including contrast sensitivity, glare tolerance and photo stress recovery [65–72,75,76].

Age-related macular degeneration is an increasing problem among the elderly and studies of the effects of lutein/zeaxanthin supplementation have produced mixed results. However, important data were provided by secondary analyses of the large Age-Related Eye Disease Study 2 (AREDS2) [77,78]. This randomized trial investigated the effect of adding lutein/zeaxanthin 10/2 mg, DHA (350 mg) + EPA (650 mg), or both to the original AREDS2 formulation (vitamin C, vitamin E, β-carotene, zinc, and copper) or to variations of this formulation (excluding β-carotene and/or with reduced zinc). Participants ($n = 4203$) were followed for a median 5 years. The primary analysis found no additional beneficial or harmful effect for lutein/zeaxanthin and/or omega-3 fatty acids on progression to late age-related macular degeneration compared with the original AREDS1 formula using β-carotene instead of lutein/zeaxanthin. However, a prespecified secondary analysis found a significant 26% risk reduction for progression to advanced age-related macular degeneration when comparing lutein/zeaxanthin supplementation with no lutein/zeaxanthin supplementation in the quintile with the lowest dietary intake of these two carotenoids (median 0.7 mg/day), as indicated by a hazard ratio of 0.74 (95% confidence interval 0.59–0.94, $p = 0.01$). In addition, a post hoc analysis showed that lutein/zeaxanthin (excluding β-carotene) was more effective than the original AREDS formulation containing β-carotene but no lutein/zeaxanthin for reducing progression to advanced age-related macular degeneration (hazard ratio 0.82, 95% CI 0.69–0.96, $p = 0.02$) [77].

There is also some evidence suggesting there is a relationship between lutein/zeaxanthin status and the risk of developing nuclear cataracts [79], and in the AREDS2 trial the addition of lutein/zeaxanthin supplementation reduced the risk of cataract surgery in the quintile with the lowest dietary intake of these carotenoids (hazard ratio 0.68, 95% CI 0.48–0.96, $p = 0.03$) [80].

If the AREDS2 complex (i.e., vitamin C and E, zinc, copper, lutein/zeaxanthin and omega-3 fatty acids) was used by all adults aged >55 years, it has been estimated this would result in an average of about 1 million avoided age-related macular degeneration and cataract events per year in the USA (based on a risk reduction of 23.6% for age-related macular degeneration and 16.2% for cataracts). This would result in a net annual cost saving of US$1.2 billion, mostly as a consequence of reduced healthcare expenditure [81]. Establishing intake recommendations for lutein is an important step forward to support optimal visual performance and reduce the risk of age-related macular eye disease in the general population. This would be a relevant contribution to public health in the face of a globally aging population.

Future studies may include additional assessments of the relationship between macular pigment and different genotypic and phenotypic forms of age-related macular degeneration, the optimum dosages of lutein, zeaxanthin, and the possible effects when combined with other nutrients.

5. Cardiovascular Disease

Despite the global decline in cardiovascular mortality, cardiovascular diseases remain the leading cause of morbidity and mortality, contributing to escalating health care cost [82]. Cardiovascular aging progresses over decades, influenced by risk factors such as tobacco use, poor physical activity and diet, resulting in hypertension, dyslipidemia (high triglycerides and lower HDL), elevated fasting blood glucose, and central obesity [83]. Cardiovascular disease is the major clinical problem in the older population, with 68% of adults 60–79 years having cardiovascular disease and this increases to 85% after the age of 80 years [84].

Good nutrition plays an important role in delaying the progression of cardiovascular disease [85,86]. The adverse effects of excess intakes of saturated and trans fats, cholesterol, added sugars, and salt in relation to cardiovascular disease progression has been relatively well-established whereas the effect of addressing inadequate essential nutrients is less well-known. Older adults are highly susceptible to undernutrition due to the various physiological and socioeconomic factors [87]. In contrast to overnutrition, the potential of addressing undernutrition to optimize cardiovascular health in older adults has received inadequate attention [88]. Evidence for nutrition in reducing the risk for cardiovascular aging mostly derives from epidemiological studies, whereas fewer interventions studies have been performed. The RCTs addressing cardiovascular disease generally have included, but not exclusively, older adults, not allowing generalizability of results to typical older adults. The authors have therefore focused on nutrition interventions addressing cardiovascular aging progress, not restricted to elderly.

5.1. Cardiovascular Events

5.1.1. Diets

Lifestyle changes, including dietary modifications, are recommended as part of the management strategy to improve lipid profiles and reduce the risk of cardiovascular disease [89–91]. The primary emphasis of dietary interventions has been on changing dietary macronutrient and salt composition. The effect of improving micronutrient-richness of the diet in cardiovascular disease control has been less-well studied. A diet rich in fruits, vegetables, wholegrains, legumes, nuts, fish, poultry, and low-fat dairy products, and limited consumption of red meat, saturated fat, and added sugar is advocated, mostly based on positive associations with cardiovascular health [89–91]. Dietary patterns that follow these principles include the Dietary Approaches to Stop Hypertension (DASH) diet, a diet rich in fiber, protein, magnesium, calcium, and potassium, and low in total and saturated fats, which has been shown to reduce low-density lipoprotein (LDL)-cholesterol levels [91], and the Mediterranean diet, which has been shown to reduce the risk for cardiovascular disease in both primary and secondary settings [92,93]. Regression of coronary artery atherosclerosis has been demonstrated with a program of intensive lifestyle changes that included a vegetarian diet, exercise, and smoking cessation [94]. In addition to dietary interventions, there has been research into the effects of individual nutrients. While the evidence for some of these is limited, several interesting findings have been published.

5.1.2. Vitamin D

Low vitamin D has been associated with cardiovascular disease in a number of studies [95]. Few studies have been targeting low vitamin D specifically in the older population. In one study with post-menopausal women randomized to Vitamin D3 2500 IU or placebo, daily for 4 months, vitamin D supplementation had no effect on endothelial function, arterial stiffness, or inflammation [96]. Results of a meta-analysis of RCT with older adult participants ($\geq$60 years) suggested that vitamin D supplementation might protect against cardiac failure but not against MI or stroke [97]. The recent results of the VITAL trial indicate that daily supplementation of 2000 IU vitamin D did not reduce the occurrence of cardiovascular events in adults aged $\geq$50 years [98].

5.1.3. B-Vitamins

B-vitamins have been the subject of substantial research because of their established effects on normalizing homocysteine levels, an important risk factor for cardiovascular disease. Figure 2 shows the risk factors including B-vitamin shortages and pathogenetic mechanisms for the effect of high homocysteine on cardiovascular disease.

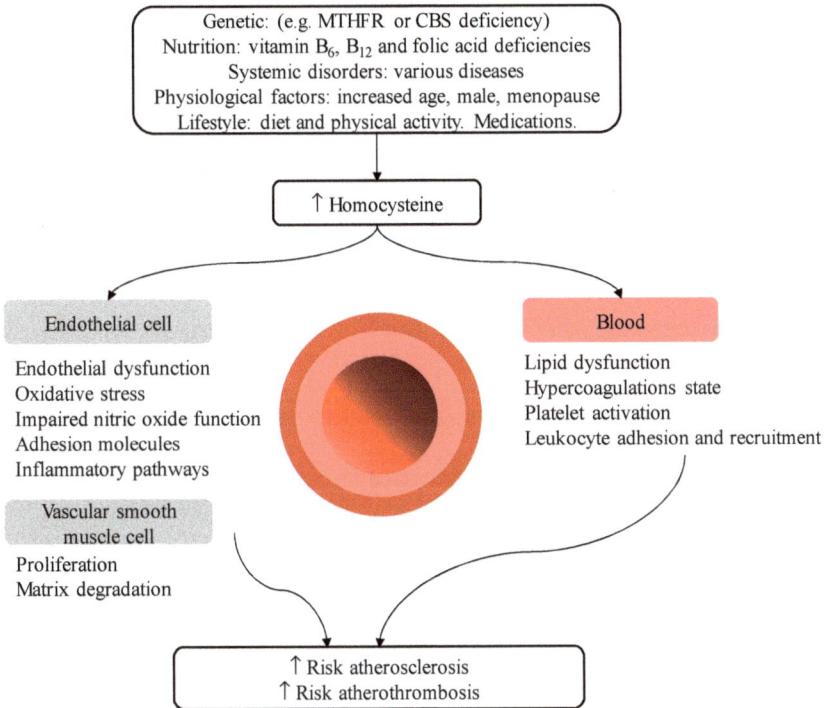

Figure 2. Risk factors and mechanisms for high homocysteine in cardiovascular disease. MTHFR: methylenetetrahydrofolate reductase, CBS: cystathionine beta-synthase.

Particularly the B-vitamins have been investigated for their potential cardiovascular benefits due to their established lowering effect on homocysteine levels, a marker for cardiovascular disease risk, including ischemic stroke. A meta-analysis of 19 RCTs of B vitamins (including folic acid, vitamin B6, vitamin B12, and B-complex vitamins) found significant reductions in homocysteine levels, however, no significant effect of vitamin B supplementation on rates of cardiovascular disease, coronary heart disease, myocardial infarction, cardiovascular death, or all-cause mortality whereas vitamin B reduced the risk of stroke by 12% [99]. Another meta-analysis of 26 RCTs found that folic acid supplementation significantly reduced the risk of stroke 7% [100].

There are various reasons for elevated blood homocysteine levels; most people have mild to moderately elevated serum homocysteine levels due to inadequate intake of folate, vitamin B_6, or vitamin B_{12} from the diet, which is reversible when intake of these vitamins is increased. Another cause are genetic variants of methylenetetrahydrofolate reductase (MTHFR) and methionine synthase reductase (MTRR) that are associated with elevated homocysteine levels. Elevated homocysteine levels are a risk factor for developing blood clots in the vasculature and have been implicated in the pathogenesis of atherosclerosis and deep vein thrombosis [101]. Given that vitamin B supplementation is associated with normalization of elevated plasma homocysteine levels, many studies have investigated whether these vitamins may decrease the risk of cardiovascular diseases. Huang and colleagues undertook a meta-analysis (19 RCTs and 47,921 participants) evaluating the effects of B vitamin supplementation (search terms: folic acid, folate, vitamin B_6, vitamin B_{12}, and B vitamins) on plasma homocysteine levels and cardiovascular and all-cause mortality [99]. The overall relative risk of a clinical outcome, versus placebo, was 0.98 for cardiovascular disease, 0.98 for CHD, 0.97 for MI, 0.97 for cardiovascular death and 0.88 for stroke; and homocysteine levels were decreased in all RCTs. Thus, B vitamin supplementation had a significant protective effect for stroke, but not for any other cardiovascular risk. A more recent meta-analysis of folic acid supplementation (30 RCTs, 82,334 participants) estimated a 10% lower risk of stroke and a 4% lower risk of overall cardiovascular disease compared with controls [102]. The greatest benefit for cardiovascular disease was observed in individuals with lower plasma folate levels at baseline and without pre-existing cardiovascular disease ($p = 0.006$ for both). While patients with a cardiovascular disease history responded to B-vitamins with normalization of homocysteine levels, those with the MTHFR 677C > T genotype were less responsive and may have greater folate requirements than do their counterparts [103].

5.1.4. Vitamin K

Vitamin K plays an important role in anticoagulation and may overcome the detrimental side effects associated with vitamin K antagonists such as warfarin. Vitamin K may also help to prevent vascular calcifications, especially in patients on warfarin [104].

5.1.5. Omega-3 LCPUFA

Supplementation of omega-3 LCPUFA increased high-density lipoprotein (HDL) cholesterol concentration, improved vascular function, and lowered heart rate and blood pressure with DHA having a greater effect than EPA while both EPA and DHA inhibited platelet activity [105]. Dietary supplementation with omega-3 LCPUFAs can reduce plasma triglyceride levels by up to 45% [106,107], with the greatest effect seen in those with the highest baseline levels [106]. Omega-3 LCPUFAs also cause a modest increase in HDL-C levels, and although they also increase LDL-C levels, this is primarily an increase in large, less atherogenic, particles [106]. In addition to improving lipid profiles, omega-3 LCPUFAs reduce inflammation, lower blood pressure (blood pressure), and have beneficial effects on endothelial function and platelet aggregation, all of which could contribute to cardioprotective effects [106]. However, despite positive effects on intermediate markers, RCTs with omega-3 LCPUFAs have produced mixed results on cardiovascular morbidity and mortality [108,109]. It must be noted that these meta-analyses included both primary and secondary prevention studies, before and after occurrence of events, respectively. One recent meta-analysis of RCTs performed reported a significant reduction in cardiovascular risk only among higher risk populations, such as those with elevated triglyceride levels (relative risk: 0.84, 95% CI 0.72–0.98) or elevated LDL-cholesterol levels (relative risk 0.86, 95% CI 0.76–0.98) [108]. Another recent Cochrane meta-analysis of RCTs found that omega3 LCPUFAs reduced cardiovascular events in the main analysis (relative risk: 0.93, 95% CI 0.88–0.97), but the result was not maintained in sensitivity analyses [109]. The failure of some trials to show effects of omega-3 LCPUFA on cardiovascular disease was explained by an insufficiently high omega-3 LCPUFA dose and/or too high omega-3 LCPUFA baseline status to demonstrate effects [110]. RCTs evaluating the effects of omega-3 LCPUFAs on cardiovascular morbidity and mortality generally enrolled a broad range of ages while only few RCTs have focused specifically on older adults. The Alpha Omega Trial that included 60–80-year-olds with previous MI and at least 50% on medication found no significant effect of approximately 400 mg of omega-3 LCPUFA on cardiovascular events [111]. In the AREDS2 study, 1 g omega-3 LCPUFA given in addition to a standard Vitamin C, Vitamin E, beta-carotene, zinc oxide, and cupric oxide supplement for 6 months to participants between 50 and 85 years had no effect on cardiovascular outcomes [112]. The recent results of the VITAL trial showed that in adults aged ≥50 y daily consuming 840 mg of omega-3 LCPUFA lowered the risk of heart attack by 28%, of fatal heart attack by 50% without significant effect on stroke or cardiovascular deaths [98]. The most pronounced benefits on major cardiovascular event reduction were found in participants who reported low fish intake at baseline. A recent meta-analysis of RCTs found that omega-3 LCPUFA supplementation caused a small, but significant, reduction in heart rate (−2.23 bpm, 95% CI −3.07 to −1.40) [113], which is considered a risk factor for cardiovascular morbidity and mortality [114].

5.1.6. Antioxidants

Inflammation and oxidative stress appear to be key drivers for a number of cardiovascular diseases and the metabolic syndrome [115,116]. Whereas observations studies suggest that antioxidant nutrient such as β-carotene and vitamin E are associated with lower cardiovascular disease, the data of RCTs on antioxidant supplements failed to confirm a significant benefit of antioxidants on atherosclerotic cardiovascular disease. For instance, supplementation with the antioxidant nutrients vitamin E, β-carotene, and vitamin C, had no significant effects on cardiovascular outcomes [117].

5.1.7. Vitamin E

A key attribute of vitamin E (a combination of 8 distinct tocopherol/tocotrienol isoforms) is its antioxidant activity and, as a consequence, its ability to protect poly-unsaturated fatty acids (PUFAs), lipoproteins, and cell membranes from oxidative damage [118]. Vitamin E has been extensively investigated for its potential to prevent cardiovascular disease events. Nevertheless, RCTs with vitamin E had mixed results on various cardiovascular disease endpoints. In the Women's Health Study, intake of 600 IU of vitamin E on alternate days in apparently healthy women non-significantly reduced the risk for cardiovascular events by 7% and significantly reduced the risk for cardiovascular death by 24% [119]. And among women ages 65 and older, vitamin E supplementation reduced the risk of major cardiac events by 26% [119]. Data from the same Women's Health Study suggested that supplementation with vitamin E may reduce the risk of venous thromboembolism in women, particularly in those with a prior history or genetic predisposition [120]. RCTs that retrospectively analyzed the data for the effect of vitamin in E in subgroups of patients with this these genotypes sometimes showed that these patients are more responsive to vitamin E supplementation [121,122].

5.1.8. Phenolics

Phenolic compounds are bioactive compounds found in plants, and there is evidence that some may be helpful for reducing cardiovascular risk factors [116]. Flavonoids are polyphenolic compounds found in fruits, vegetables, tea, and red wine [116]. Amongst the flavonoids, there is some evidence that flavonols (specifically quercetin) may be effective at reducing blood pressure in hypertensive patients; however, no effects on other cardiovascular disease risk markers such as endothelin, oxidative stress, or lipid profiles were found [116]. Although an early meta-analysis found that consumption of flavonols was associated with a lower rate of cardiovascular disease [123], a more recent meta-analysis and a systematic review do not support such an effect [116,124]. Amongst other phenolic compounds which might have beneficial cardiovascular effects, resveratrol is a stilbene found in grape skin, red wine, and peanuts [116]. A systematic review found that resveratrol was associated with reductions in total cholesterol, LDL-C, triglycerides and apolipoprotein B in a range of patients, including those with ischemic heart disease [116]. Resveratrol also reduced inflammatory and fibrinolytic biomarkers in patients with ischemic heart disease [116].

Nutrients have been investigated for their effect on cardiovascular disease progress and as such, outcomes. B-Vitamins reduced homocysteine levels, a risk factor of cardiovascular disease, without significant effects on cardiovascular disease events except for the reduced risk for stroke, which was also reduced by folic acid supplementation. Flavonoids and omega-3 LCPUFA also reduce cardiovascular disease risk factors although evidence on cardiovascular outcomes is mixed. Possible explanations include that patients enrolled in the RCTs were already at high risk of cardiovascular disease and on concomitant medications, with little opportunity for nutrition to reverse the progress. Individual nutrients like vitamin D, vitamin E and omega-3 LCPUFA on cardiovascular disease prevention have shown mixed effects. Nutrition interventions have focused mostly on primary prevention of cardiovascular aging in broad age groups and less on older adults. Recruited participants in the RCTs were often at high risk of cardiovascular risk factors or preexisting disease, a modest effect of in patients that already have heart disease or are at high risk of heart disease may be masked by effects of medication.

5.2. Hypertension

Hypertension is a major public health concern given its link to serious cardiovascular events such as stroke and ischemic heart disease, the leading causes of worldwide mortality [6]. It has been estimated that hypertension is responsible for approximately 40% of cardiovascular deaths. By the year 2025 almost 30% of the global population will be diagnosed with high blood pressure, with 25% of these cases occurring in developing countries [125]. Hypertension rises dramatically with aging due to longer exposure to age-associated alterations in vascular function and structure and cardiovascular risk factors [126].

Hypertension is a multifactorial disease with lifestyle factors such as physical activity, smoking and drinking habits, diet, bodyweight, and anxiety playing a predominant role. Management of these is the first step to achieving adequate blood pressure control. Indeed, it has been reported that two lifestyle modifications can help improve blood pressure control and decrease the number of cardiovascular outcomes [127].

5.2.1. Diets

In the current healthcare environment, lifestyle changes involving a healthy diet and increased physical activity are considered pivotal in the management of hypertension. Diets with a high nutritional value, such as the traditional Mediterranean diet, DASH and the OmniHeart (a variation of DASH with increased levels of protein) diets, can be important steps on the path to weight loss, lowering blood pressure, and prevention of hypertension [125]. The benefits of the DASH diet on blood pressure were reported in a RCT with all participants receiving graded amounts of sodium (high, intermediate, low). There were dose-response decreases in systolic and diastolic blood pressures, and age-related increases in blood pressure were blunted [128]. Both the DASH diet and low sodium markedly decreased blood pressure, and the combined effect was even greater. Findings of the DASH study also provided additional support that the sodium-to-potassium ratio is stronger associated with blood pressure outcomes than either nutrient alone among prehypertensive and hypertensive adults combined. These findings were later confirmed by a systematic review showing that the sodium-to-potassium ratio appears to be more strongly associated with blood pressure outcomes than either nutrient alone in hypertensive adults [129].

In addition to dietary control there has been research into the effects of other nutrients, including vitamins, on blood pressure and hypertension. While the evidence for some of these is limited a number of interesting findings have been published.

5.2.2. Milk peptides

A meta-analysis of 14 RCTs involving 1306 European subjects found that the milk-derived lactotripeptides isoleucine-proline-proline and valine-proline-proline produced small and statistically significant reductions in mean systolic blood pressure and diastolic blood pressure [130]. The authors noted that a similar effect had been seen in Asian populations.

5.2.3. Omega-3 LCPUFAs

The omega-3 LCPUFAs EPA and DHA found in oily fish and fish oils (including capsule preparations) have been associated with lower blood pressure levels. In a meta-analysis of 70 RCTs, EPA, and DHA reduced mean systolic blood pressure and mean diastolic blood pressure compared with placebo. The largest effect was in untreated hypertensive patients [131]. Likewise, in an earlier meta-analysis (36 trials), intake of fish oil (median dose 3.7 g/d) reduced both mean systolic and diastolic blood pressure. The antihypertensive effects of doses <0.5 g/d remains to be established [132].

5.2.4. Vitamin C

In short-term studies, vitamin C supplementation reduced systolic and diastolic blood pressure. Long-term trials on the effects of vitamin C supplementation on BP and clinical events are needed longer-term trials assessing the effects of vitamin C supplementation on blood pressure and clinical events in patients with hypertension would seem to be worthwhile [133]

5.2.5. Vitamin D

In a study involving 283 hypertensive patients, vitamin D3 (cholecalciferol) produced a modest but statistically significant reduction in systolic blood pressure compared with placebo after 3 months [134]. There was no significant effect on diastolic blood pressure.

5.2.6. Flavonols

Flavanols have also been found to lower blood pressure, and there is some evidence suggesting that they improve endothelial function in patients with ischemic heart disease, but additional studies are needed [116].

The evidence for nutrients and blood pressure is convincing for lowering sodium and sodium-to-potassium ratio. Flavanols vitamin C and D may have modest significant effects on blood pressure lowering.

5.3. Diabetes

Type 2 diabetes has become a global health-related pandemic which is forecast to rise from 425 to almost 630 million by 2045 [135]. In developing countries, the forecasted increase is more alarming, particularly in regions which are more rapidly adopting a Western lifestyle. The direct financial burden on healthcare systems and society is huge, as are the indirect costs from loss of work attendance. Intensive lifestyle modification, e.g., personalized nutrition and physical activity programs, with the goal of improving glycaemia and losing excess body weight should be the mainstay of initial management in individuals with prediabetes [136].

5.3.1. Vitamin D

Observational studies have highlighted a link between vitamin D deficiency and type 2 diabetes, as well as possible future cardiovascular events, whereas results from interventional studies have not been so conclusive [137]. A recent meta-analysis [137] including a total of 20 RCTs and 2703 participants, found that vitamin D supplementation was associated with elevated serum vitamin D levels and significantly decreased insulin resistance. Changes in other parameters such as fasting blood glucose and hemoglobin A1c (HbA1c) were relatively small and did not achieve statistical significance [137]. In a pilot study in 60 patients with co-existing type 2 diabetes and hypovitaminosis D, vitamin D improved vitamin D status and several parameters associated with glycemic control such as HbA1c, mean fasting plasma glucose, and mean post-prandial plasma glucose [138]. In addition, vitamin D in the study lowered LDL cholesterol levels, systolic blood pressure and diastolic blood pressure.

5.3.2. Vitamin E

Diabetes patients with the haptoglobin 2-2 genotype have elevated risk of cardiovascular disease events. The haptoglobin 2-2 genotype has inferior antioxidant properties as compared with other haptoglobin types resulting in elevated levels of oxidative stress, an atherogenic profile and an increased risk of cardiovascular disease events compared with other Hp genotypes [139]. The RCTs in diabetes patients that retrospectively analyzed the data for the effect of vitamin in E found that administration of vitamin E lowered the risk of cardiovascular disease events by 34% and cardiovascular-related mortality by 53% among patients with the haptoglobin 2-2 genotype [140].

5.3.3. Omega-3 LCPUFA

Cohort studies have shown that in countries where fish consumption is high the prevalence of type 2 diabetes tends to be lower and this has been attributed to the presence of omega-3 LCPUFAs [141]. However, the findings have not been conclusive with respect to providing dietary guidance and a recent systematic meta-analysis sought to provide more definitive evidence by analyzing different dosage/compositions of omega-3 LCPUFA supplementation [141]. In total, 20 RCTs recruited 1209 patients with type 2 diabetes. Overall, omega-3 LCPUFA supplementation resulted in a reduction in triglycerides with the best response with high doses for a longer duration; however, no significant changes in total cholesterol, fasting plasma glucose, post-prandial plasma glucose, HbA1c, insulin, or body mass was noted with this regimen. Interestingly, products with a relatively high ratio of EPA to DHA exhibited an increasing tendency to decrease HbA1c, insulin, total cholesterol, total triglycerides, and body mass. These findings will be helpful for clinicians and nutritionists who manage patients with diabetes to provide dietary guidance [141].

5.3.4. Vitamin K

To assess whether vitamin K is a risk factor for the development of type 2 diabetes mellitus, Beulens and colleagues analyzed a cohort of 38,094 Dutch men and women over a 10-year period [142]. The study showed that both vitamin K_1 and vitamin K_2 intake were associated with a reduced risk of type 2 diabetes mellitus. For vitamin K_1 the risk reduction occurred at the higher levels of intake, whereas for vitamin K_2 a linear inverse association was established. In older men with diabetes receiving vitamin K_1 supplementation for 36 months, vitamin K_1 significantly improved insulin sensitivity [143].

5.3.5. Chromium

Chromium plays a role in insulin metabolism by activating oligopeptide low-molecular-weight chromium (LMWCr)-binding substance and activating insulin-dependent kinase activity. A meta-analysis of the efficacy of chromium supplementation suggest that there is available evidence for chromium on glycemic control in patients with diabetes [144].

Studies in diabetes patients showed that vitamin D supplementation can improve serum vitamin D levels and significantly decrease insulin resistance. Currently, a large multicenter RCT is ongoing in the US (Vitamin D and Type 2 Diabetes Study; D2d), hypothesizing that vitamin D will enhance insulin production, glucose processing and glycemic profiles. Subgroup analyses show that vitamin E may be promising in reducing the rate of cardiovascular events among diabetes patients with haptoglobin 2-2 genotype who are at increased risk of cardiovascular events. The evidence for omega3 LCPUFA supplementation on fasting plasma glucose or HbA1C is less conclusive but omega-3 LCPUFA have promising effects for reduction of triglycerides. The evidence for chromium in glycemic control is emerging.

6. Conclusions

Inadequate or even deficient nutrient intake and status is still widely prevalent at global level and, although generally underacknowledged, is a main risk factor for NCDs [20]. Nutrient surveys indicate that the aging population is at particular risk for poor nutrient intake and status, which may result in increased risk for chronic fatigue, and cardiovascular, cognitive, and neuromuscular disorders in older adults. The present paper reviews the evidence for the role of various nutrients in modifying the risk of development of NCDs throughout aging.

Inadequate vitamin D, calcium and vitamin K intake and status are generally reported in the aging population and have been associated with musculoskeletal disorders, such as increased bone fracture risks. Increased vitamin D in combination with increased calcium and possibly also vitamin K may reduce the risk for hip fractures, thus beneficially impacting musculoskeletal health.

Inadequate B vitamins intake and status, in particular folic acid, vitamins B_6 and B_{12}, have been associated with age-related cognitive decline, while supplementation has been reported to improve cognitive performance. Similarly, evidence has been reported for vitamin C, D, and E, as well as omega-3 LCPUFAs (e.g., DHA) to slow down dementia progression.

Increased intake of lutein and zeaxanthin has been demonstrated to improve macular pigment optical density measures, a marker of age-related macular degeneration.

Various nutrients have been reported to play a role in reducing the risk for ischemic heart disease, stroke, myocardial infarction, heart failure, hypertension, and diabetes with varying levels of effect size and evidence. B-Vitamins reduced homocysteine levels and reduced the risk for stroke. Some but not all studies reported that higher omega-3 LCPUFAs intakes resulted in reduced risk of cardiovascular events; most pronounced effects being shown in subjects with low intake or status. Vitamin C and D may reduce hypertension, omega-3 LCPUFAs may have positive effect on blood lipid profiles, and omega-3 LCPUFAs, vitamin D, and chromium may reduce diabetes risk factors.

Most pronounced benefits of nutrient interventions were sometimes found in subgroups which had low baseline intake or status of the nutrient. Genetic factors can affect the status of certain nutrients, as well as contribute to increased risk for NCDs and raise the needs for certain nutrients [139,145]. Targeted supplementation with nutrients of concern to genetically predisposed subgroups has been shown to confer benefits as shown by some examples in this review. More research is needed to unravel the benefits of optimizing nutrition where it is needed, for instance by targeting those at increased risk for NCDs linked to low nutrition status or genetic profile.

Due to a growing aging global population, related NCDs including musculoskeletal disorders, dementia, loss of vision, and cardiovascular diseases will place an increasing burden on health systems and costs. Adequate nutrient status may help to improve health and wellbeing in older populations and slow the progression of NCDs. Implementing a long-term preventative strategy to promote healthy aging and break down the barriers to adequate nutrition for older adults could result in significant healthcare cost savings. Nutrition is increasingly acknowledged and integrated into public health policies and programs to manage healthy aging. Promoting nutrient-rich diets and adequate nutrient intakes for healthy aging should be considered part of an integral approach to address NCDs in health policies. There is a need for public and/or private partnerships where governments, health authorities, academics, and the food sector jointly promote the benefits of healthy nutrient-rich diets and lifestyle to manage NCDs.

In conclusion, data indicate that inadequate nutrient intake and status is common in older aged adults and represents a risk for the development of NCDs during aging. Studies for the aging population have demonstrated that optimizing nutrition can reduce the risk and progress of NCDs. Although the scientific evidence is not conclusive for all health benefits, it should not prevent health authorities from promoting balanced and adequate nutrient intakes as integral part of nutrition strategies to reduce the burden of NCDs associated with inadequate nutrition.

Author Contributions: M.J.B., M.E., and P.V.D. wrote the manuscript.

Funding: This research received no external funding.

Acknowledgments: Editorial assistance was provided by Content Ed Net (Switzerland).

Conflicts of Interest: M.J.B. and P.V.D. are employed by DSM Nutritional Products, a manufacturer of vitamins and supplier to the food, dietary supplement, and pharmaceutical industries. M.E. is a former employee of DSM Nutritional Products. There were no other conflicts of interest.

References

1. World Health Organization (WHO). Global Health Observatory (GHO) Data, Life Expectancy. Available online: http://www.who.int/gho/mortality_burden_disease/life_tables/situation_trends/en/ (accessed on 20 September 2018).
2. Figueira, I.; Fernandes, A.; Mladenovic Djordjevic, A.; Lopez-Contreras, A.; Henriques, C.M.; Selman, C.; Ferreiro, E.; Gonos, E.S.; Trejo, J.L.; Misra, J.; et al. Interventions for age-related diseases: Shifting the paradigm. *Mech. Ageing Dev.* **2016**, *160*, 69–92. [CrossRef]
3. Troesch, B.; Biesalski, H.K.; Bos, R.; Buskens, E.; Calder, P.C.; Saris, W.H.; Spieldenner, J.; Verkade, H.J.; Weber, P.; Eggersdorfer, M. Increased Intake of Foods with High Nutrient Density Can Help to Break the Intergenerational Cycle of Malnutrition and Obesity. *Nutrients* **2015**, *7*, 6016–6037. [CrossRef]
4. World Health Organization (WHO). Global Action Plan for the Prevention and Control of NCDs 2013–2020. 2018. Available online: https://www.who.int/nmh/publications/ncd-action-plan/en/ (accessed on 3 January 2019).
5. United Nations Economic and Social Council (ECOSOC). ECOSOC 2018 Task Force Resolution Urges Partners to Mobilize Resources for the Work of the Task Force. Available online: http://www.who.int/ncds/un-task-force/events/ecosoc-report-2018/en/ (accessed on 20 September 2018).
6. World Health Organization (WHO). Health Statistics and Information Systems. Disease Burden and Mortality Estimates. Global Health Estimates 2016: DALYs by Age, Sex and Cause. Available online: http://www.who.int/healthinfo/global_burden_disease/estimates/en/index1.html (accessed on 20 September 2018).
7. Eggersdorfer, M.; Walter, P. Emerging nutrition gaps in a world of affluence—Micronutrient intake and status globally. *Int. J. Vitam. Nutr. Res.* **2011**, *81*, 238–239. [CrossRef]
8. Hoeft, B.; Weber, P.; Eggersdorfer, M. Micronutrients—A global perspective on intake, health benefits and economics. *Int. J. Vitam. Nutr. Res.* **2012**, *82*, 316–320. [CrossRef]
9. Global Nutrition Report 2017, Nourishing the SDGs. Available online: http://165.227.233.32/wp-content/uploads/2017/11/Report_2017-2.pdf (accessed on 20 September 2018).
10. Drewnowski, A. Nutrient density: Addressing the challenge of obesity. *Br. J. Nutr.* **2018**, *120*, S8–S14. [CrossRef]
11. Mozaffarian, D.; Rosenberg, I.; Uauy, R. History of modern nutrition science-implications for current research, dietary guidelines, and food policy. *BMJ* **2018**, *361*, k2392. [CrossRef]
12. Mertens, E.; Kuijsten, A.; Dofkova, M.; Mistura, L.; D'Addezio, L.; Turrini, A.; Dubuisson, C.; Favret, S.; Havard, S.; Trolle, E.; et al. Geographic and socioeconomic diversity of food and nutrient intakes: A comparison of four European countries. *Eur. J. Nutr.* **2018**. [CrossRef]
13. Candari, C.J.; Cylus, J.; Nolte, E. Assessing the Economic Costs of Unhealthy Diets and low Physical Activity: An Evidence Review and Proposed Framework. Available online: http://www.euro.who.int/en/publications/abstracts/assessing-the-economic-costs-of-unhealthy-diets-and-low-physical-activity-an-evidence-review-and-proposed-framework-2017 (accessed on 3 January 2019).

14. Peter, S.; Saris, W.H.; Mathers, J.C.; Feskens, E.; Schols, A.; Navis, G.; Kuipers, F.; Weber, P.; Eggersdorfer, M. Nutrient Status Assessment in Individuals and Populations for Healthy Aging-Statement from an Expert Workshop. *Nutrients* **2015**, *7*, 10491–10500. [CrossRef]

15. De Groot, L.C. Nutritional issues for older adults: Addressing degenerative ageing with long-term studies. *Proc. Nutr. Soc.* **2016**, *75*, 169–173. [CrossRef]

16. Siddique, N.; O'Donoghue, M.; Casey, M.C.; Walsh, J.B. Malnutrition in the elderly and its effects on bone health—A review. *Clin. Nutr. ESPEN* **2017**, *21*, 31–39. [CrossRef]

17. Leslie, W.; Hankey, C. Aging, Nutritional Status and Health. *Healthcare (Basel)* **2015**, *3*, 648–658. [CrossRef]

18. Arnim, C.A.F. Nutrition security in older adults: Status quo and future development. In *Sustainable Nutrition in a Changing World*; Biesalski, H.K., Drewnowski, A., Dwyer, J.T., Strain, J.J., Weber, P., Eggersdorfer, M., Eds.; Springer International Publishing: Basel, Switzerland, 2017; pp. 61–73.

19. Kimokoti, R.W.; Millen, B.E. Nutrition for the Prevention of Chronic Diseases. *Med. Clin. N. Am.* **2016**, *100*, 1185–1198. [CrossRef]

20. Bruins, M.J.; Bird, J.K.; Aebischer, C.P.; Eggersdorfer, M. Considerations for Secondary Prevention of Nutritional Deficiencies in High-Risk Groups in High-Income Countries. *Nutrients* **2018**, *10*, 47. [CrossRef]

21. Wong, C.W. Vitamin B12 deficiency in the elderly: Is it worth screening? *Hong Kong Med. J.* **2015**, *21*, 155–164. [CrossRef]

22. Bendik, I.; Friedel, A.; Roos, F.F.; Weber, P.; Eggersdorfer, M. Vitamin D: A critical and essential micronutrient for human health. *Front. Physiol.* **2014**, *5*, 248. [CrossRef]

23. Stover, P.J. Influence of human genetic variation on nutritional requirements. *Am. J. Clin. Nutr.* **2006**, *83*, 436S–442S. [CrossRef]

24. Prince, M.J.; Wu, F.; Guo, Y.; Gutierrez Robledo, L.M.; O'Donnell, M.; Sullivan, R.; Yusuf, S. The burden of disease in older people and implications for health policy and practice. *Lancet* **2015**, *385*, 549–562. [CrossRef]

25. Avenell, A.; Mak, J.C.; O'Connell, D. Vitamin D and vitamin D analogues for preventing fractures in post-menopausal women and older men. *Cochrane Database Syst. Rev.* **2014**, *14*, CD000227. [CrossRef]

26. Johnell, O.; Kanis, J.A. An estimate of the worldwide prevalence and disability associated with osteoporotic fractures. *Osteoporos. Int.* **2006**, *17*, 1726–1733. [CrossRef]

27. World Health Organization (WHO). *WHO Scientific Group on the Assessment of Osteoporosis at Primary Health Care Level*; Summary Meeting Report, Brussels, Belgium, 5–7 May 2004; WHO: Geneva, Switzerland, 2004.

28. Hernlund, E.; Svedbom, A.; Ivergard, M.; Compston, J.; Cooper, C.; Stenmark, J.; McCloskey, E.V.; Jonsson, B.; Kanis, J.A. Osteoporosis in the European Union: Medical management, epidemiology and economic burden. A report prepared in collaboration with the International Osteoporosis Foundation (IOF) and the European Federation of Pharmaceutical Industry Associations (EFPIA). *Arch. Osteoporos.* **2013**, *8*, 136. [CrossRef]

29. Beaudart, C.; Buckinx, F.; Rabenda, V.; Gillain, S.; Cavalier, E.; Slomian, J.; Petermans, J.; Reginster, J.Y.; Bruyere, O. The effects of vitamin D on skeletal muscle strength, muscle mass, and muscle power: A systematic review and meta-analysis of randomized controlled trials. *J. Clin. Endocrinol. Metab.* **2014**, *99*, 4336–4345. [CrossRef]

30. Thiering, E.; Bruske, I.; Kratzsch, J.; Hofbauer, L.C.; Berdel, D.; von Berg, A.; Lehmann, I.; Hoffmann, B.; Bauer, C.P.; Koletzko, S.; et al. Associations between serum 25-hydroxyvitamin D and bone turnover markers in a population based sample of German children. *Sci. Rep.* **2015**, *5*, 18138. [CrossRef]

31. Quesada-Gomez, J.M.; Bouillon, R. Is calcifediol better than cholecalciferol for vitamin D supplementation? *Osteoporos. Int.* **2018**, *29*, 1697–1711. [CrossRef]

32. Sai, A.J.; Walters, R.W.; Fang, X.; Gallagher, J.C. Relationship between vitamin D, parathyroid hormone, and bone health. *J. Clin. Endocrinol. Metab.* **2011**, *96*, E436–E446. [CrossRef]

33. Heaney, R.P. Functional indices of vitamin D status and ramifications of vitamin D deficiency. *Am. J. Clin. Nutr.* **2004**, *80*, 1706S–1709S. [CrossRef]

34. Cauley, J.A.; Parimi, N.; Ensrud, K.E.; Bauer, D.C.; Cawthon, P.M.; Cummings, S.R.; Hoffman, A.R.; Shikany, J.M.; Barrett-Connor, E.; Orwoll, E.; et al. Serum 25-hydroxyvitamin D and the risk of hip and nonspine fractures in older men. *J. Bone Miner. Res.* **2010**, *25*, 545–553. [CrossRef]

35. Looker, A.C.; Mussolino, M.E. Serum 25-hydroxyvitamin D and hip fracture risk in older U.S. white adults. *J. Bone Miner. Res.* **2008**, *23*, 143–150. [CrossRef]

36. Cashman, K.D.; Dowling, K.G.; Skrabakova, Z.; Gonzalez-Gross, M.; Valtuena, J.; De Henauw, S.; Moreno, L.; Damsgaard, C.T.; Michaelsen, K.F.; Molgaard, C.; et al. Vitamin D deficiency in Europe: Pandemic? *Am. J. Clin. Nutr.* **2016**, *103*, 1033–1044. [CrossRef]

37. Hilger, J.; Friedel, A.; Herr, R.; Rausch, T.; Roos, F.; Wahl, D.A.; Pierroz, D.D.; Weber, P.; Hoffmann, K. A systematic review of vitamin D status in populations worldwide. *Br. J. Nutr.* **2014**, *111*, 23–45. [CrossRef]

38. Wahl, D.A.; Cooper, C.; Ebeling, P.R.; Eggersdorfer, M.; Hilger, J.; Hoffmann, K.; Josse, R.; Kanis, J.A.; Mithal, A.; Pierroz, D.D.; et al. A global representation of vitamin D status in healthy populations: Reply to comment by Saadi. *Arch. Osteoporos.* **2013**, *8*, 122. [CrossRef]

39. Spiro, A.; Buttriss, J.L. Vitamin D: An overview of vitamin D status and intake in Europe. *Nutr. Bull.* **2014**, *39*, 322–350. [CrossRef]

40. Van Ballegooijen, A.J.; Pilz, S.; Tomaschitz, A.; Grubler, M.R.; Verheyen, N. The Synergistic Interplay between Vitamins D and K for Bone and Cardiovascular Health: A Narrative Review. *Int. J. Endocrinol.* **2017**, *2017*, 7454376. [CrossRef]

41. Cockayne, S.; Adamson, J.; Lanham-New, S.; Shearer, M.J.; Gilbody, S.; Torgerson, D.J. Vitamin K and the prevention of fractures: Systematic review and meta-analysis of randomized controlled trials. *Arch. Intern. Med.* **2006**, *166*, 1256–1261. [CrossRef]

42. Bolton-Smith, C.; McMurdo, M.E.; Paterson, C.R.; Mole, P.A.; Harvey, J.M.; Fenton, S.T.; Prynne, C.J.; Mishra, G.D.; Shearer, M.J. Two-year randomized controlled trial of vitamin K1 (phylloquinone) and vitamin D3 plus calcium on the bone health of older women. *J. Bone Miner. Res.* **2007**, *22*, 509–519. [CrossRef]

43. Je, S.H.; Joo, N.S.; Choi, B.H.; Kim, K.M.; Kim, B.T.; Park, S.B.; Cho, D.Y.; Kim, K.N.; Lee, D.J. Vitamin K supplement along with vitamin D and calcium reduced serum concentration of undercarboxylated osteocalcin while increasing bone mineral density in Korean postmenopausal women over sixty-years-old. *J. Korean Med. Sci.* **2011**, *26*, 1093–1098. [CrossRef]

44. Moore, K.; Hughes, C.F.; Ward, M.; Hoey, L.; McNulty, H. Diet, nutrition and the ageing brain: Current evidence and new directions. *Proc. Nutr. Soc.* **2018**, *77*, 152–163. [CrossRef]

45. Prince, M.; Bryce, R.; Albanese, E.; Wimo, A.; Ribeiro, W.; Ferri, C.P. The global prevalence of dementia: A systematic review and metaanalysis. *Alzheimers Dement.* **2013**, *9*, 63–75. [CrossRef]

46. World Health Organization (WHO). Fact Sheets: Dementia. Available online: http://www.who.int/news-room/fact-sheets/detail/dementia (accessed on 12 December 2017).

47. Jiang, T.; Yu, J.T.; Tian, Y.; Tan, L. Epidemiology and etiology of Alzheimer's disease: From genetic to non-genetic factors. *Curr. Alzheimer Res.* **2013**, *10*, 852–867. [CrossRef]

48. Antal, M.; Péter, S.; Eggersdorfer, M. Alzheimer's Disease: An epidemiologic disaster from nutritional perspective. *Nutr. Health Food Sci.* **2017**, *5*, 1–4.

49. Reynolds, E. Vitamin B12, folic acid, and the nervous system. *Lancet Neurol.* **2006**, *5*, 949–960. [CrossRef]

50. Reynolds, E.H. Folic acid, ageing, depression, and dementia. *BMJ* **2002**, *324*, 1512–1515. [CrossRef]

51. McCleery, J.; Abraham, R.P.; Denton, D.A.; Rutjes, A.W.; Chong, L.Y.; Al-Assaf, A.S.; Griffith, D.J.; Rafeeq, S.; Yaman, H.; Malik, M.A.; et al. Vitamin and mineral supplementation for preventing dementia or delaying cognitive decline in people with mild cognitive impairment. *Cochrane Database Syst. Rev.* **2018**, *11*, CD011905. [CrossRef]

52. Smith, A.D.; Refsum, H.; Bottiglieri, T.; Fenech, M.; Hooshmand, B.; McCaddon, A.; Miller, J.W.; Rosenberg, I.H.; Obeid, R. Homocysteine and Dementia: An International Consensus Statement. *J. Alzheimers Dis.* **2018**, *62*, 561–570. [CrossRef]

53. Douaud, G.; Refsum, H.; de Jager, C.A.; Jacoby, R.; Nichols, T.E.; Smith, S.M.; Smith, A.D. Preventing Alzheimer's disease-related gray matter atrophy by B-vitamin treatment. *Proc. Natl. Acad. Sci. USA* **2013**, *110*, 9523–9528. [CrossRef]

54. Troesch, B.; Hoeft, B.; McBurney, M.; Eggersdorfer, M.; Weber, P. Dietary surveys indicate vitamin intakes below recommendations are common in representative Western countries. *Br. J. Nutr.* **2012**, *108*, 692–698. [CrossRef]

55. Gugliandolo, A.; Bramanti, P.; Mazzon, E. Role of Vitamin E in the Treatment of Alzheimer's Disease: Evidence from Animal Models. *Int. J. Mol. Sci.* **2017**, *18*, 2504. [CrossRef]

56. Salem, N., Jr.; Vandal, M.; Calon, F. The benefit of docosahexaenoic acid for the adult brain in aging and dementia. *Prostaglandins Leukot. Essent. Fatty Acids* **2015**, *92*, 15–22. [CrossRef]

57. Zhang, Y.J.; Gan, R.Y.; Li, S.; Zhou, Y.; Li, A.N.; Xu, D.P.; Li, H.B. Antioxidant Phytochemicals for the Prevention and Treatment of Chronic Diseases. *Molecules* **2015**, *20*, 21138–21156. [CrossRef]

58. GBD 2015 DALYs and Hale Collaborators. Global, regional, and national disability-adjusted life-years (DALYs) for 315 diseases and injuries and healthy life expectancy (HALE), 1990–2015: A systematic analysis for the Global Burden of Disease Study 2015. *Lancet* **2016**, *388*, 1603–1658. [CrossRef]

59. Quillen, D.A. Common causes of vision loss in elderly patients. *Am. Fam. Physician* **1999**, *60*, 99–108.

60. Chen, Y.; Bedell, M.; Zhang, K. Age-related macular degeneration: Genetic and environmental factors of disease. *Mol. Interv.* **2010**, *10*, 271–281. [CrossRef]

61. Tosini, G.; Ferguson, I.; Tsubota, K. Effects of blue light on the circadian system and eye physiology. *Mol. Vis.* **2016**, *22*, 61–72.

62. Demmig-Adams, B.; Adams, R.B. Eye nutrition in context: Mechanisms, implementation, and future directions. *Nutrients* **2013**, *5*, 2483–2501. [CrossRef]

63. Bernstein, P.S.; Li, B.; Vachali, P.P.; Gorusupudi, A.; Shyam, R.; Henriksen, B.S.; Nolan, J.M. Lutein, zeaxanthin, and meso-zeaxanthin: The basic and clinical science underlying carotenoid-based nutritional interventions against ocular disease. *Prog. Retin. Eye Res.* **2016**, *50*, 34–66. [CrossRef]

64. Barker, F.M., II; Snodderly, D.M.; Johnson, E.J.; Schalch, W.; Koepcke, W.; Gerss, J.; Neuringer, M. Nutritional manipulation of primate retinas, V: Effects of lutein, zeaxanthin, and n-3 fatty acids on retinal sensitivity to blue-light-induced damage. *Investig. Ophthalmol. Vis. Sci.* **2011**, *52*, 3934–3942. [CrossRef]

65. Hammond, B.R.; Fletcher, L.M.; Roos, F.; Wittwer, J.; Schalch, W. A double-blind, placebo-controlled study on the effects of lutein and zeaxanthin on photostress recovery, glare disability, and chromatic contrast. *Investig. Ophthalmol. Vis. Sci.* **2014**, *55*, 8583–8589. [CrossRef]

66. Yao, Y.; Qiu, Q.H.; Wu, X.W.; Cai, Z.Y.; Xu, S.; Liang, X.Q. Lutein supplementation improves visual performance in Chinese drivers: 1-year randomized, double-blind, placebo-controlled study. *Nutrition* **2013**, *29*, 958–964. [CrossRef]

67. Loughman, J.; Nolan, J.M.; Howard, A.N.; Connolly, E.; Meagher, K.; Beatty, S. The impact of macular pigment augmentation on visual performance using different carotenoid formulations. *Investig. Ophthalmol. Vis. Sci.* **2012**, *53*, 7871–7880. [CrossRef]

68. Nolan, J.M.; Loughman, J.; Akkali, M.C.; Stack, J.; Scanlon, G.; Davison, P.; Beatty, S. The impact of macular pigment augmentation on visual performance in normal subjects: COMPASS. *Vision Res.* **2011**, *51*, 459–469. [CrossRef]

69. Richer, S.P.; Stiles, W.; Graham-Hoffman, K.; Levin, M.; Ruskin, D.; Wrobel, J.; Park, D.W.; Thomas, C. Randomized, double-blind, placebo-controlled study of zeaxanthin and visual function in patients with atrophic age-related macular degeneration: The Zeaxanthin and Visual Function Study (ZVF) FDA IND #78, 973. *Optometry* **2011**, *82*, 667–680.

70. Stringham, J.M.; Hammond, B.R. Macular pigment and visual performance under glare conditions. *Optom. Vis. Sci.* **2008**, *85*, 82–88. [CrossRef]

71. Wenzel, A.J.; Fuld, K.; Stringham, J.M.; Curran-Celentano, J. Macular pigment optical density and photophobia light threshold. *Vision Res.* **2006**, *46*, 4615–4622. [CrossRef]

72. Kvansakul, J.; Rodriguez-Carmona, M.; Edgar, D.F.; Barker, F.M.; Kopcke, W.; Schalch, W.; Barbur, J.L. Supplementation with the carotenoids lutein or zeaxanthin improves human visual performance. *Ophthalmic. Physiol. Opt.* **2006**, *26*, 362–371. [CrossRef]

73. Feeney, J.; Finucane, C.; Savva, G.M.; Cronin, H.; Beatty, S.; Nolan, J.M.; Kenny, R.A. Low macular pigment optical density is associated with lower cognitive performance in a large, population-based sample of older adults. *Neurobiol. Aging* **2013**, *34*, 2449–2456. [CrossRef]

74. Johnson, E.J.; Maras, J.E.; Rasmussen, H.M.; Tucker, K.L. Intake of lutein and zeaxanthin differ with age, sex, and ethnicity. *J. Am. Diet. Assoc.* **2010**, *110*, 1357–1362. [CrossRef]

75. Nolan, J.M.; Power, R.; Stringham, J.; Dennison, J.; Stack, J.; Kelly, D.; Moran, R.; Akuffo, K.O.; Corcoran, L.; Beatty, S. Author Response: Comments on Enrichment of Macular Pigment Enhances Contrast Sensitivity in Subjects Free of Retinal Disease: CREST—Report 1. *Investig. Ophthalmol. Vis. Sci.* **2016**, *57*, 5416. [CrossRef]

76. Olmedilla, B.; Granado, F.; Blanco, I.; Vaquero, M. Lutein, but not alpha-tocopherol, supplementation improves visual function in patients with age-related cataracts: A 2-y double-blind, placebo-controlled pilot study. *Nutrition* **2003**, *19*, 21–24. [CrossRef]

77. Age-Related Eye Disease Study 2 Research Group. Lutein + zeaxanthin and omega-3 fatty acids for age-related macular degeneration: The Age-Related Eye Disease Study 2 (AREDS2) randomized clinical trial. *JAMA* **2013**, *309*, 2005–2015. [CrossRef]

78. Age-Related Eye Disease Study 2 Research Group; Chew, E.Y.; Clemons, T.E.; Sangiovanni, J.P.; Danis, R.P.; Ferris, F.L., III; Elman, M.J.; Antoszyk, A.N.; Ruby, A.J.; Orth, D.; et al. Secondary analyses of the effects of lutein/zeaxanthin on age-related macular degeneration progression: AREDS2 report No. 3. *JAMA Ophthalmol.* **2014**, *132*, 142–149. [CrossRef]

79. Liu, X.H.; Yu, R.B.; Liu, R.; Hao, Z.X.; Han, C.C.; Zhu, Z.H.; Ma, L. Association between lutein and zeaxanthin status and the risk of cataract: A meta-analysis. *Nutrients* **2014**, *6*, 452–465. [CrossRef]

80. Age-Related Eye Disease Study 2 Research Group; Chew, E.Y.; SanGiovanni, J.P.; Ferris, F.L.; Wong, W.T.; Agron, E.; Clemons, T.E.; Sperduto, R.; Danis, R.; Chandra, S.R.; et al. Lutein/zeaxanthin for the treatment of age-related cataract: AREDS2 randomized trial report no. 4. *JAMA Ophthalmol.* **2013**, *131*, 843–850. [CrossRef]

81. Shanahan, C. The Economic Benefits of Using Lutein and Zeaxanthin Food Supplements in the European Union. Available online: https://ww2.frost.com/files/7015/0772/2735/HCCS_Lutein_AMD.2017.10.12.pdf (accessed on 3 January 2019).

82. GBD Causes of Death Collaborators. Global, regional, and national age-sex specific mortality for 264 causes of death, 1980–2016: A systematic analysis for the Global Burden of Disease Study 2016. *Lancet* **2017**, *390*, 1151–1210. [CrossRef]

83. Mozaffarian, D. Dietary and Policy Priorities for Cardiovascular Disease, Diabetes, and Obesity: A Comprehensive Review. *Circulation* **2016**, *133*, 187–225. [CrossRef]

84. Leening, M.J.; Ferket, B.S.; Steyerberg, E.W.; Kavousi, M.; Deckers, J.W.; Nieboer, D.; Heeringa, J.; Portegies, M.L.; Hofman, A.; Ikram, M.A.; et al. Sex differences in lifetime risk and first manifestation of cardiovascular disease: Prospective population based cohort study. *BMJ* **2014**, *349*, g5992. [CrossRef]

85. The Institute for Health Metrics and Evaluation (IHME). Global Burden of Disease (GBD). GBD Data Visualizations. Available online: http://www.healthdata.org/gbd (accessed on 20 September 2018).

86. Hankey, G.J. The Role of Nutrition in the Risk and Burden of Stroke: An Update of the Evidence. *Stroke J. Cereb. Circ.* **2017**, *48*, 3168–3174. [CrossRef]

87. Van Staveren, W.A.; de Groot, L.C. Evidence-based dietary guidance and the role of dairy products for appropriate nutrition in the elderly. *J. Am. Coll. Nutr.* **2011**, *30*, 429S–437S. [CrossRef]

88. Fleg, J.L.; Forman, D.E.; Berra, K.; Bittner, V.; Blumenthal, J.A.; Chen, M.A.; Cheng, S.; Kitzman, D.W.; Maurer, M.S.; Rich, M.W.; et al. Secondary prevention of atherosclerotic cardiovascular disease in older adults: A scientific statement from the American Heart Association. *Circulation* **2013**, *128*, 2422–2446. [CrossRef]

89. Catapano, A.L.; Graham, I.; De Backer, G.; Wiklund, O.; Chapman, M.J.; Drexel, H.; Hoes, A.W.; Jennings, C.S.; Landmesser, U.; Pedersen, T.R.; et al. 2016 ESC/EAS Guidelines for the Management of Dyslipidaemias. *Rev. Esp. Cardiol. (Engl. Ed.)* **2017**, *70*, 115.

90. Jellinger, P.S. American Association of Clinical Endocrinologists/American College of Endocrinology Management of Dyslipidemia and Prevention of Cardiovascular Disease Clinical Practice Guidelines. *Diabetes Spectr.* **2018**, *31*, 234–245. [CrossRef]

91. Eckel, R.H.; Jakicic, J.M.; Ard, J.D.; de Jesus, J.M.; Houston Miller, N.; Hubbard, V.S.; Lee, I.M.; Lichtenstein, A.H.; Loria, C.M.; Millen, B.E.; et al. 2013 AHA/ACC guideline on lifestyle management to reduce cardiovascular risk: A report of the American College of Cardiology/American Heart Association Task Force on Practice Guidelines. *Circulation* **2014**, *129*, S76–S99. [CrossRef]

92. Estruch, R.; Ros, E.; Salas-Salvado, J.; Covas, M.I.; Corella, D.; Aros, F.; Gomez-Gracia, E.; Ruiz-Gutierrez, V.; Fiol, M.; Lapetra, J.; et al. Primary Prevention of Cardiovascular Disease with a Mediterranean Diet Supplemented with Extra-Virgin Olive Oil or Nuts. *N. Engl. J. Med.* **2018**, *378*, e34. [CrossRef]

93. De Lorgeril, M.; Salen, P.; Martin, J.L.; Monjaud, I.; Delaye, J.; Mamelle, N. Mediterranean diet, traditional risk factors, and the rate of cardiovascular complications after myocardial infarction: Final report of the Lyon Diet Heart Study. *Circulation* **1999**, *99*, 779–785. [CrossRef]

94. Ornish, D.; Scherwitz, L.W.; Billings, J.H.; Brown, S.E.; Gould, K.L.; Merritt, T.A.; Sparler, S.; Armstrong, W.T.; Ports, T.A.; Kirkeeide, R.L.; et al. Intensive lifestyle changes for reversal of coronary heart disease. *JAMA* **1998**, *280*, 2001–2007. [CrossRef]

95. Kheiri, B.; Abdalla, A.; Osman, M.; Ahmed, S.; Hassan, M.; Bachuwa, G. Vitamin D deficiency and risk of cardiovascular diseases: A narrative review. *Clin. Hypertens.* **2018**, *24*, 9. [CrossRef]

96. Gepner, A.D.; Ramamurthy, R.; Krueger, D.C.; Korcarz, C.E.; Binkley, N.; Stein, J.H. A prospective randomized controlled trial of the effects of vitamin D supplementation on cardiovascular disease risk. *PLoS ONE* **2012**, *7*, e36617. [CrossRef]
97. Ford, J.A.; MacLennan, G.S.; Avenell, A.; Bolland, M.; Grey, A.; Witham, M.; Group, R.T. Cardiovascular disease and vitamin D supplementation: Trial analysis, systematic review, and meta-analysis. *Am. J. Clin. Nutr.* **2014**, *100*, 746–755. [CrossRef]
98. Vitamin D and Omega-3 Trial (VITAL). Available online: https://www.vitalstudy.org/findings.html (accessed on 20 December 2018).
99. Huang, T.; Chen, Y.; Yang, B.; Yang, J.; Wahlqvist, M.L.; Li, D. Meta-analysis of B vitamin supplementation on plasma homocysteine, cardiovascular and all-cause mortality. *Clin. Nutr.* **2012**, *31*, 448–454. [CrossRef]
100. Yang, H.T.; Lee, M.; Hong, K.S.; Ovbiagele, B.; Saver, J.L. Efficacy of folic acid supplementation in cardiovascular disease prevention: An updated meta-analysis of randomized controlled trials. *Eur. J. Intern. Med.* **2012**, *23*, 745–754. [CrossRef]
101. Wald, D.S.; Law, M.; Morris, J.K. Homocysteine and cardiovascular disease: Evidence on causality from a meta-analysis. *BMJ* **2002**, *325*, 1202. [CrossRef]
102. Li, Y.; Huang, T.; Zheng, Y.; Muka, T.; Troup, J.; Hu, F.B. Folic Acid Supplementation and the Risk of Cardiovascular Diseases: A Meta-Analysis of Randomized Controlled Trials. *J. Am. Heart Assoc.* **2016**, *5*, e003768. [CrossRef]
103. Fezeu, L.K.; Ducros, V.; Gueant, J.L.; Guilland, J.C.; Andreeva, V.A.; Hercberg, S.; Galan, P. MTHFR 677C→T genotype modulates the effect of a 5-year supplementation with B-vitamins on homocysteine concentration: The SU.FOL.OM3 randomized controlled trial. *PLoS ONE* **2018**, *13*, e0193352. [CrossRef]
104. DiNicolantonio, J.J.; Bhutani, J.; O'Keefe, J.H. The health benefits of vitamin K. *Open Heart* **2015**, *2*, e000300. [CrossRef]
105. Innes, J.K.; Calder, P.C. The Differential Effects of Eicosapentaenoic Acid and Docosahexaenoic Acid on Cardiometabolic Risk Factors: A Systematic Review. *Int. J. Mol. Sci.* **2018**, *19*, 532. [CrossRef]
106. Thota, R.N.; Ferguson, J.J.A.; Abbott, K.A.; Dias, C.B.; Garg, M.L. Science behind the cardio-metabolic benefits of omega-3 polyunsaturated fatty acids: Biochemical effects vs. clinical outcomes. *Food Funct.* **2018**, *9*, 3576–3596. [CrossRef]
107. Karalis, D.G. A Review of Clinical Practice Guidelines for the Management of Hypertriglyceridemia: A Focus on High Dose Omega-3 Fatty Acids. *Adv. Ther.* **2017**, *34*, 300–323. [CrossRef]
108. Alexander, D.D.; Miller, P.E.; Van Elswyk, M.E.; Kuratko, C.N.; Bylsma, L.C. A Meta-Analysis of Randomized Controlled Trials and Prospective Cohort Studies of Eicosapentaenoic and Docosahexaenoic Long-Chain Omega-3 Fatty Acids and Coronary Heart Disease Risk. *Mayo Clin. Proc.* **2017**, *92*, 15–29. [CrossRef]
109. Abdelhamid, A.S.; Brown, T.J.; Brainard, J.S.; Biswas, P.; Thorpe, G.C.; Moore, H.J.; Deane, K.H.; AlAbdulghafoor, F.K.; Summerbell, C.D.; Worthington, H.V.; et al. Omega-3 fatty acids for the primary and secondary prevention of cardiovascular disease. *Cochrane Database Syst. Rev.* **2018**, *7*, CD003177.
110. Meyer, B.J.; Groot, R.H.M. Effects of Omega-3 Long Chain Polyunsaturated Fatty Acid Supplementation on Cardiovascular Mortality: The Importance of the Dose of DHA. *Nutrients* **2017**, *9*, 1305. [CrossRef]
111. Kromhout, D.; Giltay, E.J.; Geleijnse, J.M.; Alpha Omega Trial, G. n-3 fatty acids and cardiovascular events after myocardial infarction. *N. Engl. J. Med.* **2010**, *363*, 2015–2026. [CrossRef]
112. Writing Group for the AREDS2 Research Group; Bonds, D.E.; Harrington, M.; Worrall, B.B.; Bertoni, A.G.; Eaton, C.B.; Hsia, J.; Robinson, J.; Clemons, T.E.; Fine, L.J.; et al. Effect of long-chain omega-3 fatty acids and lutein + zeaxanthin supplements on cardiovascular outcomes: Results of the Age-Related Eye Disease Study 2 (AREDS2) randomized clinical trial. *JAMA Intern. Med.* **2014**, *174*, 763–771.
113. Hidayat, K.; Yang, J.; Zhang, Z.; Chen, G.C.; Qin, L.Q.; Eggersdorfer, M.; Zhang, W. Effect of omega-3 long-chain polyunsaturated fatty acid supplementation on heart rate: A meta-analysis of randomized controlled trials. *Eur. J. Clin. Nutr.* **2018**, *72*, 805–817. [CrossRef]
114. Zhang, G.Q.; Zhang, W. Heart rate, lifespan, and mortality risk. *Ageing Res. Rev.* **2009**, *8*, 52–60. [CrossRef]
115. Chen, Y.; Michalak, M.; Agellon, L.B. Importance of Nutrients and Nutrient Metabolism on Human Health. *Yale J. Biol. Med.* **2018**, *91*, 95–103.
116. Rangel-Huerta, O.D.; Pastor-Villaescusa, B.; Aguilera, C.M.; Gil, A. A Systematic Review of the Efficacy of Bioactive Compounds in Cardiovascular Disease: Phenolic Compounds. *Nutrients* **2015**, *7*, 5177–5216. [CrossRef]

117. Ye, Y.; Li, J.; Yuan, Z. Effect of antioxidant vitamin supplementation on cardiovascular outcomes: A meta-analysis of randomized controlled trials. *PLoS ONE* **2013**, *8*, e56803. [CrossRef]

118. Raederstorff, D.; Wyss, A.; Calder, P.C.; Weber, P.; Eggersdorfer, M. Vitamin E function and requirements in relation to PUFA. *Br. J. Nutr.* **2015**, *114*, 1113–1122. [CrossRef]

119. Lee, I.M.; Cook, N.R.; Gaziano, J.M.; Gordon, D.; Ridker, P.M.; Manson, J.E.; Hennekens, C.H.; Buring, J.E. Vitamin E in the primary prevention of cardiovascular disease and cancer: The Women's Health Study: A randomized controlled trial. *JAMA* **2005**, *294*, 56–65. [CrossRef]

120. Glynn, R.J.; Ridker, P.M.; Goldhaber, S.Z.; Zee, R.Y.; Buring, J.E. Effects of random allocation to vitamin E supplementation on the occurrence of venous thromboembolism: Report from the Women's Health Study. *Circulation* **2007**, *116*, 1497–1503. [CrossRef]

121. Farbstein, D.; Levy, A.P. The genetics of vascular complications in diabetes mellitus. *Cardiol. Clin.* **2010**, *28*, 477–496. [CrossRef]

122. He, H.Y.; Liu, M.Z.; Zhang, Y.L.; Zhang, W. Vitamin Pharmacogenomics: New Insight into Individual Differences in Diseases and Drug Responses. *Genom. Proteom. Bioinform.* **2017**, *15*, 94–100. [CrossRef]

123. Huxley, R.R.; Neil, H.A. The relation between dietary flavonol intake and coronary heart disease mortality: A meta-analysis of prospective cohort studies. *Eur. J. Clin. Nutr.* **2003**, *57*, 904–908. [CrossRef] [PubMed]

124. Wang, Z.M.; Nie, Z.L.; Zhou, B.; Lian, X.Q.; Zhao, H.; Gao, W.; Wang, Y.S.; Jia, E.Z.; Wang, L.S.; Yang, Z.J. Flavonols intake and the risk of coronary heart disease: A meta-analysis of cohort studies. *Atherosclerosis* **2012**, *222*, 270–273. [CrossRef] [PubMed]

125. Castro, I.; Waclawovsky, G.; Marcadenti, A. Nutrition and physical activity on hypertension: Implication of current evidence and guidelines. *Curr. Hypertens. Rev.* **2015**, *11*, 91–99. [CrossRef] [PubMed]

126. Miller, A.P.; Navar, A.M.; Roubin, G.S.; Oparil, S. Cardiovascular care for older adults: Hypertension and stroke in the older adult. *J. Geriatr. Cardiol.* **2016**, *13*, 373–379. [PubMed]

127. James, P.A.; Oparil, S.; Carter, B.L.; Cushman, W.C.; Dennison-Himmelfarb, C.; Handler, J.; Lackland, D.T.; LeFevre, M.L.; MacKenzie, T.D.; Ogedegbe, O.; et al. 2014 evidence-based guideline for the management of high blood pressure in adults: Report from the panel members appointed to the Eighth Joint National Committee (JNC 8). *JAMA* **2014**, *311*, 507–520. [CrossRef] [PubMed]

128. Nguyen, H.; Odelola, O.A.; Rangaswami, J.; Amanullah, A. A review of nutritional factors in hypertension management. *Int. J. Hypertens.* **2013**, *2013*, 698940. [CrossRef] [PubMed]

129. Perez, V.; Chang, E.T. Sodium-to-potassium ratio and blood pressure, hypertension, and related factors. *Adv. Nutr.* **2014**, *5*, 712–741. [CrossRef]

130. Cicero, A.F.; Colletti, A.; Rosticci, M.; Cagnati, M.; Urso, R.; Giovannini, M.; Borghi, C.; D'Addato, S. Effect of Lactotripeptides (Isoleucine-Proline-Proline/Valine-Proline-Proline) on Blood Pressure and Arterial Stiffness Changes in Subjects with Suboptimal Blood Pressure Control and Metabolic Syndrome: A Double-Blind, Randomized, Crossover Clinical Trial. *Metab. Syndr. Relat. Disord.* **2016**, *14*, 161–166. [CrossRef]

131. Miller, P.E.; Van Elswyk, M.; Alexander, D.D. Long-chain omega-3 fatty acids eicosapentaenoic acid and docosahexaenoic acid and blood pressure: A meta-analysis of randomized controlled trials. *Am. J. Hypertens.* **2014**, *27*, 885–896. [CrossRef]

132. Geleijnse, J.M.; Giltay, E.J.; Grobbee, D.E.; Donders, A.R.; Kok, F.J. Blood pressure response to fish oil supplementation: Metaregression analysis of randomized trials. *J. Hypertens.* **2002**, *20*, 1493–1499. [CrossRef]

133. Juraschek, S.P.; Guallar, E.; Appel, L.J.; Miller, E.R., III. Effects of vitamin C supplementation on blood pressure: A meta-analysis of randomized controlled trials. *Am. J. Clin. Nutr.* **2012**, *95*, 1079–1088. [CrossRef] [PubMed]

134. Forman, J.P.; Scott, J.B.; Ng, K.; Drake, B.F.; Suarez, E.G.; Hayden, D.L.; Bennett, G.G.; Chandler, P.D.; Hollis, B.W.; Emmons, K.M.; et al. Effect of vitamin D supplementation on blood pressure in blacks. *Hypertension* **2013**, *61*, 779–785. [CrossRef] [PubMed]

135. International Diabetes Federation (IDF). IDF Diabetes Atlas 8th Edition. Available online: http://www.diabetesatlas.org/ (accessed on 20 September 2018).

136. Samocha-Bonet, D.; Debs, S.; Greenfield, J.R. Prevention and Treatment of Type 2 Diabetes: A Pathophysiological-Based Approach. *Trends Endocrinol. Metab.* **2018**, *29*, 370–379. [CrossRef] [PubMed]

137. Li, X.; Liu, Y.; Zheng, Y.; Wang, P.; Zhang, Y. The Effect of Vitamin D Supplementation on Glycemic Control in Type 2 Diabetes Patients: A Systematic Review and Meta-Analysis. *Nutrients* **2018**, *10*, 375. [PubMed]

138. Upreti, V.; Maitri, V.; Dhull, P.; Handa, A.; Prakash, M.S.; Behl, A. Effect of oral vitamin D supplementation on glycemic control in patients with type 2 diabetes mellitus with coexisting hypovitaminosis D: A parellel group placebo controlled randomized controlled pilot study. *Diabetes Metab. Syndr.* **2018**, *12*, 509–512. [CrossRef] [PubMed]

139. Milman, U.; Blum, S.; Shapira, C.; Aronson, D.; Miller-Lotan, R.; Anbinder, Y.; Alshiek, J.; Bennett, L.; Kostenko, M.; Landau, M.; et al. Vitamin E supplementation reduces cardiovascular events in a subgroup of middle-aged individuals with both type 2 diabetes mellitus and the haptoglobin 2-2 genotype: A prospective double-blinded clinical trial. *Arterioscler. Thromb. Vasc. Biol.* **2008**, *28*, 341–347. [CrossRef] [PubMed]

140. Asleh, R.; Briasoulis, A.; Berinstein, E.M.; Wiener, J.B.; Palla, M.; Kushwaha, S.S.; Levy, A.P. Meta-analysis of the association of the haptoglobin genotype with cardiovascular outcomes and the pharmacogenomic interactions with vitamin E supplementation. *Pharmacogenom. Pers. Med.* **2018**, *11*, 71–82. [CrossRef]

141. Chen, C.; Yu, X.; Shao, S. Effects of Omega-3 Fatty Acid Supplementation on Glucose Control and Lipid Levels in Type 2 Diabetes: A Meta-Analysis. *PLoS ONE* **2015**, *10*, e0139565. [CrossRef]

142. Beulens, J.W.; van der, A.D.; Grobbee, D.E.; Sluijs, I.; Spijkerman, A.M.; van der Schouw, Y.T. Dietary phylloquinone and menaquinones intakes and risk of type 2 diabetes. *Diabetes Care* **2010**, *33*, 1699–1705. [CrossRef]

143. Yoshida, M.; Jacques, P.F.; Meigs, J.B.; Saltzman, E.; Shea, M.K.; Gundberg, C.; Dawson-Hughes, B.; Dallal, G.; Booth, S.L. Effect of vitamin K supplementation on insulin resistance in older men and women. *Diabetes Care* **2008**, *31*, 2092–2096. [CrossRef]

144. Suksomboon, N.; Poolsup, N.; Yuwanakorn, A. Systematic review and meta-analysis of the efficacy and safety of chromium supplementation in diabetes. *J. Clin. Pharm. Ther.* **2014**, *39*, 292–306. [CrossRef] [PubMed]

145. Blum, S.; Vardi, M.; Brown, J.B.; Russell, A.; Milman, U.; Shapira, C.; Levy, N.S.; Miller-Lotan, R.; Asleh, R.; Levy, A.P. Vitamin E reduces cardiovascular disease in individuals with diabetes mellitus and the haptoglobin 2-2 genotype. *Pharmacogenomics* **2010**, *11*, 675–684. [CrossRef] [PubMed]

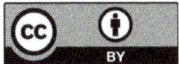

MDPI

St. Alban-Anlage 66

4052 Basel

Switzerland

Tel. +41 61 683 77 34

Fax +41 61 302 89 18

www.mdpi.com

Nutrients Editorial Office

E-mail: nutrients@mdpi.com

www.mdpi.com/journal/nutrients

9 7 8 3 0 3 8 9 7 6 0 2 8